T0190295

Communications
in Computer and Information Science 1814

Rationale

The CCIS series is devoted to the publication of proceedings of computer science conferences. Its aim is to efficiently disseminate original research results in informatics in printed and electronic form. While the focus is on publication of peer-reviewed full papers presenting mature work, inclusion of reviewed short papers reporting on work in progress is welcome, too. Besides globally relevant meetings with internationally representative program committees guaranteeing a strict peer-reviewing and paper selection process, conferences run by societies or of high regional or national relevance are also considered for publication.

Topics

The topical scope of CCIS spans the entire spectrum of informatics ranging from foundational topics in the theory of computing to information and communications science and technology and a broad variety of interdisciplinary application fields.

Information for Volume Editors and Authors

Publication in CCIS is free of charge. No royalties are paid, however, we offer registered conference participants temporary free access to the online version of the conference proceedings on SpringerLink (http://link.springer.com) by means of an http referrer from the conference website and/or a number of complimentary printed copies, as specified in the official acceptance email of the event.

CCIS proceedings can be published in time for distribution at conferences or as postproceedings, and delivered in the form of printed books and/or electronically as USBs and/or e-content licenses for accessing proceedings at SpringerLink. Furthermore, CCIS proceedings are included in the CCIS electronic book series hosted in the SpringerLink digital library at http://link.springer.com/bookseries/7899. Conferences publishing in CCIS are allowed to use Online Conference Service (OCS) for managing the whole proceedings lifecycle (from submission and reviewing to preparing for publication) free of charge.

Publication process

The language of publication is exclusively English. Authors publishing in CCIS have to sign the Springer CCIS copyright transfer form, however, they are free to use their material published in CCIS for substantially changed, more elaborate subsequent publications elsewhere. For the preparation of the camera-ready papers/files, authors have to strictly adhere to the Springer CCIS Authors' Instructions and are strongly encouraged to use the CCIS LaTeX style files or templates.

Abstracting/Indexing

CCIS is abstracted/indexed in DBLP, Google Scholar, EI-Compendex, Mathematical Reviews, SCImago, Scopus. CCIS volumes are also submitted for the inclusion in ISI Proceedings.

How to start

To start the evaluation of your proposal for inclusion in the CCIS series, please send an e-mail to ccis@springer.com.

Ana Cecília A. Roque · Denis Gracanin ·
Ronny Lorenz · Athanasios Tsanas ·
Nathalie Bier · Ana Fred · Hugo Gamboa
Editors

Biomedical Engineering Systems and Technologies

15th International Joint Conference, BIOSTEC 2022
Virtual Event, February 9–11, 2022
Revised Selected Papers

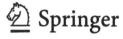 Springer

Editors
Ana Cecília A. Roque
Universidade Nova de Lisboa
Caparica, Portugal

Ronny Lorenz
University of Vienna
Vienna, Austria

Nathalie Bier
Université de Montréal
Montréal, QC, Canada

Hugo Gamboa
Nova School of Science and Technology
and University of Lisbon
Caparica, Portugal

Denis Gracanin
Virginia Tech
Blacksburg, VA, USA

Athanasios Tsanas ⓘ
University of Edinburgh
Edinburgh, UK

Ana Fred
Instituto de Telecomunicações and Instituto
Superior Técnico - Lisbon University
Lisbon, Portugal

ISSN 1865-0929   ISSN 1865-0937 (electronic)
Communications in Computer and Information Science
ISBN 978-3-031-38853-8   ISBN 978-3-031-38854-5 (eBook)
https://doi.org/10.1007/978-3-031-38854-5

This Springer imprint is published by the registered company Springer Nature Switzerland AG
The registered company address is: Gewerbestrasse 11, 6330 Cham, Switzerland

Preface

The present book includes extended and revised versions of a set of selected papers from the 15th International Joint Conference on Biomedical Engineering Systems and Technologies (BIOSTEC 2022), exceptionally held as an online event, due to covid-19, from the 9th to the 11th of February.

BIOSTEC is composed of co-located conferences, each specialized in a different knowledge area, namely BIODEVICES, BIOIMAGING, BIOINFORMATICS, BIOSIGNALS and HEALTHINF.

BIOSTEC 2022 received 262 paper submissions from 49 countries, of which 8% were included in this book.

The papers were selected by the event chairs and their selection is based on a number of criteria that include the classifications and comments provided by the program committee members, the session chairs' assessment and also the program chairs' global view of all papers included in the technical program. The authors of selected papers were then invited to submit a revised and extended version of their papers having at least 30% innovative material.

The purpose of BIOSTEC is to bring together researchers and practitioners, including engineers, biologists, health professionals and informatics/computer scientists, interested in both theoretical advances and applications of information systems, artificial intelligence, signal processing, electronics and other engineering tools in knowledge areas related to biology and medicine.

The papers selected to be included in this book contribute to the understanding of relevant trends of current research on Biomedical Engineering Systems and Technologies, including: eHealth Applications, Pattern Recognition and Machine Learning, Decision Support Systems, Application of Health Informatics in Clinical Cases, eHealth, Medical Signal Acquisition, Analysis and Processing, Mobile Technologies for Healthcare Applications, Evaluation and Use of Healthcare IT, Medical Informatics and Pattern Recognition & Machine Learning for Biosignal Data.

We would like to thank all the authors for their contributions and also the reviewers who have helped to ensure the quality of this publication.

February 2022

Ana Cecília A. Roque
Denis Gracanin
Ronny Lorenz
Athanasios Tsanas
Nathalie Bier
Ana Fred
Hugo Gamboa

Preface

Organization

Conference Co-chairs

Ana Fred   Instituto de Telecomunicações and University of Lisbon, Portugal

Hugo Gamboa   Nova University of Lisbon, Portugal

Program Co-chairs

BIODEVICES

Ana Roque   Universidade Nova de Lisboa, Portugal

BIOIMAGING

Denis Gracanin   Virginia Tech, USA

BIOINFORMATICS

Ronny Lorenz   University of Vienna, Austria

BIOSIGNALS

Athanasios Tsanas   University of Edinburgh, UK

HEALTHINF

Nathalie Bier   Université de Montréal and Research Center of the Institut universitaire de gériatrie de Montréal, Canada

BIODEVICES Program Committee

Carlos Abreu   Instituto Politécnico de Viana do Castelo, Portugal

Steve Beeby   University of Southampton, UK

Youngjae Chun	University of Pittsburgh, USA
Alberto Cliquet Jr.	University of São Paulo & University of Campinas, Brazil
Maria Evelina Fantacci	University of Pisa and INFN, Italy
Mireya Fernández Chimeno	Universitat Politècnica de Catalunya, Spain
Juan Carlos Garcia	University of Alcala, Spain
Miguel García Gonzalez	Universitat Politècnica de Catalunya, Spain
Javier Garcia-Casado	Universitat Politècnica de València, Spain
Dean Krusienski	Virginia Commonwealth University, USA
Hiroshi Kumagai	Kitasato University, Japan
Jarmo Malinen	Aalto University, Finland
Simona Miclaus	Nicolae Balcescu Land Forces Academy, Romania
Ana Moita	Instituto Superior Técnico and Academia Militar, Portugal
Robert Newcomb	University of Maryland, USA
Abraham Otero	Universidad San Pablo CEU, Spain
Zafer Ziya Öztürk	Gebze University of Technology, Turkey
Wim Rutten	University of Twente, The Netherlands
Seonghan Ryu	Hannam University, South Korea
Michael Schöning	FH Aachen, Germany
Mauro Serpelloni	University of Brescia, Italy
Dong Ik Shin	Asan Medical Center, South Korea
Filomena Soares	Universidade do Minho, Portugal
John Tudor	University of Southampton, UK
Pankaj Vadgama	Queen Mary University of London, UK
Duarte Valério	Instituto Superior Técnico - Universidade de Lisboa, Portugal
Renato Varoto	Independent Researcher, Brazil

BIOIMAGING Program Committee

Peter Balazs	University of Szeged, Hungary
Virginia Ballarín	Universidad Nacional de Mar del Plata, Argentina
Richard Bayford	Middlesex University London, UK
Alpan Bek	Middle East Technical University, Turkey
Alberto Bravin	Università Milano-Bicocca, Italy
Heang-Ping Chan	University of Michigan, USA
Mostafa Charmi	University of Zanjan, Iran
Jyh-Cheng Chen	National Yang-Ming University, Taiwan, Republic of China

Costel Flueraru	National Research Council of Canada, Canada
Carlos Geraldes	Universidade de Coimbra, Portugal
Dimitris Gorpas	Technical University of Munich, Germany
Tzung-Pei Hong	National University of Kaohsiung, Taiwan, Republic of China
Xiaoyi Jiang	University of Münster, Germany
Algimantas Krisciukaitis	Lithuanian University of Health Sciences, Lithuania
Hongen Liao	Tsinghua University, China
Ivan Lima Jr.	North Dakota State University, USA
Lucia Maddalena	ICAR, National Research Council (CNR), Italy
Vaidotas Marozas	Kaunas University of Technology, Lithuania
Joanna Isabelle Olszewska	University of the West of Scotland, UK
Kalman Palagyi	University of Szeged, Hungary
George Panoutsos	University of Sheffield, UK
Tae Jung Park	Chung-Ang University, South Korea
Vadim Perez	Instituto Mexicano del Seguro Social, Mexico
Gregory Sharp	Massachusetts General Hospital, USA
Leonid Shvartsman	Hebrew University, Israel
Arkadiusz Tomczyk	Lodz University of Technology, Poland
Carlos Travieso-González	Universidad de Las Palmas de Gran Canaria, Spain
Benjamin Tsui	Johns Hopkins University, USA
Vladimír Ulman	Masaryk University, Czech Republic
Yuanyuan Wang	Fudan University, China

BIOINFORMATICS Program Committee

Mohamed Abouelhoda	Nile University, Egypt
Tatsuya Akutsu	Kyoto University, Japan
Payam Behzadi	Shahr-e-Qods Branch, Islamic Azad University, Iran
Shifra Ben-Dor	Weizmann Institute of Science, Israel
Gilles Bernot	Université Côte d'Azur, France
Jean-Paul Comet	Université Côte d'Azur, France
Keith Crandall	George Washington University, USA
Thomas Dandekar	University of Würzburg, Germany
Maria Evelina Fantacci	University of Pisa and INFN, Italy
Alexandru Floares	SAIA, Romania
Dmitrij Frishman	Technical University of Munich, Germany
Giuseppe Jurman	Fondazione Bruno Kessler, Italy

Jirí Kléma	Czech Technical University in Prague, Czech Republic
Ivan Kulakovskiy	IPR RAS, Russian Federation
Yinglei Lai	George Washington University, USA
Man-Kee Lam	Universiti Teknologi PETRONAS, Malaysia
Carlile Lavor	University of Campinas, Brazil
Giancarlo Mauri	Università di Milano-Bicocca, Italy
Paolo Milazzo	Università di Pisa, Italy
Jason Miller	Shepherd University, USA
Chilukuri Mohan	Syracuse University, USA
José Molina	Universidad Carlos III de Madrid, Spain
Jean-Christophe Nebel	Kingston University London, UK
Matteo Pellegrini	University of California, Los Angeles, USA
Graziano Pesole	University of Bari, Italy
Javier Reina-Tosina	University of Seville, Spain
Laura Roa	University of Seville, Spain
Vincent Rodin	University of Brest/CNRS, France
Ulrich Rückert	Bielefeld University, Germany
J. Cristian Salgado	University of Chile, Chile
Andrew Schumann	University of Information Technology and Management in Rzeszow, Poland
João Setubal	Universidade de São Paulo, Brazil
Sylvain Soliman	Inria Saclay, France
Peter F. Stadler	University of Leipzig, Germany
Peter Sykacek	University of Natural Resources and Life Sciences, Vienna, Austria
Y-H. Taguchi	Chuo University, Japan

BIOINFORMATICS Additional Reviewers

Sergey Abramov	VIGG RAS, Russian Federation
Artem Kasianov	IITP RAS, Russian Federation

BIOSIGNALS Program Committee

Eda Akman Aydin	Gazi University, Turkey
Raul Alcaraz	University of Castilla-La Mancha, Spain
Robert Allen	University of Southampton, UK
Jesús B. Alonso	Universidad de Las Palmas de Gran Canaria, Spain

Eberhard Beck	Brandenburg University of Applied Sciences, Germany
Guy Carrault	University of Rennes 1, France
Maria Claudia Castro	Centro Universitário FEI, Brazil
Adam Czajka	University of Notre Dame, USA
Petr Dolezel	University of Pardubice, Czech Republic
Javier Garcia-Casado	Universitat Politècnica de València, Spain
Pedro Gómez Vilda	Independent Researcher, Spain
Inan Güler	Gazi University, Turkey
Thomas Hinze	Friedrich Schiller University Jena, Germany
Roberto Hornero	University of Valladolid, Spain
Akos Jobbagy	Budapest Univ. of Tech. and Econ., Hungary
Gordana Jovanovic Dolecek	Institute INAOE, Mexico
Natalya Kizilova	Warsaw University of Technology, Poland
Lenka Lhotska	Czech Technical University in Prague, Czech Republic
Harald Loose	Brandenburg University of Applied Sciences, Germany
S. Maheswaran	Kongu Engineering College, India
Luca Mainardi	Politecnico di Milano, Italy
Jirí Mekyska	Brno University of Technology, Czech Republic
Fernando Monteiro	Polytechnic Institute of Bragança, Portugal
Mihaela Morega	University Politehnica of Bucharest, Romania
Joanna Isabelle Olszewska	University of the West of Scotland, UK
Rui Pedro Paiva	University of Coimbra, Portugal
George Panoutsos	University of Sheffield, UK
Riccardo Pernice	University of Palermo, Italy
Vitor Pires	Escola Superior de Tecnologia de Setúbal - Instituto Politécnico de Setúbal, Portugal
Fabienne Poree	Université de Rennes 1, France
Shitala Prasad	A*Star, Singapore
José Joaquín Rieta	Universidad Politécnica de Valencia, Spain
Pedro Rodrigues	Universidade Católica Portuguesa, Porto, Portugal
Giovanni Saggio	Tor Vergata University of Rome, Italy
Andrews Samraj	Mahendra Engineering College, India
Reinhard Schneider	Fachhochschule Vorarlberg, Austria
Lotfi Senhadji	University of Rennes 1, France
Zdenek Smekal	Brno University of Technology, Czech Republic
H. So	City University of Hong Kong, China
Wallapak Tavanapong	Iowa State University, USA
António Teixeira	University of Aveiro, Portugal
Carlos Thomaz	Centro Universitário FEI, Brazil

Hua-Nong Ting	University of Malaya, Malaysia
Carlos Travieso-González	Universidad de Las Palmas de Gran Canaria, Spain
Egon L. van den Broek	Utrecht University, The Netherlands
Yuanyuan Wang	Fudan University, China
Didier Wolf	Université de Lorraine, France
Rafal Zdunek	Politechnika Wroclawska, Poland

BIOSIGNALS Additional Reviewers

Rafael Orsi	FEI, Brazil

HEALTHINF Program Committee

Carlos Abreu	Instituto Politécnico de Viana do Castelo, Portugal
Luca Anselma	Università degli Studi di Torino, Italy
Payam Behzadi	Shahr-e-Qods Branch, Islamic Azad University, Iran
José Alberto Benítez-Andrades	Universidad de León, Spain
Jon Bird	University of Bristol, UK
Sorana Bolboaca	Iuliu Hatieganu University of Medicine and Pharmacy, Romania
Silvia Bonfanti	University of Bergamo, Italy
Alessio Bottrighi	Università del Piemonte Orientale, Italy
Andrew Boyd	University of Illinois at Chicago, USA
Klaus Brinker	Hamm-Lippstadt University of Applied Sciences, Germany
Federico Cabitza	Università degli Studi di Milano-Bicocca and IRCCS Ospedale Galeazzi, Italy
Andrea Campagner	University of Milano-Bicocca, Italy
Manuel Campos-Martinez	University of Murcia, Spain
Davide Ciucci	Università degli Studi di Milano-Bicocca, Italy
Malcolm Clarke	Ondokuz Mayis University, Turkey
Mihail Cocosila	Athabasca University, Canada
Emmanuel Conchon	XLIM, France
Carlos Costa	Universidade de Aveiro, Portugal
Liliana Dobrica	University Politehnica of Bucharest, Romania
George Drosatos	Athena Research Center, Greece
Farshideh Einsele	Berne University of Applied Sciences, Switzerland

Arkalgud Ramaprasad	University of Illinois at Chicago, USA
Grzegorz Redlarski	Gdansk University of Technology, Poland
Alejandro Rodríguez González	Centro de Tecnología Biomédica, Spain
George Sakellaropoulos	University of Patras, Greece
Ovidio Salvetti	National Research Council of Italy - CNR, Italy
Akio Sashima	AIST, Japan
Carla Simone	University of Milano-Bicocca, Italy
Åsa Smedberg	Stockholm University, Sweden
Francesco Tiezzi	University of Camerino, Italy
Marie Travers	University of Limerick, Ireland
Yi-Ju Tseng	National Yang Ming Chiao Tung University, Taiwan, Republic of China
Lauri Tuovinen	University of Oulu, Finland
Mohy Uddin	King Abdullah International Medical Research Center, Saudi Arabia
Gary Ushaw	Newcastle University, UK
Egon L. van den Broek	Utrecht University, The Netherlands
Francisco Veredas	Universidad de Málaga, Spain
Ghada Zamzmi	National Institutes of Health, USA
Dimitrios Zarakovitis	University of the Peloponnese, Greece

HEALTHINF Additional Reviewers

Felix Beierle	University of Wuerzburg, Germany
Belkacem Chikhaoui	Computer Research Institute of Montreal, Canada
Sebastien Gaboury	Université du Québec à Chicoutimi, Canada
Varvara Kalokyri	FORTH-ICS, Greece

Invited Speakers

Federico Cabitza	Università degli Studi di Milano-Bicocca and IRCCS Ospedale Galeazzi, Italy
Katja Bühler	VRVis, Austria
Ana Rita Londral	Universidade NOVA de Lisboa, Portugal

Contents

First Version of a Support System for the Medical Diagnosis of Pathologies in the Larynx

Joana Fernandes[1,2]([envelope]) [iD], Diamantino Freitas[2]([envelope]) [iD], and João Paulo Teixeira[3]([envelope]) [iD]

[1] Research Centre in Digitalization and Intelligent Robotics (CeDRI), Instituto Politecnico de Braganca (IPB), 5300 Braganca, Portugal
joana.fernandes@ipb.pt
[2] Faculdade de Engenharia da Universidade do Porto (FEUP), 4200-465 Porto, Portugal
dfreitas@fe.up.pt
[3] Research Center in Digitalization and Intelligent Robotics (CeDRI), Associate Laboratory for Sustainability and Technology (SusTEC), Polytechnic Institute of Bragança (IPB), Campus de Santa Apolónia, 5300-253 Bragança, Portugal
joaopt@ipb.pt

Abstract. Voice pathologies are widespread in society. However, the exams are invasive and uncomfortable for the patient, depending on the doctor's experience doing the evaluation. Classifying and recognizing speech pathologies in a non-invasive way using acoustic analysis saves time for the patient and the specialist while allowing analyzes to be objective and efficient. This work presents a detailed description of an aid system for diagnosing speech pathologies associated with the larynx. The interface displays the parameters that physicians use most to classify subjects: absolute Jitter, relative Jitter, absolute Shimmer, relative Shimmer, Harmonic to Noise Ratio (HNR) and autocorrelation. The parameters used for the classification of the model are also presented (relative Jitter, absolute Jitter, RAP jitter, PPQ5 Jitter, absolute Shimmer, relative Shimmer, shimmer APQ3, shimmer APQ5, fundamental frequency, HNR, autocorrelation, Shannon entropy, entropy logarithmic and subject's sex), as well as the description of the entire pre-processing of the data (treatment of Outliers using the quartile method, then data normalization and, finally, application of Principal Component Analysis (PCA) to reduce the dimension). The selected classification model is Wide Neural Network, with an accuracy of 98% and AUC of 0.99.

Keywords: System for diagnosing speech pathologies · Wide neural network · Speech features · Vocal acoustic analysis

1 Introduction

Vocal pathologies are quite common in the population, with about 10% of the population suffering from vocal pathologies [1, 2] in different stages of evolution and severity. Vocal pathologies directly affect vocal quality, causing disorders in people's daily lives since

A. C. A. Roque et al. (Eds.): BIOSTEC 2022, CCIS 1814, pp. 1–15, 2023.
https://doi.org/10.1007/978-3-031-38854-5_1

they alter phonation. These pathologies can result in serious social problems, leading to mental problems, depression and other related illnesses [3]. Harmful habits such as smoking, excessive consumption of alcoholic beverages, persistent inhalation of air contaminated by dust and voice abuse have led to a drastic increase in these pathologies in recent times [4].

Several tests can be performed to detect vocal pathologies, such as stroboscopy, laryngoscopy and endoscopy. However, these methods require a specialist, are time intensive, invasive and uncomfortable for patients. The Consensus Auditory Perceptive Assessment (CAPE-V) scale and degree, roughness, breathiness, asthenia and tension (GRBAS) are used in auditory acoustic analyses. Nevertheless, these assessments are subjective and depend on the physician's experience who does the evaluation [5]. Developing techniques that automatically allow the acoustic analysis to be carried out saves the patient and the specialist time. It can also jeopardize the accuracy of the assessments [6].

Artificial intelligence technology in medical diagnosis has accelerated the transformation from traditional clinical diagnosis to automatic detection of voices with pathologies. However, automatically recognizing vocal pathologies is still at an early stage. The test signal is classified as having or not having the pathology or by classifying a specific pathology. Most of the published works use binary classifiers. We have as an example the work of Pakravan and Jahed, 2022 [7], Saad Darouiche et al. 2022 [8], Zhang et al. 2021 [9], Castellana et al. 2018 [10], Omeroglu et al., 2022 [11] where the classification between healthy and pathological voice is made.

The literature regarding the recognition of voice pathologies, which is intended to identify the specific pathology that affects the patient's voice, still presents few contributions and a limited group of distinct pathologies. Thus, the results do not allow these systems to be used for clinical evaluations, requiring a more profound investigation with different pathologies.

Salehi, 2015 [12], Ankışhan, 2018 [13] and Rabeh et al., 2018 [14] worked with binary classification (healthy/pathological) and obtained an accuracy of 100%. Chen and Chen 2022 [15] got an accuracy of 99.4% in distinguishing between healthy and pathological. Mohammed et al., 2020 [16], to differentiate between healthy and pathological, also obtained an accuracy of 95.41% and 94.22% and 96.13% for F1-Score and Recall. Zakariah et al. 2022 [17] got an accuracy of 77.49% without distinction of sex in the classification between healthy and pathological. A binary classification was also performed by the same authors between healthy and each pathology (Dysphonia, chronic laryngitis, dysody, functional dysphonia, vocal cord cordectomy and leukoplakia) and obtained an accuracy of 85.71%, 93.87%, 81.25%, 86.04%, 96.77% and 89.06% respectively. Ali et al., 2018 [18], in their work, used a binary classification between healthy and pathological, where they obtained an accuracy of 99.72%. However, in the binary classification between 5 pathologies (polyp × spasmodic dysphonia, polyp × keratosis, polyp × nodules, spasmodic dysphonia × nodules, spasmodic dysphonia × keratosis, keratosis × nodules and paralysis × others) accuracies of 97.54%, 99.08%, 96.75%, 98.65%, 95.83%, 97.10% and 99.13% were obtained, respectively. Hammami et al., 2020 [19], in the classification between healthy and pathological, got an accuracy of 99.26%. However, when they distinguished between hyperfunctional dysphonia and recurrent paralysis, the accuracy was 90.32%.

Observing the state of the art, it is possible to perceive that classifying between healthy and pathological speech is already possible with a high degree of accuracy. However, in these works, it is also noticed that the number of pathologies is not very wide. In general, the same authors are almost always used (vocal cord paralysis, hyperfunctional dysphonia, polyps), leaving the possibility of being more difficult for other pathologies such as Reinke's Edema, laryngeal and hypopharyngeal tumor, for example.

The reduced number of databases and subjects in the databases also means that when trying to classify different pathologies, a reduced number of pathologies is used, and the accuracies are also low.

This work will present the first version of a system to aid the diagnosis of speech pathologies associated with the larynx. This system is intended to be put into operation in clinics so that specialists collect signals from patients with diagnostic pathologies to increase the database of signals, with more subjects and vocal pathologies.

2 Materials

This section presents the database used, where the number of pathologies and the subjects used by pathological condition are mentioned. The groups of voice disorders used are also presented.

2.1 Database

The German Saarbrucken Voice Database (SVD) was used. This database is available online by the Institute of Phonetics at the University of Saarland (Pützer and Barry 2007).

The database consists of voice signals of more than 2000 subjects with several diseases and controls/healthy subjects. Each person has the recording of phonemes /a/, /i/ and /u/ in the low, neutral and high tones, swipe along tones, and the German phrase "Guten Morgen, wie geht es Ihnen?" ("Good morning, how are you?"). The size of the sound files is between 1 and 3 s and has a sampling frequency of 50 kHz.

To carry out the training to classify between healthy and pathological, 194 control subjects and 350 pathological subjects distributed across 17 pathologies were used. In the description of the curated database by Fernandes et al. 2019 [37], the total number of subjects is 901. However, since some sound files had some noise, these were excluded. Dysphonia was also excluded, as it is not a pathology but a voice disorder. Thus, the number of subjects used and its distribution among the various pathologies can be seen in Table 1.

Table 1. Table captions should be placed above the tables.

Test Groups	Sample Size
Control	194
Hyperfunctional Dysphonia	89
Vocal Cord Paralysis	74
Functional Dysphonia	51
Psychogenic Dysphonia	31
Spasmodic Dysphonia	24
Chronic Laryngitis	23
Vocal Cord Polyp	14
Reinke's Edema	14
Hypofunctional Dysphonia	9
Carcinoma of Vocal Cord	7
Hypopharyngeal Tumor	4
Cyst	3
Granuloma	2
Hypotonic Dysphonia	2
Laryngeal Tumor	1
Intubation Granuloma	1
Fibroma	1

2.2 Voice Pathologies

This section describes shortly the voice pathologies used in the database.

Chronic Laryngitis. Chronic laryngitis is characterized by inflammation that causes swelling of the laryngeal mucosa and abundant production of secretions, factors responsible for practically permanent tenacious hoarseness [20]. It corresponds to an inflammation of the laryngeal mucosa, persistent over time, sometimes with many years of evolution. As a rule, this disease is developed by several acute infections, repeated over time. People more exposed to risk factors such as tobacco, alcohol, environments contaminated by dust, smoke and irritating vapors, and abuse or misuse of the voice are usually more affected.

Vocal Cord Paralysis. It is considered a voice disorder that happens when the larynx muscles cannot perform their function. This disease can be unilateral; only one of the vocal cords is paralyzed, or bilateral when both vocal cords are paralyzed. Bilateral is rarer and more severe, as it is life-threatening, while unilateral is more common [20].

Laryngeal Tumor. It is a tumor that originates in the mucous membranes that line the larynx [21].

Carcinoma of Vocal Cord. It is a malignant laryngeal cancer that is located in the vocal cords. Usually, this tumor is associated with harmful habits such as smoking, excessive consumption of alcoholic beverages, and persistent inhalation of air contaminated by dust or irritating vapors; Also, repeated acute infections can lead to this tumor [22].

Cyst. It is a rounded body with end walls filled with fluid that can be found in the larynx or pharynx [23].

Spasmodic Dysphonia. Neurological disease involving the vocal cords. This disease conditions the quality and fluency of the voice since the voice becomes "tense" and "fragmented" as the muscles contract intensely and irregularly [24].

Functional Dysphonia. Vocal alteration is due to the use of the voice, which is when a vocal behavior disorder occurs. The incorrect use of the voice, abusive use of the voice, vocal inadaptations and psychogenic alterations can cause this disease alone or in combination [25].

Hyperfunctional Dysphonia. The symptoms of this disease are a hoarse and strained voice, with a feeling of clearing the throat and a foreign body sensation in the pharynx [27]. It is due to an excessive involuntary contraction of the phonatory muscles due to the misuse of the voice.

Hypofunctional Dysphonia. In this disease, the glottis does not close completely due to weak generalized or laryngeal muscles. In this form, the voice becomes hushed and muted. Subjects with this disease need throat clearing and the sensation of a foreign body and neck pain [26].

Psychogenic Dysphonia. It is characterized by a disorder of a psychological nature, in which voice alterations occur without laryngeal structural damage or neurological disease. In this disease, voice, articulation and fluency are sensitive to psychological oscillations. Thus, stressing factors may be related to vocal alterations [27].

Reinke's Edema. It corresponds to a chronic larynx disease that affects Reinke's space, occupied by thick mucus. As the mucus accumulates, the space increases and the vocal folds increase in thickness, heading towards the interior of the larynx. In this disease, the voice becomes hoarse and with a more severe tone since the disease causes changes in the elasticity of the vocal folds. Due to these alterations, as a rule, the patient makes a greater vocal effort, which causes an excessive opening of the glottis and an asymmetric, irregular and aperiodic vibration of the vocal folds [30]. In more extreme cases, it can make it difficult for air to pass.

Fibroma. It is a benign tumor, one of the most common in the throat area. It can be found in various parts of the throat. However, the most frequent location is the vocal cords. People who use their voices more for work, such as teachers and singers, are more likely to develop this disease due to vocal overload. Smokers or people who stay for a long time in places with dust, dry air or dangerous vapors can also develop this disease [28].

Hypopharyngeal Tumor. It corresponds to a highly differentiated neoplasm located in the back of the pharynx and usually occurs in people who systematically consume alcoholic beverages or smokers [29].

Vocal Cord Polyp. They correspond to a non-cancerous mass due to excessive use of the voice, chronic allergic reactions in the larynx or chronic inhalation of irritating substances such as tobacco or industrial pollutants. As a rule, this mass expands during growth until it is joined to the surface by a pendulum. Usually, only an isolated polyp is formed. However, there are cases where more than one formation can occur [30].

Granuloma. It is a non-neoplastic lesion that usually develops in the vicinity of the posterior vocal folds. The granuloma may look like an ulcerated lesion. It may appear as an epithelial ulceration region or take the form of a nodular or exophytic mass lesion. This disease can arise from gastric reflux, intubation trauma or vocal abuse [34]. These injuries can affect one or both vocal cords.

Intubation Granuloma. They correspond to a complication that can arise when endo-tracheal intubation occurs. This condition is increasingly common due to intubation in modern surgery [31].

Hypotonic Dysphonia. It corresponds to a voice disorder caused by a decrease in the muscle tone of the vocal folds and other muscles involved in voice formation. This pathology is a violation of the adaptive-trophic function of the autonomic nervous system [32].

3   Methods

This section describes the parameters that are used as an input matrix for a neural network that allows classifying between healthy and pathological, as well as the procedure for training the network.

3.1   Feature Extraction

This section describes all the features used.

Jitter. It is defined as the measure of the glottal variation between the vibration cycles of the vocal cords. As a rule, individuals who cannot control vocal cord vibration tend to have higher jitter values [33, 34].

Absolute Jitter (jitta) Is the variation of the glottal period between cycles, that is, the average absolute difference between consecutive periods, expressed by Eq. 1.

$$jitta = \frac{1}{N-1} \sum_{i=2}^{N} |T_i - T_{i-1}| \tag{1}$$

Relative Jitter (Jitter) Is the mean absolute difference between the consecutive glottal periods divided by the mean period and expressed as a percentage (Eq. 2).

$$jitter = \frac{\frac{1}{N-1}\sum_{i=2}^{N}|T_i - T_{i-1}|}{\frac{1}{N}\sum_{i=1}^{N}T_i} \times 100 \tag{2}$$

Relative Average Perturbation Jitter (RAP) Is the average absolute difference between a period and the average of it and its two neighbors, divided by the average period, in percentage (Eq. 3).

$$RAP = \frac{\frac{1}{N-2}\sum_{i=2}^{N-1}\left|T_i - \left(\frac{1}{3}\sum_{n=i-1}^{i+1}T_n\right)\right|}{\frac{1}{N}\sum_{i=1}^{N}T_i} \times 100 \tag{3}$$

Five-point Period Perturbation Quotients Jitter (PPQ5) Is the average absolute difference between a period and the average of it and its four closet neighbors, divided by the average period in percentage, expressed by Eq. 4.

$$PPQ5 = \frac{\frac{1}{N-4}\sum_{i=3}^{N-2}\left|T_i - \left(\frac{1}{5}\sum_{n=i-2}^{i+2}T_n\right)\right|}{\frac{1}{N}\sum_{i=1}^{N}T_i} \times 100 \tag{4}$$

Shimmer. It is defined as the variation in magnitude over glottal periods. The main reasons for the glottal magnitude variation are injuries and reduced glottal resistance [33, 34].

Absolute Shimmer (ShdB) Is expressed as the peak-to-peak magnitude variation in decibel, i.e., the base 10 algorithm of the absolute mean of the magnitude ratio between consecutive periods multiplied by 20. It is expressed in decibels by Eq. 5.

$$ShdB = \frac{1}{N-1}\sum_{i=2}^{N}\left|20 \times log\left(\frac{A_{i+1}}{A_i}\right)\right| \tag{5}$$

Relative Shimmer (shim) Is the mean absolute difference between the magnitudes of consecutive periods, divided by the mean magnitude, expressed as a percentage by Eq. 6.

$$shim = \frac{\frac{1}{N-1}\sum_{i=2}^{N}|A_i - A_{i-1}|}{\frac{1}{N}\sum_{i=1}^{N}A_i} \times 100 \tag{6}$$

Three-point Amplitude Perturbation Quotient Shimmer (APQ3) Is the average absolute difference between the amplitude of a period and the average of the amplitudes of it and its neighbor, divided by the average amplitude, expressed by Eq. 7.

$$APQ3 = \frac{\frac{1}{N-2}\sum_{i=2}^{N-1}\left|A_i - \left(\frac{1}{3}\sum_{n=i-1}^{i+1}A_n\right)\right|}{\frac{1}{N}\sum_{i=1}^{N}A_i} \times 100 \tag{7}$$

Five-point Amplitude Perturbation Quotient Shimmer (APQ3) Is the average absolute difference between the amplitude of a period and the average of the amplitudes of it and its four closest neighbors, divided by the average amplitude, expressed by Eq. 8.

$$APQ5 = \frac{\frac{1}{N-4}\sum_{i=3}^{N-2}\left|A_i - \left(\frac{1}{5}\sum_{n=i-2}^{i+2}A_n\right)\right|}{\frac{1}{N}\sum_{i=1}^{N}A_i} \times 100 \tag{8}$$

Fundamental Frequency (F0). In a speech signal, the vocal cords' vibration frequency corresponds to the fundamental frequency [35]. The F0 is determined using the Auto-correlation method with a frame window length of 100 ms and considering a minimum F0 of 50 Hz.

Harmonic to Noise Ratio (HNR). It allows measuring the relationship between a speech signal's harmonic and noise components, indicating the signal's general period-icity. The relationship between the periodic component (harmonic part) and the aperiodic component (noise) is quantified. The overall HNR value of a signal varies because dif-ferent vocal tract configurations provide different amplitudes for harmonics. The HNR is vowel sensitive, so for different vowels, one should not compare the HNR. Vowels with higher frequency components, such as the vowel 'u', are expected to have lower HNR [40–42]. The determination of HNR uses algorithms in the time domain. The first peak of the normalized autocorrelation is considered the energy of the harmonic compo-nent of the signal, and the remaining energy is regarded as the noise energy. The noisy component is given by the difference between 1 and the harmonic energy as represented in Eq. 9. In this equation, H is the harmonic component provided by the energy of the first peak of the normalized autocorrelation of the signal. The final HNR value is the average HNR over successive segments.

$$HNR(dB) = 10 \times log_{10} \frac{H}{1 - H} \qquad (9)$$

Autocorrelation. Allows similar parts of speech repeated along the signal to be mea-sured. The more similar repetitions along the signal, the greater the autocorrelation value [34, 36]. The autocorrelation of a signal is determined by dividing the normalized auto-correlation of the speech signal by the normalized autocorrelation of a window used to segment the speech signal (Hanning). Thus, the magnitude of the signal segment's first peak is considered the autocorrelation value. This process is repeated, segment by segment, until the end of the signal. Finally, the signal autocorrelation is the average of all the segments' autocorrelations.

Entropy. It considers the amount of energy present in a complex system, as it allows quantitative assessment of the degree of randomness and uncertainty of a given sequence of data. In Eq. 10, the Shannon entropy is observed, and in Eq. 11, the Logarithmic Entropy. Entropy analysis will enable you to accurately assess the characteristic nonlinear behavior of speech signals [44].

$$ShE = -\sum_{n=1}^{N} |x(n)|^2 log\left[|x(n)|^2\right] \qquad (10)$$

$$LE = \sum_{n=1}^{N} log\left[|x(n)|^2\right] \qquad (11)$$

3.2 Classification Procedure

For the network training, 13 parameters were used (relative Jitter, absolute Jitter, RAP jit-ter, PPQ5 Jitter, absolute Shimmer, relative Shimmer, APQ3 Shimmer, APQ5 Shimmer, fundamental frequency (F0), HNR, autocorrelation, Shannon entropy and logarithmic entropy). Since each subject has 3 tones and 3 vowels, each subject has 118 parameters once the subject's sex was also added. Thus, the input matrix comprises 118 lines x N number of subjects.

Considering the work of Silva et al. 2019 [37], where an improvement of up to 13 percentage points was obtained, as pre-processing of the input matrix data, the Outliers treatment was used using the box-plot method. This process consists of identifying outliers and changing their value by a threshold value determined according to the method used.

Then, the data were normalized using the range method where the interval between [−1, 1] is resized.

Finally, Principal Component Analysis (PCA) was used in order to reduce the dimension. This technique uses mathematical concepts such as standard deviation, covariance eigenvalues and eigenvectors. Initially, it subtracts the mean of each data dimension, producing a data set whose mean is zero, called the fitted data. Then, the eigenvectors and eigenvalues are calculated from the covariance matrix. It is necessary to decide how many main components to choose. Once the principal components are determined, at the output the eigenvalues are already sorted, it is only necessary to calculate the accumulated percentage of these values. In this way, the first eigenvectors corresponding to 90% or 95% of the accumulated percentage are selected. This means that the first eigenvectors explain 90% or 95% of the data [38]. Finally, the adjusted data are multiplied by the inverse of the selected eigenvector matrix. In this way, 21 components were kept to use as input to the network.

As classification methods, Decision Trees, Discriminant Analysis, Logistic Regression Classifiers were tried. Naive Bayes Classifiers, Support Vector Ma-chines; Nearest Neighbor Classifiers; Ensemble Classifiers; Neural Network Classifiers. The cross-validation technique with 10-fold cross-validation was applied to these classifiers.

Subjects were grouped into two groups, one group with control subjects and a second group with all subjects with some pathology. Therefore, the model is a binary classification process.

4   Results and Discussion

The following sections present the speech diagnosis aid system' interface to be used at the Centro Hospitalar Universitário de São João do Porto, Portugal. The system will allow a first introduction to the clinical environment and, at the same time, be able to collect the speech signal dataset.

Figure 1 shows the system's initial screen.

Figure 1 shows two options: "Record Sound" allows the acquisition of speech signals at the moment and the option "Open File" where it is possible to select pre-recorded sounds.

If the option "Record Sound" is selected, an interface like the one in Fig. 2 is obtained.

In this interface, it is possible to hear an example of the sounds intended to be recorded in the various vowels and tones. When recording the sound, it is possible to observe the representation of the sound. Finally, it is possible to listen to the signals,

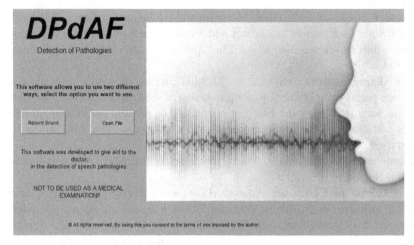

Fig. 1. Home screen of the medical decision support system.

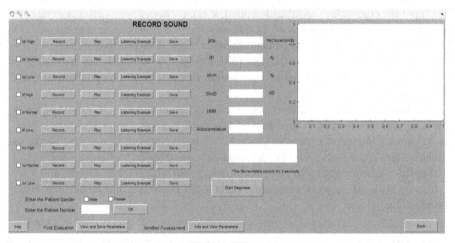

Fig. 2. Record Sound interface when we press the "Record Sound" button from the home interface. The blank places are because there is no recording yet.

redo the recording, view the signal, obtain acoustic parameters of each signal, create a database with the acoustic parameters, or add a new measurement to an already existing patient. Finally, there is the possibility to record these sounds as audio files and make a pre-diagnosis between healthy and pathological. Figure 3 shows the "Record Sound" interface when sounds were recorded to perform the diagnosis.

As seen in Fig. 3, the signals were recorded, and when the vowel /a/ Normal is selected, the parameters jitta, jitt, shim, ShdB, HNR, NHR and autocorrelation and the representation of this signal can be observed. When the button to perform the diagnosis is selected, this subject is indicated as being healthy.

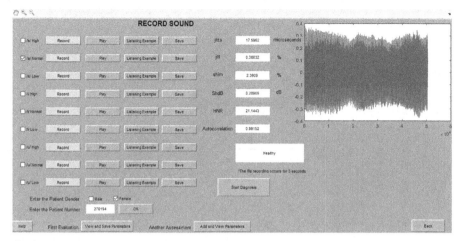

Fig. 3. Record Sound interface with a subject diagnosis with sounds available for analysis, and the subject diagnosis is already presented. The displayed signal and the parameters correspond to the Normal/Neutral /a/ signal.

The patient's database is created by selecting the 'View and Save Parameters' button, and the parameters are displayed, as shown in Fig. 4.

Date	Jitta_a_High	Jitt_a_High	Shim_a_High	ShdB_a_High	HNR_a_High	Autocorrelation_a_High	Jitta_a_Normal	Jitt_a_Normal	Shim_a_Normal	ShdB_a_Normal	H
27-Jul-2022	57.1930	1.2675	1.8002	0.1648	19.5356	0.9819	18.9862	0.4103	1.4128	0.1229	

Fig. 4. Subject parameters for all vowels in all keys.

Selecting the 'View and Save Parameters' button must happen on the patient's first consultation; otherwise, the 'Add and View Parameters' button must be selected as it will update the parameters in the database to the date of the current patient and show the results that are previously recorded (Fig. 5).

Date	Jitta_a_High	Jitt_a_High	Shim_a_High	ShdB_a_High	HNR_a_High	Autocorrelation_a_High	Jitta_a_Normal	Jitt_a_Normal	Shim_a_Normal	ShdB_a_Normal	
23-Jun-2022	22.1970	0.7282	1.6987	0.1479	29.5358	0.9986	16.6667	0.4030	1.8773	0.1658	
27-Jul-2022	22.1970	0.7282	1.6987	0.1479	29.5358	0.9986	16.6667	0.4030	1.8773	0.1658	

Fig. 5. Patient history where it is possible to observe two dates, that is, the first and second evaluation.

As it can be see in Fig. 5, when selecting 'Add and View Parameters', will update the parameters in the database and show the results that are previously registered. It is possible to observe the dates when those parameters were extracted and the parameters for all vowels and tones.

If the "Open File" option is selected, an interface like the one in Fig. 6 is obtained.

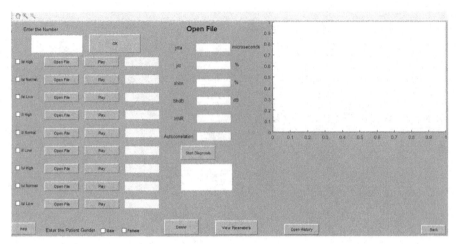

Fig. 6. Open File interface when we click the "Open File" button on the home interface. The blank places are because there is no file for analysis yet.

This interface is the same as the "Record Sound" interface. In that, it is possible to use previously recorded files, while in the "Record Sound", audio files are recorded. It does not allow for storing new data in the database but only consulting it.

In Fig. 7, it is possible to observe the "Open File" interface when a subject is selected to perform the diagnosis.

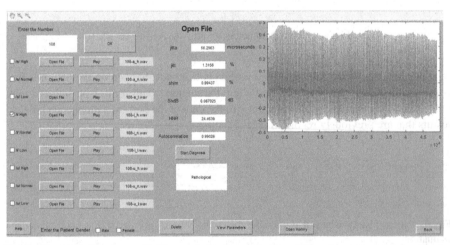

Fig. 7. Open File interface with files available for analysis and the subject diagnosis is already displayed. The displayed signal, as well as the parameters, corresponding to the /i/ High signal.

As can be seen in Fig. 7, subject 108 was selected. When the vowel /i/ High is selected, the parameters jitta, jitt, shim, ShdB, HNR, Autocorrelation and NHR can be observed, and the representation of this signal. When making the diagnosis, this signal is indicated as being pathological.

If the "View Parameters" button is pressed, the parameters will appear with the same organization described in Fig. 4. When the "Open History" button is selected, the database created for that subject will appear, as shown in Fig. 5.

The network used for the classification was a Wide Neural Network, with an accuracy of 98% and an AUC of 0.99 to distinguish between healthy and pathological subjects. This model has 100 nodes in the hidden layer, and the activation function used was ReLU. Considering the classification performance presented in the state of the art, the results obtained are at the same level. However, these results are obtained by taking into account more pathologies.

5   Conclusions

In this work, a detailed description of the first version of a system to aid the diagnosis of speech pathologies associated with the larynx was made.

In the first experimental phase, this system will collect the voices of new subjects, increasing the database with more subjects and pathologies. At the same time, it suggests to the doctor if the subject is healthy or pathological and shows evidence for the classification given by the value of the parameters presented. It also sensitizes the health professionals/clinics to use the system.

Considering the state of the art, it is easy to see that there are several works where this topic is addressed. However, these works use few pathologies. This work includes 17 pathologies in the training of the network.

The Wide Neural Network model was used to classify healthy and pathological subjects. It achieved an accuracy of 98% and an AUC of 0.99. This value is among the best performances described in state of the art.

In this way, it is possible to put this system into operation at the Hospital to follow up on improvements to the system through contact with health professionals.

Acknowledgments. The authors are grateful to the Foundation for Science and Technology (FCT, Portugal) for financial support through national funds FCT/MCTES (PIDDAC) to CeDRI (UIDB/05757/2020 and UIDP/05757/2020), SusTEC (LA/P/0007/2021) and 2021.04729.BD.

References

1. Reid, J., Parmar, P., Lund, T., Aalto, D.K., Jeffery, C.C.: Development of a machine-learning based voice disorder screening tool. Am. J. Otolaryngol. **43**(2), 103327 (2022). https://doi.org/10.1016/J.AMJOTO.2021.103327
2. Martins, R.H.G., Santana, M.F., Tavares, E.L.M.: Vocal cysts: clinical, endoscopic, and surgical aspects. J. Voice **25**(1), 107–110 (2011). https://doi.org/10.1016/J.JVOICE.2009.06.008
3. Ding, H., Gu, Z., Dai, P., Zhou, Z., Wang, L., Wu, X.: Deep connected attention (DCA) ResNet for robust voice pathology detection and classification. Biomed. Signal Process. Control **70**, 102973 (2021). https://doi.org/10.1016/J.BSPC.2021.102973

4. Godino-Llorente, J.I., Gomez-Vilda, P., Blanco-Velasco, M.: Dimensionality reduction of a pathological voice quality assessment system based on Gaussian mixture models and short-term cepstral parameters. IEEE Trans. Biomed. Eng. **53**(10), 1943–1953 (2006). https://doi.org/10.1109/TBME.2006.871883

5. Gidaye, G., Nirmal, J., Ezzine, K., Frikha, M.: Unified wavelet-based framework for evaluation of voice impairment. Int. J. Speech Technol.**25**(3), 527–548 (2022)https://doi.org/10.1007/s10772-022-09969-6

6. Hegde, S., Shetty, S., Rai, S., Dodderi, T.: A survey on machine learning approaches for automatic detection of voice disorders. J. Voice **33**(6), 947.e11-947.e33 (2019). https://doi.org/10.1016/J.JVOICE.2018.07.014

7. Pakravan, M., Jahed, M.: Significant pathological voice discrimination by computing posterior distribution of balanced accuracy. Biomed. Signal Process. Control **73**, 103410 (2022). https://doi.org/10.1016/J.BSPC.2021.103410

8. Darouiche, M.S., El Moubtahij, H., Yakhlef, M.B., Tazi, E.B.: An automatic voice disorder detection system based on extreme gradient boosting classifier; an automatic voice disorder detection system based on extreme gradient boosting classifier. In: 2022 2nd International Conference on Innovative Research in Applied Science, Engineering and Technology (2022) https://doi.org/10.1109/IRASET52964.2022.9737980

9. Zhang, X.J., Zhu, X.C., Wu, D., Xiao, Z.Z., Tao, Z., Zhao, H.M.: Nonlinear features of bark wavelet sub-band filtering for pathological voice recognition. Eng. Lett. **29**(1), 49–60 (2021)

10. Castellana, A., Carullo, A., Corbellini, S., Astolfi, A.: Discriminating pathological voice from healthy voice using cepstral peak prominence smoothed distribution in sustained vowel. IEEE Trans. Instrum. Meas. **67**(3), 646–654 (2018). https://doi.org/10.1109/TIM.2017.2781958

11. Omeroglu, A.N., Mohammed, H.M.A., Oral, E.A.: Multi-modal voice pathology detection architecture based on deep and handcrafted feature fusion. Eng. Sci. Technol. an Int. J. **36**, 101148 (2022). https://doi.org/10.1016/J.JESTCH.2022.101148

12. Salehi, P.: The separation of multi-class pathological speech signals related to vocal cords disorders using adaptation wavelet transform based on lifting scheme. Cumhur. Üniversitesi Fen Edeb. Fakültesi Fen Bilim. Derg. **36**(6), 2371–2382 (2015)

13. Ankışhan, H.: A new approach for detection of pathological voice disorders with reduced parameters. Electrica **18**(1), 60–71 (2018)

14. Hamdi, R., Hajji, S., Cherif, A.: Voice pathology recognition and classification using noise related features. Int. J. Adv. Comput. Sci. Appl. **9**(11), 82–87 (2018). https://doi.org/10.14569/IJACSA.2018.091112

15. Chen, L., Chen, J.: Deep neural network for automatic classification of pathological voice signals. J. Voice **36**(2), 288.e15-288.e24 (2022). https://doi.org/10.1016/J.JVOICE.2020.05.029

16. Mohammed, M.A., et al.: Voice pathology detection and classification using convolutional neural network model. Appl. Sci. **10**(11), 3723 (2020). https://doi.org/10.3390/app10113723

17. Zakariah, M., Ajmi Alotaibi, Y., Guo, Y., Tran-Trung, K., Elahi, M.M.: An analytical study of speech pathology detection based on MFCC and deep neural networks (2022) https://doi.org/10.1155/2022/7814952

18. Ali, Z., Hossain, M.S., Muhammad, G., Sangaiah, A.K.: An intelligent healthcare system for detection and classification to discriminate vocal fold disorders. Futur. Gener. Comput. Syst. **85**, 19–28 (2018). https://doi.org/10.1016/J.FUTURE.2018.02.021

19. Hammami, I., Salhi, L., Labidi, S.: Voice Pathologies classification and detection using EMD-DWT analysis based on higher order statistic features. IRBM **41**(3), 161–171 (2020). https://doi.org/10.1016/J.IRBM.2019.11.004

20. Toutounchi, S.J.S., Eydi, M., Golzari, S.E., Ghaffari, M.R., Parvizian, N.: Vocal cord paralysis and its etiologies: a prospective study. J. Cardiovasc. Thorac. Res. **6**(1), 47–50 (2014). https://doi.org/10.5681/jcvtr.2014.009

21. Moorthy, S.S., Gupta, S., Laurent, B., Weisberger, E.C.: Management of airway in patients with laryngeal tumors. J. Clin. Anesth. **17**(8), 604–609 (2005). https://doi.org/10.1016/J.JCL INANE.2004.12.019
22. Trotti, A., et al.: Randomized trial of hyperfractionation versus conventional fractionation in T2 squamous cell carcinoma of the vocal cord (RTOG 9512). Int. J. Radiat. Oncol. **89**(5), 958–963 (2014). https://doi.org/10.1016/J.IJROBP.2014.04.041
23. Arens, C., Glanz, H., Kleinsasser, O.: Clinical and morphological aspects of laryngeal cysts (1997)
24. Aminoff, M.J., Dedo, H.H., Izdebski, K.: Clinical aspects of spasmodic dysphonia. Neurosurgery Psychiatry **41**, 361–365 (1978). https://doi.org/10.1136/jnnp.41.4.361
25. Roy, N.: Functional dysphonia. Curr Opin Otolaryngol Head Neck Surg **11**(3), 144–148 (2003). https://doi.org/10.1097/00020840-200306000-00002
26. Kosztyla-Hojna, B., Rogowski, M., Ruczaj, J., Pepinski, W., Lobaczuk-Sitnik, A.: An analysis of occupational dysphonia diagnosed in the North-East of Poland. Int. J. Occup. Med. Environ. Health **17**(2) 2004
27. Sudhir, P.M., Chandra, P.S., Shivashankar, N., Yamini, B.K.: Comprehensive management of psychogenic dysphonia: a case illustration. J. Commun. Disord. **42**(5), 305–312 (2009). https://doi.org/10.1016/J.JCOMDIS.2009.04.003
28. Karki, P., Gurung, U., Baskota, D.: Fibroma of epiglottis. Nepal. J. ENT Head Neck Surg. **1**(1), 19–20 (2010). https://doi.org/10.3126/njenthns.v1i1.4733
29. Wycliffe, N.D., Grover, R.S., Kim, P.D., Simental, A., Jr.: Hypopharyngeal cancer. Top Magn Reson Imaging **18**(4), 243–258 (2007). https://doi.org/10.1097/RMR.0b013e3181570c3f
30. Epstein, S.S., Winston, P., Friedmann, I., Ormerod, F.C.: The vocal cord polyp. J. Laryngol. Otol. **71**(10), 673–688 (1957). https://doi.org/10.1017/S0022215100052312
31. Epstein, S.S., Winston, P.: Intubation Granuloma. J. Laryngol. Otol. **71**(1), 37–48 (1957). https://doi.org/10.1017/S0022215100051549
32. Jurkov, A.Y., Bahilin, V.M., Shustova, T.I., Alekseeva, N.S.: A crosscorrelation analysis of fluctuations in heart rate and breathing when diagnosing the autonomic disorders in patients with hypotonic type of functional dysphonia. Zhurnal Nevrol. i Psihiatr. Im. S.S. Korsakova **120**(5), 60–66 (2020) https://doi.org/10.17116/jnevro202012005160
33. Teixeira, J.P., Gonçalves, A.: Algorithm for jitter and shimmer measurement in pathologic voices. Procedia Comput. Sci. **100**, 271–279 (2016). https://doi.org/10.1016/J.PROCS.2016.09.155
34. Fernandes, J., Silva, L., Teixeira, F., Guedes, V., Santos, J., Teixeira, J.P.: Parameters for vocal acoustic analysis - cured database. Procedia Comput. Sci. **164**, 654–661 (2019). https://doi.org/10.1016/J.PROCS.2019.12.232
35. Hamdi, R., HAJJI, S., Cherif, A., Processing, S.: Recognition of pathological voices by Human Factor Cepstral Coefficients (HFCC). J. Comput. Sci. (2020)https://doi.org/10.3844/jcssp.2020.1085.1099
36. Boersma, P.: Stemmen meten met Praat. Stem-, Spraak- en Taalpathologie **12**(4), 237–251 (2004)
37. Silva, L., et al.: Outliers treatment to improve the recognition of voice pathologies. Procedia Comput. Sci. **164**, 678–685 (2019). https://doi.org/10.1016/J.PROCS.2019.12.235
38. Teixeira, J.P., Alves, N., Fernandes, P.O.: Vocal acoustic analysis: ANN versos SVM in classification of dysphonic voices and vocal cords paralysis. Int. J. E-Health Med. Commun. **11** (2020) https://doi.org/10.4018/IJEHMC.2020010103

Analysis of Extracellular Vesicle Data on Fluorescence and Atomic Force Microscopy Images

Hannah Janout[1,2(✉)]⬤, Jonas Schurr[1,2]⬤, Andreas Haghofer[1,2]⬤, Fabian Hauser[3], Jaroslaw Jacak[3]⬤, and Stephan Winkler[1,2]⬤

[1] Bioinformatics, University of Applied Sciences Upper Austria, Hagenberg, Austria
Hannah.Janout@fh-hagenberg.at
[2] Institute of Symbolic AI, Johannes Kepler University Linz, Linz, Austria
[3] Nano Structuring and Bio-Analytics, University of Applied Sciences Upper Austria, Linz, Austria

Abstract. Extracellular vesicles (EV) enable cell-to-cell communication in the body of an organism and carry significant potential in the medical field as disease indicators, tissue regeneration, and drug carriers. We developed two workflows to analyze EV data based on microscopy images reliably. The first workflow enables determining the total number of fluorophores per EV by analyzing the photobleaching step counts in a stepwise photobleaching experiment recorded through fluorescence microscopy. Furthermore, we present a workflow for the quality assessment of EV populations through multimodal imaging. Thus, enabling quantification of the purification quality (differentiation between EVs and other components) and the labeling ratio. Both workflows have shown excellent results on various data sets and under various conditions.

Keywords: Extracellular vesicle · Green fluorescent protein · Image analysis · Multimodal imaging · Bioinformatics · Fluorescence microscopy · Atomic force microscopy

1 Introduction

Extracellular vesicles (EV) were first described in 1946 [14]. They are found in eukaryotes and prokaryotes and consist of cell-derived membranous structures. EVs are used as cell-to-cell communicators as they are naturally shed or produced by cells at various stages of their life cycle under pathological and physiological conditions. They can later be absorbed by other cells and allow the transfer of proteins, lipids, or nucleic acids. Thus, EVs play an essential role in an organism's body's overall function and well-being and offer a direct way of determining the (patho)physiological state of cells and influencing cell behavior.

Since their discovery in 1946, several biological functions have been attributed to EVs. One study shows that specific types of cancer and kidney diseases significantly impact the EVs composition [2,3]. Additionally, studies show a significant potential

A. C. A. Roque et al. (Eds.): BIOSTEC 2022, CCIS 1814, pp. 16–33, 2023.
https://doi.org/10.1007/978-3-031-38854-5_2

of EVs in regenerative medicine due to their ability to promote cell survival to restore damaged or diseased cells, and tissues [1].

Henceforth, EV research has become a hot topic in the last few years, and the importance of this field is ever-growing. Nevertheless, EVs and their behavior research lack a universal standard for labeling and analysis. Consequently, accumulated EV experiment data and its analysis results vary greatly, complicating their analysis and comparison between data of different institutes. Furthermore, there is no general software available for the analysis of EV data; thus, institutes often require tailored software programs to analyze their data.

Therefore, we present two highly flexible workflows for quantifying, standardizing, and assessing the quality of EV populations displayed on microscopy images. Therefore easing the current research setback by providing a standardized and customizable way of analyzing different sorts of EV images disregardless of their type, origin, and composure.

The first workflow utilizes the principle of fluorescence and clustering methodologies to determine labeling proteins contained in EVs and the localization of EVs inside cells. Thus, allowing the evaluation of modification procedures on EV and enabling observation of EV ability to infiltrate cells.

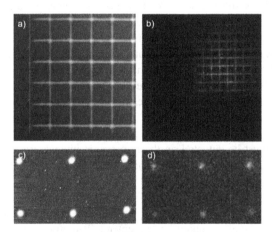

Fig. 1. Input data for quality assessment of an EV population. The first column displays the atomic force microscope and the second fluorescence microscope image data. Image a) and b) display a grid structure as orientation for image alignment. The circles are used for orientation in images c) and d), with image d) not displaying any EVs. Image taken from [16].

With the precarious quality of EV populations, consistency in EV-related experiments is hardly maintained. Thus, the second workflow presented focuses on EV colocalization and assessing a population's quality through multimodal imaging. Instead of measuring a population with one microscope, multiple are used, enhancing the obtained information and enabling different ways of analysis. Figure 1 presents an example data set for the second workflow. The images display the measurements of the atomic force microscope (AFM) in the first and fluorescence microscope (FM) in the second column. a) and b) display data sets with a grid structure used as anchor points for the alignment, while c) and d) show circular markings.

The described subject matter is based on the paper "Data Platform for the Unification and Analysis of Extracellular Vesicle Data" presented by Hannah Janout at the Doctoral Consortium of the Biostec 2022. This paper gives a more detailed view of the preliminary works proposed in the original. It provides a more detailed description of the scientific problem of extracellular vesicle research and the implemented solutions. Furthermore, it provides insight on improving and combining the implemented workflows to create better solutions to day-to-day EV problems and drive the research forward.

1.1 Goal

A common problem in EV research is the invisibility of pure EVs on fluorescent microscopy images since EVs are too small for detection and do not emit any detectable light on their own. Therefore, EVs are labeled with fluorescent substances, such as green fluorescent proteins (GFP). Through labeling, EVs become traceable, and further analysis is enabled. An example of fluorescence images with labeled EVs is shown in Fig. 2.

Before the analysis and evaluation of EVs and the whole population are possible, the modification process to carry their labeling agent must be stable and reliable. The number of labeling agents per EV directly impacts its visibility and behavior. Furthermore, the exact intensity of one labeling protein can be determined and used for further analysis through knowledge about the number of labeling proteins per EV. Labeling proteins lose their fluorescence after repeated activation due to an effect named photobleaching [9]. Thus taking a series of images of a single EV population over a specific time frame will display failed protein activation as intensity fluctuation. By analyzing this fluctuation, a conclusion can be drawn on the number of labels per EV. To enable the analysis, EVs must be detected on the fluorescent images, tracked throughout the time series, and their intensity fluctuation analyzed to determine the ultimate number of labeling and their intensity correctly.

EVs can be cultivated and modified through different procedures and utilized substance mixtures. This causes a great variety in the outcoming population quality, and consistent population quality cannot be guaranteed. Therefore, we aim to address and solve this problem by developing specialized algorithms for quality assessment in a population. One way to reliably assess the quality is by analyzing a population's life and death status and the number of successfully labeled and functioning EVs. However, with the currently available workflows, gaining the entirety of this information through one type of measurement is not possible. We aim to utilize multimodal imaging with fluorescence and atomic force microscopy for information gain and new ways to filter noise and unwanted measurements. Therefore, before a final quality assessment of the population is made, a tailored workflow must be implemented to align the different types of images through image registration techniques and enable colocalization. Furthermore, EV numbers and their properties must be analyzed for the final evaluation. While these steps seem simple, differences in data format, size, resolution, coloration, and region of interest selection complicate the process.

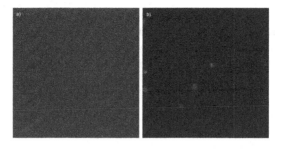

Fig. 2. First frame of two input data sets, a) displays data with only EVs. b) displays EVs contained in yeast cells. Image taken from [16].

2   State of the Art

Storing detailed research information and sharing it between institutes and researchers is a big part of driving research forward. Vesiclepedia [4] is a well-known compendium of EVs, providing free access to studies from different institutes and detailed information about EVs, such as their type of composition. Through providing the possibility of manual curation and through cooperation with EV research facilities, Vesiclepedia is ever-growing.

Advancement in EV analysis and the sheer possibility of different research methodologies have led to various algorithms and methodologies for detecting, tracking, and characterizing EVs. Some of these methodologies, such as enzyme-linked immunosorbent assay (ELISA), rely on chemical reactions for analysis. While others, such as nanoparticle tracking analysis (NTA), take a more mathematical approach [5]. While methods like ELISA allow for simple and reliable detection and quantification of EVs, no further analysis of the EVs in the population can be made unless they are processed with additional methods. Thus, requiring further expert knowledge for their complete analysis.

This paper's described goals require many solutions for commonly known challenges, such as EV detection and tracking, segmentation of cells, and the alignment of multimodal images. Detecting particles, not limited to EVs, is an indispensable step in data analysis as it lays the fundamentals for further steps. Over the years, various analysis methods have been developed, manual and automated. Typically, detection algorithms consist of three steps: preprocessing, signal enhancement, and object extraction, with varying implementations of the individual steps [6]. Wilson et al. [7] developed a workflow for the automated detection and tracking of large fluorescence microscopy data sets. They describe a new way of signal enhancement by creating a particle probability image based on calculated multi-scale Haar-like features and detecting particles through the thresholding of this image. Their workflow's automation increases its versatility and ease of use, making it a great asset. The tracking particles utilize interacting multiple model filter [8] designed for tracking highly maneuverable objects. These filters predict an object's future location, helping to associate multiple objects and reducing noise in tracking [7, 12].

The demand for neural networks for segmentation is constantly growing as use cases increase. Especially Unets, introduced by Ronneberger et al. in 2015 [10], have become a staple in biomedical image segmentation, with the original and alternative architecture defining the state-of-the-art approach. Figure 3 shows the original architecture proposed by Ronneberger et al.

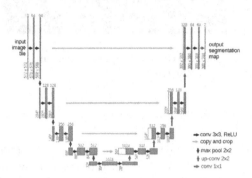

Fig. 3. U-net architecture. Each blue box corresponds to a multi-channel feature map. The number of channels is denoted on top of the box. The x-y-size is provided at the lower-left edge of the box. White boxes represent copied feature maps. The arrows denote the different operations. Reprinted and cited from U-Net: Convolutional Networks for Biomedical Image Segmentation by Ronneberger et al. [10] (Color figure online).

Enhancement of image data through the usage of multiple images, differentiated by their timestamp, viewpoint, or module, is widely used in data analysis. Over years, many algorithms for image registration, including image matching, alignment, and overlay, have been developed over the years. The Scale Invariant Feature Transform (SIFT), developed in 2004 by D.G. Lowe [11], has become the most renowned feature-detection-description algorithm. SIFT solves image rotation, affine transformation, intensity, and viewpoint changes in matching features, allowing for a precise alignment of images.

3   Methods

3.1   Determination of Green Fluorescent Proteins in Extracellular Vesicles

The base for our workflow tailored for quantifying green fluorescent proteins (GFP) in EV is made by the principle of fluorescence and stepwise photobleaching. The input data consists of a series of fluorescence microscopy images saved as SPE files. These SPE fils are a Princeton Instruments WinView CCD image file format.

As the initial intensity of a single GFP is unknown prior to the analysis, quantifying with a single fluorescence image is impossible. Thus, our workflow takes a series of images as input. These images display the same EV population at different time stamps, allowing for tracking their intensity fluctuations. In some cases, the images display not only single EVs but also cells that contain labeled EVs. This allows for the observation and evaluation of EVs in their natural environment.

The following methodologies describe how a series of fluorescence images are analyzed by detecting and tracking EVs and determining the GFP quantity through clustering principles. A more detailed description of the methodology is given in "Analysis of Extracellular Vesicles on the Basis of Nanoscale Fluorescence and Atomic Force Microscopy Images" by Janout et al.

Extracellular Vesicle Detection. EVs are expressed as small, circular blobs of higher intensity with a diameter of only a few pixels on the input images. The illumination of a fluorescence microscope is inconsistent with the whole image, creating a brighter hot spot in one image region and darker spots in another. Furthermore, EVs contained in cells lay on a brighter background than those outside of cells. Thus, the appearance and expression of EVs on these two application types may vary considerably, making the application of conventional segmentation techniques, such as thresholding, not feasible.

Therefore, we developed a specialized filter kernel for detecting EVs, which relies on the intensity difference between EV and their surrounding background. The EV detection is executed separately for each image of the series, and the kernel processes each pixel individually. The kernel's size and function depends on three parameters, *FG_kernel*, *BG_kernel* and *Delta_kernel*. *FG_kernel* covers the directly neighboring pixels of the current center pixel and describes the potential area of detectable EVs. *BG_kernel* describes the area of the background surrounding the EV. *Delta_kernel* determines the distance in pixels between *FG_kernel* and *BG_kernel*, assuring that the higher intensity of the foreground does not influence the surroundings and cause miscalculations in the background. The intensities of the foreground and background regions are averaged and compared. If the average foreground intensity is higher than the background and the difference is above a user-defined threshold, the kernel's center pixel is labeled as a potential EV. These labeled pixel locations are considered in further processing. Figure 4 shows a schematic representation of the kernel, the light gray area in the middle highlighting the foreground and potential area of the EV. The dark gray area displays the spacing determined through the delta, and black displays the pixels used for the background calculation.

Neighboring pixels labeled as EV are combined by applying a tailored floodfill algorithm. This algorithm moves over the image and connects neighboring EV pixels to one element before moving on to the next. In a grouping of EV pixels, the pixel with the highest intensity is selected as the EV center.

Due to an EV's small size, circular form, and high contrast to the surrounding background, additional calculations, as seen in the state-of-the-art approaches, Sect. 2, are not necessary. Furthermore, the algorithm's simplicity quickly accomplishes adaptations to new data.

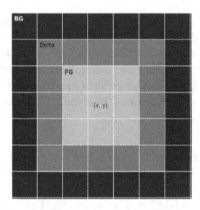

Fig. 4. Schematic representation of the detection kernel with a *FG_kernel* of size 3 and *Delta_kernel* of size 1. Image taken from [16].

Extracellular Vesicle Tracking. Once the EV detection is complete for each image of the series, a relation between the individual data of each image must be established. Hence, a so-called *track* is started for each EV found on the first image. From then on, each EV on image i, starting from the second image, has its distance calculated to all EV on image i-1. Is the distance between the EVs below a set maximum displacement, they are associated with each other. In the case of multiple matches, the closest one is chosen. By choosing a maximum displacement value, slight movement in the EV position is enabled. This is significant as the center of EVs can move minimally throughout the measurement, either naturally or through minimal miscalculations of the EVs center pixel. Figure 5 shows a schematic representation of an EVs movement over 6 frames, highlighting the importance of enabling movement between images.

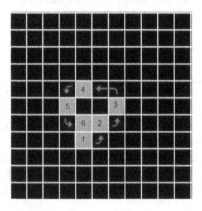

Fig. 5. Schematic representation of an EV movement throughout six frames. Image taken from [16].

Quantification of Green Fluorescent Proteins. Green fluorescent proteins express themselves in EVs through light emission when exposed to excitation light; GFPs of the same type emit light of the same wavelength. Hence, the intensity of an EV is determined by the number of contained GFPs and is always a multitude of a single GFP's intensity, only minimally influenced by noise and uneven illumination through the microscope. Through the experiment and generation of the image series, GFPs are activated repeatedly, which results in failure of their fluorophores and loss of detectable intensity. Hence, through repeated exposure, more and more GFPs lose fluorescence, and the intensity of the shown EVs fades. This phenomenon is known as stepwise photobleaching [9].

The effect of stepwise photobleaching is evident in the tracked EVs in the form of equally spaced intensity drops. Whereas the intensity drop is equivalent to the intensity of a single GFP's fluorophore. By applying the principle of clustering methodologies, the exact intensity of a single GFP and, ultimately, the total number of GFPs is determined.

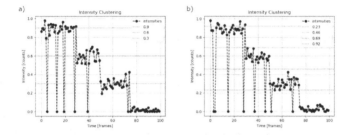

Fig. 6. Schematic representation of a tracked EV's intensities and two types of equidistant cluster centers applied. a) shows a delta of 0.3 with 3 centers, while b) shows a delta of 0.23 with 4 centers.

The clustering step is called after the tracking of EVs and is applied individually to each track. Since each EV entry of the track consists of multiple pixels, either the average or maximum intensity of an entry is used. Which of these is considered in further calculations is determined by the user. Afterward, these intensities are filtered, so only the peak values remain. These peaks are defined as intensities higher or lower than their predecessor and successor. This step is performed to eliminate the influence of noise. Then, an iterative search for the best fitting, equidistant cluster centers is started with these peak intensities. These centers are equally spaced from each other, whereas the spacing distance is equivalent to the intensity of a single GFP. Each peak entry is assigned to its closest cluster center. Therefore, no peak entry is outside of a center, but a cluster center can be without peaks. Figure 6 shows a schematic representation of an EVs track and two types of delta values used as equidistant cluster centers. The left image depicts a distance of 0.3 between the centers, with a total of 3 centers able to fit the data. For this case, the intensity of a single fluorophore is seen as equivalent to 0.3 and can be fit into the given data 3 times. Thus, this EV contains a total of 3 GFPs. The right image depicts a smaller distance of 0.23, equal to a single GFP's intensity. In total, 4 cluster centers fit into the given data, whereas one center is almost empty.

The fit of the equidistant centers to the peaks is comprised through the Davies Bouldin index (DBI). The Davies Bouldin index is a cluster validity index and is a metric to evaluate the fit between cluster data and centers. The Davies Bouldin index computes the average similarity of each cluster with its most similar one, aiming to minimize it. The closer the index is to zero, the better the fit. The formula is defined as follows.

$$DBI(S, M) = \frac{1}{N} \sum_{i=1}^{N} max_{i \neq j}(\frac{S_i + S_j}{M_{ij}}) \qquad (1)$$

whereas S describes the dispersion of the respective clusters i and j. M is the separation between the clusters i and j. S and M are listed below, where $d(u, w)$ is defined as the Euclidean distance between the points u and w.

$$S(x) = \max_{u, w \in x} d(u, w) \qquad (2)$$

$$M(i, j) = \min_{u \in i, w \in j} d(u, w) \qquad (3)$$

Cell Segmentation. Specific input images do not contain EV alone but also cells, such as yeast. In these images, EVs are not freely floating but are confined to cells and accumulated there. Their number, location, and functionality can be analyzed by analyzing EVs inside cells. In these application cases, only vesicles contained in cells are of interest, and thus, cells must be segmented before the EV detection.

We implemented two approaches for cell detection. On the one hand, a custom filter algorithm was developed, which computes the density distribution on the original image and a blurred version modified with a conventional Gaussian blur. These images are subtracted from each other, resulting in only the high-intensity regions of the cells remaining on the image and all types of noise and single EV disappearing. The filtering result is highly dependent on the chosen parameters, such as sigma for the Gaussian blur and the window size used for the density computation. On the other hand, this filter is highly adaptable through parameter changes, and its implementation was not dependent on the pre-existence of labeled data. Nevertheless, this approach is not without fault, and wrong parameter settings can result in segmentation errors and make the application overly complicated for inexperienced users. Therefore, an alternative was introduced as an Unet, a convolutional neural network developed for biomedical image segmentation [10]. The input for this Unet comprises image files of yeast cells with contained EV and a matching binary mask, highlighting the position of each cell. To ensure proper training and prevent overfitting of the network, the original input images are divided into subimages of a specific size and augmented to increase the data. The Unet trained on this data produces an image of the same size as its input, with each pixel containing the model's confidence that it belongs to a cell. Thus, by thresholding the returned image, a mask is created. The advantages of the network lie in its ease of application, as no parameters must be tuned beforehand. Consequently, this makes the Unet prone to mislabeling pixels on data with a significant difference from the images it was trained on, unlike the filtering algorithm, which can be adapted to fit several types of images. Furthermore, like almost all cell segmentation models, cells close to each other are often connected through a thin bridge, fusing them. Thus, closing is necessary, eroding and dilating the image multiple times to split these bridges. Consequently, the original shape of cells is altered, and smaller cells become more rectangular due to the mask used for the closing.

3.2 Quality Assessment of Extracellular Vesicle Populations

Using a single input image for quality assessment is not possible due to its limited information gain. Therefore, we measure EVs twice, once with a fluorescence microscope (FM) to gain information about the number of live, fluorescent EVs, and a second time through an atomic force microscope (AFM), which informs about every EV in the population, regardless of its condition. These images must be associated to enable a correct evaluation and ultimate quality assessment.

The mustering of data results in images of different sizes, formats, orientations, intensity, and regions without any prominent features for automatic extraction. Therefore, conventional image registration algorithms are not feasible. Instead, we designed a specialized workflow to extract prominent features from the measurements and compute a transformation matrix, enabling alignment, EV colocalization, and statistical evaluation.

A more detailed description of the methodology is given in "Analysis of Extracellular Vesicles on the Basis of Nanoscale Fluorescence and Atomic Force Microscopy Images" by Janout et al.

Anchor Point Extraction. The AFM and FM images contain specific structures applied to the medium in the form of either a grid or circles. These structures serve as points of orientation and anchor points for the alignment between image formats. The images are processed separately as the FM and AFM differ in intensity, size, and quality.

On the AFM images, the structures are largely pronounced and visible due to the AFMs high resolution. Therefore, conventional thresholding and Houghline algorithms suffice to extract the grid structure. For the circular anchor points, the workflow is more complicated. These points are more similar to the detected EVs and vary in size and number depending on the images. Furthermore, horizontal artifacts and uneven illumination alter the shape and intensity of points. Therefore, these images have a threshold applied to filter out lower intensity regions and convert the image to binary. Next, a connected component algorithm detects all groups of pixels not separated by a boundary. The quantified components are then filtered by their size and circularity. Thus, bright artifacts, EVs, and noise are singled out, and only the anchor points remain.

For the FM images, the workflow is not as clean due to lower image resolution and higher image noise. For the grid structure, the workflow of the AFM images is augmented by enhancing all tubular structures of the images. As a result, the grid lines are enhanced while noise and EV signals are reduced. Thus, the lines become prominent enough for a Houghline algorithm, and the grid can be extracted. However, due to uneven illumination on the FM images, part of the grid structure are not visible or oversaturated. Therefore, the last step consists of a grid reconstruction by analyzing the positioning and spacing between the lines and repositioning them. This process corrects false detected lines and fills in missing ones, reconstructing the whole grid. The intersections of grid lines are then used as anchor points for alignment. The extraction of the circular objects follows the same routine as for AFM, only with a Gaussian blur to eliminate noise and smaller EVs.

Image Alignment. Once anchor points are extracted from each image type, an affine transformation matrix is calculated by overlapping the points and determining the required transformations. An affine transformation is a linear type of transformation. It is a composition of rotations, translations, scale, and shears. Thus, image lines remain straight, contrary to nonlinear transformation types. Figure 7 shows geometric transformation and the effect the individual transformation steps have on an image [13].

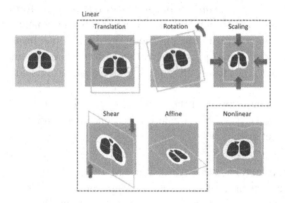

Fig. 7. Schematic display of a geometric transformation. It displays how the original image is individually transformed by rotation, translation, scaling, and shearing to form the affine transformation ultimately. Furthermore, it shows how linear transformations retain an object's straight line while nonlinear transformations alter them. Reprinted from Image processing and recognition for biological images by Uchida Seiichi [13].

Extracellular Vesicle Extraction. In both image types, extracellular vesicles express themselves as dots of higher intensity in the images. For the FM images, an additional file is available prior to analysis. This file contains the nanometer position of EV on the medium and is computed through an external software named 2Calm [15].

A topographical view of the measured medium is seen on the AFM image. Hence, regions of higher intensity are comparable to an incline and local maxima on the medium. Thus, the most efficient way of extracting EVs is through thresholding, as the nanometer height of an EV is known prior to the analysis. Hence, by converting a known nanometer scale to a range from 0 to 255, EVs are segmented based on their height.

Colocalization. The colocalization of EVs on FM and AFM images is based on the same principle as the tracking step described in Sect. 3.1. The affine transformation points from one image can accurately be mapped to the other and enable the quantification of the Euclidean distance between each point. Their distance is calculated for every EV on the FM image to those on the AFM image. If their distance is below a specific threshold, they are seen as a match and, thus, must describe the same EV. In the case of several matches, the closest one is chosen.

Statistical Evaluation. The statistical evaluation is key to assessing a population's quality as it provides necessary information about each EV group. The workflow provides information regarding the found EV on AFM and FM images and colocalized EVs. Regardless of its origin, each EV has information about its pixel, nanometer, and transformed position next to its intensity and nanometer height. Lastly, the full width at half maximum (FWHM) is calculated. This value describes the width of a spectrum curve, such as a Gaussian distribution, at half its maximum. This value requires a spectrum curve as a basis. Hence, a Gaussian distribution is fit for each EV, and based on the resulting sigma, the full width at half maximum is calculated with the following equation.

$$FWHM = 2 * \sqrt{2 * \ln 2} * \sigma \qquad (4)$$

4 Results

4.1 Determination of Green Fluorescent Protein in Extracellular Vesicle

Researchers at the University of Applied Sciences in Linz have used the first workflow described in the paper for several months and tested it thoroughly. The program's workflow begins by loading a series of images from an SPE file, a Princeton Instruments WinView CCD image format file. An example is seen in Fig. 2, a) displays the first frame of a series with only EVs, while b) shows a data set with yeast cells. The images display a visible difference in intensity of the background and the contained EVs. Furthermore, the EVs in image a) are barely visible due to their small size and noise content.

To ensure an accurate assessment of the image seen in b), a mask segmenting the cells must be computed. Figure 8 displays the outcomes of the employed strategies.

The image in a) displays the outcome of the specially developed filter, which computed a Gaussian blur and finalized the image's binarization using the standard parameters *gaussianSigma = 32* and *threshold = 0.1*. Although the low-intensity cells' edges are ragged and only half complete, the image reveals how the filter segmented each enclosing cell. These small errors can lead to miscalculation if EVs are located at the edge of a cell and only emit low light. To counteract this error, the parameters must be adapted slightly. To counteract this error, the parameters must be adapted slightly. In this case, decreasing the thresholding may result in a better result but risks introducing noise. Therefore, image b) shows the Unet result, specifically trained to segment yeast cells on fluorescence images. The model can segment the cells much cleaner than the filter, and even cells of low intensity are segmented accurately. Despite the great advantages, the Unet has its problems as well. Due to the limited training data, the model is

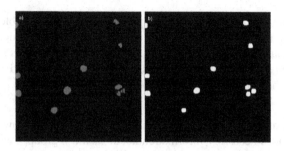

Fig. 8. Mask result of the image shown in Fig. 2. a) shows the result of the implemented filter and b) the output mask of the Unet. Image taken from [16].

slightly overfitted to the current data, making it prone to error on newly required data sets.

Each data set has its EVs recognized and tracked on each frame, regardless of the cell segmentation technique utilized. A delta value, or the determined intensity of one specific GFP's fluorescence, is computed by analyzing the intensity fluctuation for the tracked EV and clustering them according to their value.

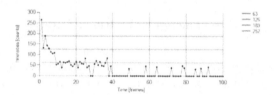

Fig. 9. Visualization of the intensity fluctuation and best fitting delta of an EV. The best delta was determined to be at 63 and can be fit 4 times into the data, resulting in a total of four GFPs. Image taken from [16].

An example is shown in Fig. 9, where the result of an EV's intensity tracking is visualized. The graph displays the individual intensities to each timestamp, in total over a time of 100 frames. The graph shows that the intensity declines over time, especially during the first 15 frames. GFP failure is exhibited through the sudden loss of intensity, which occurs between frames 1 and 15 and later in frame 39. As the graph on the figure shows, the best GFP intensity for the given intensity profile lies at 63, with a total of 4 GFPs able to fit in the data. This value reached the lowest Davies Bouldin index, indicating that the distance from cluster values to their center is minimal, with the distance between cluster centers being maximal.

A graph is created with the delta values on the x-axis and the Davies Bouldin indices on the y-axis, as shown in Fig. 10, to allow for an overview of the algorithm's workflow and the ability to reason with the outcome. The graph highlights the specified delta value in orange while displaying all valid delta values in blue. Some delta values are shown in black, and the returned index is set to a magic number as cluster validation

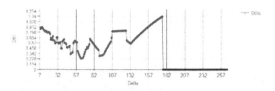

Fig. 10. Graph displaying the resulting Davies-Bouldin indices for every delta value tried on the data seen in Fig. 9. The best delta is marked in orange, while invalid tries are shown in black. Image taken from [16].

is not possible with a single cluster. Although an increase in delta causes the index to rise and become worse, it does not increase monotonously and instead exhibits a variety of local minima and maxima. Given that the delta determination shows no discernible pattern, it emphasizes the value of a thorough, iterative search.

So far, the workflow has produced fantastic outcomes. However, mistakes can always be made when detecting, tracking, or calculating delta due to noise and other factors. Thus, the workflow allows for high parameter flexibility for adapting to distinct data sets and updating EV listings following detection and tracking with an extra option to change the delta value, incorporating a user's expertise and knowledge into the workflow's decision-making.

4.2 Quality Assessment of Extracellular Vesicle Populations

Four input files are needed for the quality assessment, two for each microscope measurement. For the AFM measurements, the original JPK-QI-IMAGE and a PNG file are necessary. Information about the executed experiment, including dimension and resolution, is contained in the JPK-QI-IMAGE file. A PNG file is used as the image source since some experiments call for preprocessing to get rid of noise or artifacts.

For the FM measurements, between one and two TIFFs and one LOC file are needed. The measured fluorescence image is present in the TIFF. In earlier experiments, only one TIFF file was needed because the marks distinguished the EVs from one another well enough. Later studies replaced the marks with circles that closely resembled EVs. Thus, these experiments were enhanced with fluorescent markers that activate on a different wavelength than the GFPs. The LOC file originates from software developed at the University of Applied Sciences in Linz named 2Calm [15]. It is used for the exact localization of EV on the FM image, containing information about their position in nanometer, Gaussian sigma, resolution, etc.

Figure 1 displays the input images from the PNG and TIFF files. The first row depicts data with a grid structure as markings, a) displaying the AFM and b) the FM image. AFM measurement is too resource expensive and becomes too inaccurate for larger areas. Thus, only a medium's region of interest (ROI) is measured. The FM image displays the whole medium and has an overall lower resolution. Images c) and d) display input images from more recent experiments. Both images' grid structure was replaced by circles enhanced with fluorescence activated by the light of a specific wavelength.

c) shows the AFM measurement with high resolution, while d) displays the FM image with only the markings.

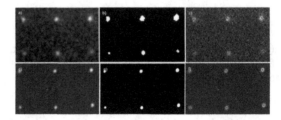

Fig. 11. Intermediate and end result of circular marking detection. The upper row displays the FM, and the lower row the AFM images. Image a) displays the original image after applying a Gaussian blur. Image b) shows the binary image created from a) with only the largest 6 elements present, and c) highlights the found markings on the original image in blue. Image d) displays the AFM image after filtering for the markings. Image e) shows the binary image with the 6 largest elements generated from d), and image f) shows the original image with the markings highlighted in blue. Image taken from [16] (Color figure online).

The following figures display the marking extraction for circular objects and a grid structure. The intermediate results of extracting circular objects are shown in Fig. 11. AFM workflow is shown in the bottom row and the FM workflow in the top row.

The images in columns a) and d) show the image after filtering, whereas columns b) and e) reveal the binary image with the 6 greatest components in the foreground. The original image is shown in c) and f) with the calculated anchor points highlighted.

Fig. 12 depicts intermediate results for the grid reconstruction and base of anchor point calculation. a) and d) display the binary images after applying connected component algorithms and filtering to the images. b) and e) display detected Houghlines of the grid structure.

Lastly, c) and f) show the reconstructed grid structure based on the Houghlines, the intersections of the reconstruction are used as anchor points in further analysis.

The images are modified to segment the shown markings and extract anchor points regardless of the present markings. For each image, the number of extracted anchor points can differ. In the case of Fig. 12 c), the number of points is higher than in f) since the whole grid structure is visible. The calculation of a transformation matrix requires the same number of points; thus, in selected cases, the anchor points must be filtered through user input to assure proper alignment. Their affine transformation matrix is calculated with the anchor points computed for each measurement. This matrix informs about the necessary rotation, scale, shear, and translation to map the points of image A to image B.

Extraction of the EVs comes after the images have been successfully aligned. EV coordinates are supplied in a LOC file for the FM images. Since there is no such data for AFM pictures, the procedure must identify the EVs. The nanometer height of EVs is known for this set of data. As a result, only the EVs are left after segmenting the image by establishing a higher and lower nanometer threshold.

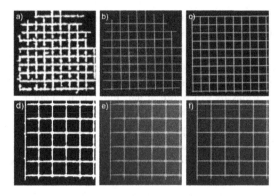

Fig. 12. Intermediate results of the grid reconstruction step necessary for anchor point extraction. The top row depicts the results for the FM data, while the bottom row shows AFM. Image a) and d) display the binary image after applying a connected component algorithm and filtering the largest objects on the original image. Images b) and e) show computed Houghlines from the binary image. Finally, images c) and f) show the reconstructed grid structure based on the computed Hough lines. The reconstruction is shown in green, and the original image is magenta. The FM images were cropped to display the grid structure for easier visualization. Image taken from [16] (Color figure online).

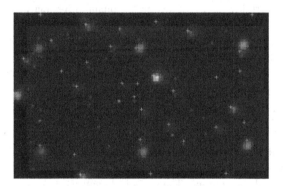

Fig. 13. Aligned images and their corresponding EVs. AFM is shown in magenta, with the EVs represented as blue crosses. FM data is visualized in green, with the EVs shown as a green asterisk. Image taken from [16] (Color figure online).

For the AFM image, EVs were found on the original image, and their locations were provided in their original format. They are brought into the same dimension as the FM EVs to enable a proper colocalization using forwarding mapping through the determined transformation matrix. Figure 13 shows a visualization of the aligned images and the results of their associated EV detection. AFM is displayed in magenta, with blue crosses representing the EVs. Green asterisks are used to represent the EVs in the FM image. As the image shows, numerous EVs were found on both the AFM and FM images. However, despite their abundance, only a small percentage of EVs can be colocalized. Colocalization is accomplished by measuring the separation between the AFM and FM's EVs. EVs that are close together and fall under a particular distance criterion are connected as the data set, and image resolution affects the threshold value. User input is therefore necessary.

For each EV present on the images, statistical information is provided in a table. These include their area, nanometer, pixel, mapping coordinates, and colocalized EV. Furthermore, each EV has its full width at half maximum calculated based on a fitted Gaussian distribution. As some of the detected EVs are only a few pixels in size, computation of this value is not always possible, and the value -1 is returned. By analyzing the given statistics, especially the number of EVs on the individual images and the percentage of colocalized EVs, the ultimate quality of the population can be assessed and used to improve EV research.

5   Conclusion

Extracellular vesicles have a crucial impact on a variety of physiological processes and cellular behavior within an organism. Due to their high potential and research value, EV processes and populations require proper analysis, evaluation, and quality assessment workflows.

We created two procedures to analyze and assess EV data based on microscope images. The first workflow concentrates on the quantitative analysis of GFP labeling in EVs using the concepts of stepwise photobleaching and clustering techniques. This algorithm correctly quantifies the GFPs of each EV and achieves excellent accuracy in detecting and tracking EVs over a set of images. Data analysis is not hindered by variations in data resolution, form, or EV density, thanks to the workflow's strong adaptability. Additionally, the procedure exhibits the same quality with EVs contained in live cells as opposed to an empty medium.

The second workflow focuses on the multimodal imaging-based quality assessment of EV populations. A significant information gain is made possible, and each method is made more dependable by combining atomic force and fluorescence microscopy. The suggested workflow has shown outstanding results for colocalizing EVs and extracting anchor points for each image type. The statistical analysis makes it possible to distinguish between EVs and other components, giving a reliable technique to measure the process of EV data purification.

When these analysis methods are combined, data on the labeling ratio and purification quality (difference between EVs and other components) is obtained. The evaluation of taken-up loads, medicines, RNAs, and other factors in constructed EV-nano-vessels will be done in the future using atomic force microscopy and stepwise photobleaching.

Acknowledgments. The work described in this paper is supported by the Center of Excellence for Technical Innovation in Medicine (TIMED, project BioCETA) and cooperation with the nanostructuring and bio-analytics (NASAN) research group at the University of Applied Sciences campus Linz.

References

1. Yáñez-Mó, M., Siljander, P.: Biological properties of extracellular vesicles and their physiological functions. J. Extracellular Vesicles **4**, 27066 (2015). https://doi.org/10.3402/jev.v4. 27066
2. Park, Y., Shin, H.: Prostate-specific extracellular vesicles as a novel biomarker in human prostate cancer. Sci. Rep. **6**, 30386 (2016). https://doi.org/10.1038/srep30386
3. Zhou, H., Pisitkun, T., et al.: Exosomal fetuin-a identified by proteomics: a novel urinary biomarker for detecting acute kidney injury. Kidney Int. **70**, 1847–1857 (2006). https://doi.org/10.1038/sj.ki.5001874
4. Kalra, R., et al.: Vesiclepedia: a compendium for extracellular vesicles with continuous community annotation. PLOS Biology. **10**, 1–5 (2012). https://doi.org/10.1371/journal.pbio. 1001450
5. Serrano-Pertierra, E., Oliveira-Rodríguez, M.: Extracellular vesicles: current analytical techniques for detection and quantification. Biomolecules **10**, 824 (2020). https://doi.org/10. 3390/biom10060824, biom10060824[PII]
6. Mabaso, M., Withey, D., et al.: Spot detection methods in fluorescence microscopy imaging: a review. Image Anal. Stereol. **37**, 173–190 (2018). https://www.ias-iss.org/ojs/IAS/article/ view/1690
7. Wilson, R., Yang, L.: Automated single particle detection and tracking for large microscopy datasets. R. Soc. Open Sci. **3**, 160225 (2016). https://doi.org/10.1098/rsos.160225
8. Godinez, W., Lampe, M., et al.: Deterministic and probabilistic approaches for tracking virus particles in time-lapse fluorescence microscopy image sequences. Med. Image Anal. **13**, 325–342 (2009). https://www.sciencedirect.com/science/article/pii/S1361841508001412, Includes Special Section on Functional Imaging and Modelling of the Heart
9. Surat, P.: Photobleaching in Fluorescence Microscopy. News-Medical.net. (2021). https:// www.azolifesciences.com/article/Photobleaching-in-Fluorescence-Microscopy.aspx
10. Ronneberger, O., Fischer, P., Brox, T.: U-Net: convolutional networks for biomedical image segmentation. In: Navab, N., Hornegger, J., Wells, W.M., Frangi, A.F. (eds.) MICCAI 2015. LNCS, vol. 9351, pp. 234–241. Springer, Cham (2015). https://doi.org/10.1007/978-3-319-24574-4_28
11. Lowe, D.: Distinctive image features from scale-invariant keypoints. Int. J. Comput. Vis. **60**, 91–110 (2004). https://doi.org/10.1023/B:VISI.0000029664.99615.94
12. Chenouard, N., Bloch, I., et al.: Multiple hypothesis tracking in microscopy images. In: 2009 IEEE International Symposium on Biomedical Imaging: From Nano To Macro, pp. 1346–1349 (2009)
13. Uchida, S.: Image processing and recognition for biological images. Dev. Growth Differ. **55**, 523–549 (2013)
14. Chargaff, R.: The biological significance of the thromboplastic protein of blood. J. Biol. Chem. **166**, 189–197 (1946). https://www.sciencedirect.com/science/article/pii/ S0021925817349979
15. Mayr, S., Hauser, F., Puthukodan, S., Axmann, M., Göhring, J., Jacak, J.: Statistical analysis of 3D localization microscopy images for quantification of membrane protein distributions in a platelet clot model. PLOS Comput. Biol. **16**, 1–34 (2020). https://doi.org/10.1371/journal. pcbi.1007902
16. Janout, H.: Data Platform for the Unification and Analysis of Extracellular Vesicle Data. (Biostec 2022). https://www.insticc.org/node/TechnicalProgram/biostec/2022/ presentationDetails/110275

Automated Segmentation of Patterned Cells in Micropatterning Microscopy Images

Jonas Schurr[1,2(✉)] , Andreas Haghofer[1,2] , Peter Lanzerstorfer[3] ,
and Stephan Winkler[1,2]

[1] University of Applied Sciences Upper Austria, Bioinformatics, Hagenberg, Austria
[2] Johannes Kepler University Linz, Linz, Austria
jonas.schurr@fh-hagenberg.at
[3] University of Applied Sciences Upper Austria, Wels, Austria

Abstract. Micropatterning in living cells is used for the analysis of protein-protein interactions. The quantitative analysis of images produced within this process is time-consuming and non-trivial task. For the simplification and speedup of such analyses, we describe a method for fully automated analysis of micro-patterned cells in fluorescence microscopy images. An approach based on an evolution strategy allows the grid extraction of the assays to estimate the pattern on the cells. We outline a workflow for the segmentation of these patterned cells based on a Unet. We also show the efficiency of different data augmentations applied to different patterning setups. A Dice score of 0.89 with 3 μm patterns and 0.79 with 1 μm patterns could be achieved. As we demonstrate in this study, we can provide thorough micropatterning studies, by automating the cell segmentation process.

Keywords: Image processing methods · Fluorescence microscopy · Image analysis · Bioinformatics · Image segmentation

1 Background

The analysis of molecule interactions is usually not a simple task. Interactions between a membrane protein and a cytosolic interaction partner are of critical importance for cell signaling. They are often involved in the first steps conveying information across the plasma membrane. It has been shown that subcellular μ-patterning, is a flexible and straightforward method for the analysis of these protein-protein interactions in living cells. [1] By using subcellular μ-patterning protein interactions cannot only be observed in the cell membrane but also in the cytosol of living cells [1, 3]. With this approach, images of living cells are generated, which allows a simplified characterization of protein interactions. Especially quantification and intensity analysis are of high interest and can provide valuable insights. Further developments in medical and biological experiments, automated analysis, simplified evaluation, and reliable extraction of important measures are important for the use and development of new and improved microarrays and biochips.

A. C. A. Roque et al. (Eds.): BIOSTEC 2022, CCIS 1814, pp. 34–52, 2023.
https://doi.org/10.1007/978-3-031-38854-5_3

With this in mind, we here present a framework for automated cell segmentation and quantitative analysis of fluorescence-microscopy images for the analysis of protein µ-patterning experiments. By providing framework features such as automated object identification and segmentation, a straightforward quantitation process of recorded microscopy images (as shown in Fig. 1) was realized.

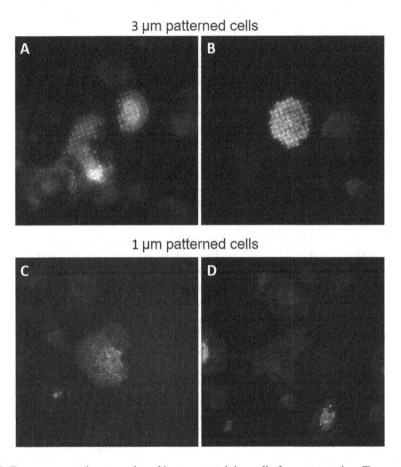

Fig. 1. Four representative examples of images containing cells for segmentation. Two samples for 3 µm patterning and two samples for 1 µm patterning. In sub-figure B and C a lower number of cells are shown with high intensity. While in sub-figure D an image with multiple unsegmented patterned cells is shown with low intensity.

During the process of image acquisition, a vast number of single images as well as image stacks (representing respective time-resolved image series), are generated. Therefore, easy-to-use tools and algorithms are required for faster and simple image processing and evaluation. Due to the high amount of data, automation of the cell segmentation steps is of critical importance. A higher degree of automation allows higher comparability, objectivity, and reproducibility also by the reduction of manual steps performed by humans. Manual analyses require domain knowledge and are time-consuming. Even with a high variance within and between images of patterned cells, an accurate characterization regarding quantification and intensity is important [1].

For the quantification and intensity analysis of single patterns on patterned cells, an automated extraction of the patterns is of high interest. Besides the identification of the patterns themselves, only cells with patterns are of interest for the final extraction of measures. A distinction between patterned cells and unpatterned cells must be realized to extract only valid protein-protein interactions.

For this case, we have developed and improved a software suite called Spotty [5]. Spotty is a highly modular framework and easy-to-use GUI. Spotty offers multiple dedicated bioimaging workflows with reusable generalizable algorithms for the analysis of fluorescence microscopy and intensity analysis. Also, this work is integrated into this software. The proposed approach contributes to the automation of the analysis and evaluation of these experiments. The here proposed workflow provides important metrics which are automatically extracted and analysed.

Multiple steps are required and provided for fully automated analyses of quantity, intensities, and contrasts of patterned cells. For the extraction of the patterns and their surroundings grid estimation is required. Additionally, a robust and accurate cell segmentation is necessary. One of the main goals of this work is the replacement of manual cell segmentation. It is often done manually or by semi-automated thresholding which is not accurate enough in this case. For automated patterned cell segmentation, neural network models are used. Multiple problems must be solved by an automated approach. The segmentation must be robust and has to differ between relevant patterned and unpatterned cells. It has to deal with high variability between different cells but also high variability in cells between different images. Additionally, the models must handle two different types of patterns which are 1 μm patterns and 3 μm patterns. Also problem specific experiment quality can influence the result with artifacts, cell viability, and pattern quality besides image quality problems like size, location, and noise, as shown in Fig. 1.

Parts of this work are based on the first authors' previous work [4]. In this work, the used methods and their results were extended. We additionally show the effect of data augmentation applied to different patterning setups. The difference of data based on 1 μm patterning and data based on 3 μm patterning are elaborated. We also focused on the use of additional data augmentation and sub-imaging. Multiple sizes of sub-images were tested. Additionally, new state-of-the-art neural network model architectures were used.

2   State of the Art

Advancements in microscopy and in the field of fluorescence microscopy imaging have led to an increasing amount of images and more high-quality data. This opens up the possibility to identify the behavior of cell organelles and biological processes. This also leads to more extensive analyses of protein-protein interactions through μ-patterning. Due to the rising complexity and amount of data, fast algorithms with a degree of automation can increase analysis speed. To best of the authors' knowledge, no previous publications exist providing a fully automated analysis of protein-protein interactions in living cells, which are based on μ-patterning. Similar works have been conducted before, but they often do not provide an easy-to-use workflow and require additional human intervention [10, 11].

Multiple research groups deal with the biological analysis of microarrays. Since solutions are often tailored to a single experiment, the absence of generalizable algorithms is a common issue in image analysis and bioimaging. But still, fully automated workflows for particular biological problems are often not available. General image processing tools such as ImageJ or dedicated software from microscope manufacturers can often provide limited functionality for extensive analysis including multiple steps and often require expert knowledge [12, 13].

There are many cell segmentation algorithms solving different problems [14, 16, 21]. Depending on the problem and objectives, traditional image processing methods like thresholding can deliver sufficient results. But often, especially in cell segmentation with high variability or unspecific cell characteristics they can be inaccurate or not robust enough. Therefore neural networks have recently been used as a state-of-the-art approach and provide the best overall performance on specific problems.

For cell segmentation, currently, as a basis for the architecture of models, mostly Unet-shaped neural network models are used [14]. Since then multiple improvements and adaptions have been published as state-of-the-art models for cell segmentation neural networks [2, 15, 21]. They can better generalize high variability between multiple but also within images and do not require a specific parameter tuning based on the problem, which is often carefully adjusted with domain experts. On the other side, a sufficient amount of mostly manual labeled high-quality labels is necessary. Especially for segmentation, this can be a time-consuming task. A promising technique to increase the amount of data and therefore the variability of a data set is data augmentation. Data augmentation is used for model training and can increase the performance of a model compared to the original data set [22, 23]. This work aims to solve the mentioned field-specific problems since the available state-of-the-art methods cannot provide suitable results and do have their limitations.

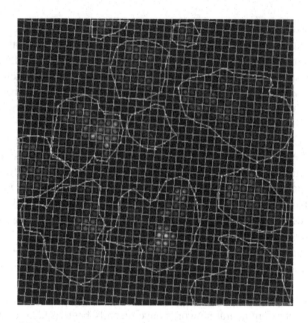

Fig. 2. Representative image of manual marking of the cells which have to be analysed. These ROIs are also used as labels for model training. Image taken from [4].

3   Methodology

The proposed workflow streamlines the study of μ-patterning data. It is specifically developed to work with μ-patterning arrays, which are used to study how proteins interact with one another in living cells. The related pattern within an assay cell (grid cell) will be more luminous if there is a contact between the cell and the examined proteins on the assay. Fluorescence microscopy is used to capture several images of μ-patterned living cells. Multiple images and image stacks can be handled using the suggested methodology. The ROIs must be extracted after performing the required grid estimation for the patterns created by an evolutionary strategy to extract the patterns on (and outside) the cells [6]. With our approach presented here, we further improve and simplify the analysis and comparison of μ-patterning data with an automated cell segmentation approach as shown in Fig. 3. For the creation and use of the model labeled data was collected in executed analyses within the previous workflow and labeled by domain experts as shown in Fig. 2. Image preprocessing steps like sub-imaging was applied before model training. Additionally, data augmentation was performed and tested to solve problems of a low amount of labeled data. After creating the model architecture and training the model, post-processing is required due to a lack of robustness in special and corner cases. After segmentation, Regions of interest (ROIs) are created and the extracted patterned cells can be used for final pattern evaluation, final characterization, and analyses.

3.1   Data and Material

The already implemented and used workflow was used for the labeling and creation of ground truth data for the training of the neural network. Currently, the labeling for a ground truth is done by domain experts where ROIs are drawn to mark wanted cells and areas. These ROIs were extracted and saved for later usage. The extracted ROIs are used as labels representing patterned cells. Unpatterned cells are not labeled and are not of interest (as shown in Fig. 5). An advantage of this procedure is, that all produced labels are real-world data and real-world labels extracted out of the used workflow for actual analyses. For the finale usage of the model for the segmentation of patterned cell small deflections are neglectable. This is due to the single patterns where only patterns in grid cells which are fully within a cell are included in the final evaluation. A full pattern for final evaluations is defined by patterns which are part of the cell and where the cell is fully within a grid cell of the detected grid. The used images and extracted labels do have a size of 512×512 pixels and are grayscale images or binary images, respectively. Additionally multiple setups in the biological experiments are used. The amount of labeled for training is 60 images (1 μm patterned) and 75 images (3 μm patterned). One major difference which can influence the results is a difference in size for the physical grid structure. In this work in the first case 1 μm structures are used and in the second case 3 μm structures are used. This is also reflected in the images resulting in much smaller grid cells for images of the 1 μm setups and therefore in a different representation of patterned cell structure in the images.

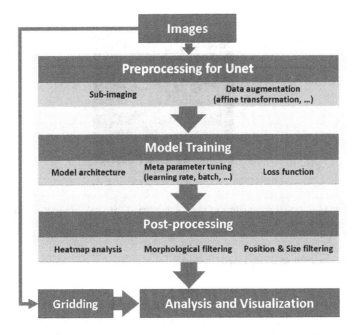

Fig. 3. The single steps of the whole analysis workflow are shown. Preprocessing for Unet, Model Training and Post-processing are part of the segmentation workflow.

3.2 Gridding

A line grid is fitted onto the image to help distinguish each signal from the array's cell-by-cell pattern. Ted fitted grid mimics the micro array's grid structure, which allows the analysis of every pattern on every cell by designating a grid cell for it. Automating this process enables a quick and easy analysis of the images. In addition, if I an image the fitted grid is not suitable enough, the grid can be manually adjusted. An evolutionary strategy was used to align the grid as accurately as feasible. The grid was defined using a number of factors, mainly affine transformation parameters. Specifically, rotation (deflection with regard to the image's edges), scaling, and translation. (vertical and horizontal offset). Scaling is defined by the grid width which defines the distance in pixels between two grid lines. The adjustable parameters are represented in Fig. 4. These parameters are optimized based on the fitness function. The fitness of a parameterset representing a grid is evaluated by the difference between the image of an expected grid and a processed version of the original image. To get an image that can be compared to an expected grid the single signals need to be extracted while the background needs to be ignored. To approach this, canny edge detection algorithm was used with additional binarization of the image and closing to improve the signal of the single array cells in the binary image. To remove noise dilation and erosion steps are performed. The image is processed in a way to reflect the signal and distinguish the signal compared to the background. The fitness is defined by the percentage of overlapping white pixels, which represent the lines between the signals defining the grid, and black pixels, which represent the signals.

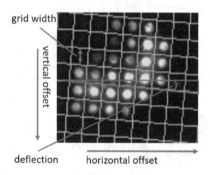

Fig. 4. Overview of the used parameters of the solution candidate representing a grid for pattern selection within a cell [6].

3.3   Automated Cell Segmentation

Since the relevant patterns that need to be extracted are on cells, relevant cells have to be found. For a fast analysis, this step must be accurate and automated. For the automated segmentation, a Unet was trained. Additionally, post-processing has to be applied to remove cells that contain less than four patterns because they can't be used for further analysis and also to exclude cells on the border of the image. Additionally, it is used to increase the accuracy of the Unet, as the mentioned encoder-decoder. By itself, the accuracy of the Unet is not high enough due to limiting factors such as constraints according to size, quality of the patterns, and location. In addition, images can be adapted manually within the GUI afterward, if needed, by manually removing unwanted cells or slightly moving or adapting the segmented regions by erosion, dilation, or translation.

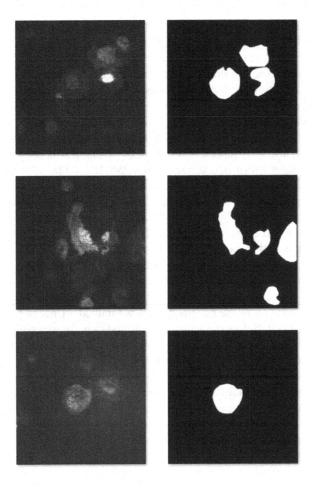

Fig. 5. Comparison of the wanted, labeled patterned cells and the corresponding raw image (right: raw image, left: labels).

Preprocessing. At first a resizing to the same size of all images is necessary to assure the same size in all single images. In our case images are 512×512 pixels. The raw input images used for this part of the analysis and the cell segmentation are grayscale images between 0 and 255 representing the intensity levels of the captured experiment. The images are grayscale and to allow a faster calculation and simple training the values are normalized to values between 0 and 1. The masks were prepared to match values of 0 or 1 per pixel, where 1 is representing a patterned cell and 0 is representing the background.

It is necessary to tackle the problem of low amounts of data. While 60 images can be enough for the learning process of a Unet, in our images, with high variability and a high amount of corner cases, it is crucial to provide a high enough amount of data with a large variety between the images to provide corresponding features of the cells. A possibility to reduce the problem of a low amount of data can be the use of sub-images. By splitting the whole image into sub-images of the same size the amount of training data for the model can be increased. We created multiple randomly cropped sub-images for each epoch. In our case factor 20 to the original amount of image was used for each epoch. The sub-images are created based on a random sub sample of the original images. Additionally, it also simplifies the learning process by providing less or even single cells within a sub-image. By doing this it has to be taken into account that there are also images with multiple cells. While a cell can lie on the border also in the original image and can be cut without being fully represented on the image, it can be necessary to keep also fully represented cells in the learning samples. For the augmentation, the sub-images with different sizes (256×256, 128×128, 64×64 and 32×32) are applied. Four kinds of augmentations were used with a given probability besides random cropping. Namely: $90°$ rotation and flipping, linear transformations (rotation, scaling and shearing), noise by Gaussian blur, and intensity alterations by changing randomly intensity and contrast. These modifications are used to give more possibilities for the position and shape of the cell within the image. While these modifications are mainly used to increase the number of images, then a shifting of the brightness was applied to increase the number of over- or underexposed images. It can also be used to improve the image quality of over- and underexposed images themselves.

For the segmentation of the patterned cells, we trained a Unet to predict the areas filled by a relevant cell. Before the actual training, additionally, we applied the augmentation to further increase the variance within the data set and increase the performance of the model. Data augmentation can increase the amount of data and therefore increase the segmentation accuracy. By applying suitable functions for multiple image modification we can also provide samples and constellations or positions of cells that were not within the training set which can also lead to an increased variance within the data set. This can lead to a more robust model and can prevent overfitting. By applying multiple modifications and combinations to a single image multiple copies of the image will be generated which increases the size of the data set multiple times. To further increase variability, for each batch original raw pictures are randomly chosen for random cropping and augmentation. Therefore on a high chance, each new sub-images is unique and the model almost never gets the exact sub-images within the whole training process. The augmentation functions are provided by a package called Albumentations are used [18]. The mentioned augmentation is only applied to the training set.

Model Training. Also in this work, the idea of a neural network, especially an encoder-decoder architecture, is used for feature extraction and final segmentation. As an increment of the original Unet, Unet++ with RegnetY120 as backbone was used in this work [20,21]. The implementation of a Unet++ with RegnetY was used besides other architectures as the standard implementation of the Unet, an Attention Unet and a Residual Unet [19,21]. Unets allow full segmentation with a single model. In some cases, especially if there is not enough data for corner cases and outliers, the performance of the model can decrease. These corner cases can be identified by the adaption of the architecture of the neural network or can be handled with post-processing. A split of 70% for training 15% for validation, and 15% for testing was used. Multiple settings for the used batch size were tested, our training showed the best results with a batch size of 32. The training of the model is stopped after 1000 epochs since the used validation loss does not further improve.

For the final prediction of the full 512×512 test images, multiple sub-images with the size of the trained sub-images are used for the prediction to reconstruct the final image. With a sliding window, multiple overlapping sub-images are created and predicted. The multiple overlapping predictions are combined within a heatmap. By thresholding with 50%, the final prediction is done.

For the creation of the model, multiple loss functions and metrics have been tested to counteract the class imbalance. Because in segmentation problems the performance measured only by the correctly identified pixels compared to all pixels is not suitable as a loss function and therefore it does not provide suitable results, because the model cannot learn or extract features. The following metrics, which are also used in literature, were used: Dice score, accuracy, sigmoid focal cross-entropy, binary cross-entropy [17]. Sigmoid focal cross-entropy was used as an improvement compared to binary cross-entropy which can be used in imbalanced data to down weight the classification of the simple class, which is normally the background. In the current model, a merged score of the Dice score weighted with 1.5 and binary cross-entropy weighted with 0.5 was used as loss function for the final results.

Post-processing. To further improve the performance of the model, heatmaps based on the output of the last layer were generated. Based on these results areas which are hard to predict can be extracted. This knowledge can be used for performance improvements in corner cases like close cells and cell borders, but it is also used for labeling the data to identify and increase the number of hard cases and corner cases.

In addition to the prediction of the model, post-processing steps are performed to further increase the accuracy and get the necessary results for the follow-up analyses, but also to further increase the Dice score of the segmentation result after the model prediction. Cells with a low linear distance between them can be merged into one single cell by small bridges within the model prediction. Therefore the model outcome is adapted by post-processing with morphological filtering. Morphological filtering is applied to solve an occurring problem of the prediction of the network to reduce the number of such bridges and to separate connected cells into two single cells. Through opening (erosion followed by dilation) with a 7×7 structuring element, we can increase the amount of separated cells. And therefore also increase the overall performance.

Additionally, a possibility for the removal of cells that are too small is necessary. Sometimes cells cannot fully grow onto the used plate within the biological experiments. Therefore the part of the cell which can be seen and has to be analysed in the image is too small and does only contain a few patterns which are also often not well-shaped or fully developed. Whereas these cells are theoretically valid cells with patterns they are not considered for further evaluation. These have to be excluded afterward which is done by a connected components algorithm and based on a threshold for the size given by the user currently it is used with a minimum size of 1% of the image. Besides the exclusion of too small cells, cells touching the border of the image also have to be excluded for final evaluations. Since the contrast is often not high enough or they interact with the edge of the plate within the biological experiments and therefore can be malformed and cannot be used for further analyses. The filtering for cells connected to the border is not included into the final results since patterned cells for model training include patterned cells which are also on the border of the image. But they are excluded afterwards since they have to be excluded for further biological analyses.

Result Analysis and Evaluation. For a final evaluation, the global background and the spot radius of a single pattern cell must be considered. The spot radius defines the circle of a pattern. This radius declares the area that is taken into account for the signal and differs between the local and global background. This difference is used for the calculation of the contrast. First, the global background needs to be subtracted to calculate the contrast of a signal and provide comparability between multiple signals. To analyse potential protein-protein interactions intensity and contrast values between foreground and background of each grid cell for each patterned cell on the image, the intensity metrics are calculated and are visualized as in an heatmap.

Implementation Details. The developed algorithms and GUI are implemented in C#. Additionally for the preprocessing and the model training Python 3.9 with OpenCV 3.5, Pytorch 1.11 and Tensorflow 2.7 with CUDA 11.6 was used [8,9]. The trained model and the segmentation workflow were integrated into our existing framework to allow a full automation and usage of the cell segmentation with all the other processing and evaluation algorithms and connect them to a full workflow for μ-patterning analyses.

4   Results

We show that the patterned cell segmentation provides useful results. We have conducted multiple tests with augmentation, different sub-images, data types, and post-processing steps for improved results and to solve the mentioned problems. As shown in Fig. 6 the presented approach can automatically select wanted cells and remove unwanted cells. The model deals with cells of different intensities and can also differ between good pattern quality and unpatterned cells and also often between insufficient pattern quality on the cells. Also, artifacts are often not included in the predicted cell segments or can be excluded in the post-processing. Even though the segmentation is not perfectly fitting all labels, most patterned cells are identified correctly and segmented fairly well. These results show that even with corresponding preprocessing segmentation by a Unet is not always enough, since it does have problems separating close cells and filtering cells by their size. We show that the proposed post-processing can be used for the problem of connected cells and too small cells or very small artifacts. We provide qualitative and quantitative results which show the suitability and limitations of the approach. Additionally results about the influence of data augmentation and different sub-images on different types of micropatterning are elaborated and discussed.

4.1   Segmentation Results

Three representative examples can be seen in Fig. 6 and Fig. 9. In Fig. 9 an example for a not perfect prediction can be seen, even if with post-processing the cells can be

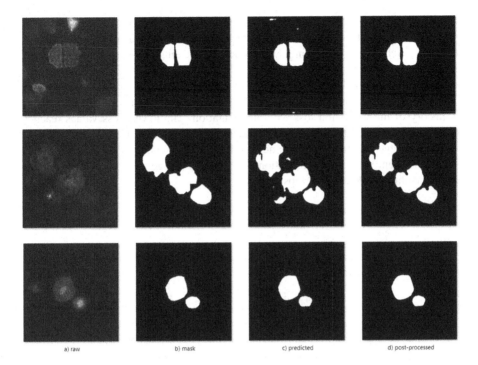

a) raw   b) mask   c) predicted   d) post-processed

Fig. 6. Three row-wise examples of unseen predicted images of the test set. Comparison of raw image, mask image, predicted image, post-processed image.

separated and small areas of false positive areas can be removed, two low-quality patterned cells remain. In the one case this can be due to the fact that one of the cells does indeed have a visible pattern but is not good enough for a final evaluation. In the second case this can be due to the fact that the wrongly segmented cell does have patterns but is too dark in comparison to the other cells. Additionally the cells are very close and connected by bright bridges in between them. In the first row of Fig. 6 a almost perfect fit can be seen. Only relevant patterned cells with a high quality pattern are included into the segmentation result. Multiple non relevant patterned cells with low quality pattern, artifacts and unpatterned cells are ignored. Additionally the wanted patterned cells are segmented correctly and separated already by the Unet. In the second image (second row) a similar result can be seen but with the problem of additionally wrongly segmented parts of a low quality patterned cell. By post-processing these wrongly segmented areas can be removed. In all three images it can be seen that the original correct predictions of the Unet remains almost untouched and does not reduce the quality of the prediction.

4.2   Model Training

Two different types of data are generated by different biological setups. The difference in these setups is defined by the grid size of the patterns, where the grid size can be 3 μm or 1 μm resulting in smaller patterns on the cell. To get high accuracy for both types of images, they are used for the training of different models to provide sufficient results on images for each type of patterning. One model is not enough to extract the differences between these two types of images. In Fig. 7 the difference in the training history of the validation can be seen in the different loss curves. The upper line is the result without additional augmentation besides cropping sub-images. The lower line shows the training history of the validation loss with augmentation. The lowest loss values reached are 0.15 with augmentation and 0.19 without augmentation. The difference between the two curves suggests a slight improvement on the test data set due to augmentation (1. It can also be seen that with augmentation the results converge earlier and therefore can reduce the amount of learning steps.

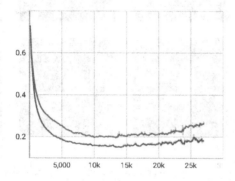

Fig. 7. Validation loss curve of two different models based on 1 μm patterning data. Comparison of curve with augmentation (lower) and without augmentation (upper). The x-axis show the number of performed training steps and the y-axis the loss value.

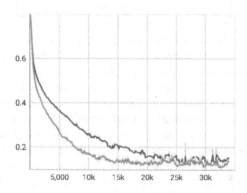

Fig. 8. Validation loss curve of two different models based on 3 μm patterning data. Comparison of curve with augmentation (lower) and without augmentation (upper). The x-axis show the number of performed training steps and the y-axis the loss value.

Figure 8 describes the validation history of the training of the models based on the 3 μm images. It shows the comparison between the curves with (lower) and without (upper) augmentation. The lowest loss values reached are 0.10 with augmentation and 0.12 without augmentation. Compared to the 1 μm results (shown in Fig. 8) for the training with 3 μm images, the 3 μm models can provide slightly better lowest loss values. The augmentation does not suggest an additional improvement but still does provide a faster convergence in the training process in the case of 3 μm images.

4.3   Prediction Results

In Table 1 the final results of the models on the unseen test set are shown. For each type of data set, the same test set is used. It can be clearly seen that there is a noticeable difference in overall performance between 1 μm and 3 μm. While the Dice score in 3 μm images reaches up to 0.84 with image size 256×256 pixels, 1 μm augmentation is lower with up to 0.78 also with an image size of 256×256 pixels. Multiple metrics were computed to show the overall performance of the models. While for 1 μm data the model shows decent performance regarding a Dice score of 0.78, some problems in the prediction with the model are clearly reflected in the precision, with a score of 0.69. On the contrary, recall and sensitivity do have a high value indicating a stable prediction regarding false and true negatives. A high value in recall and specificity indicates a good performance for finding all wanted cells without missing too many cells or without missing too many parts of a cell. The lower value in the precision is due to a higher number of false positives, which can be explained by a higher amount of falsely segmented cells without patterns. Besides a small number of false positives

Table 1. Comparison of trained models based on Dice score, precision, recall and specificity.

Pattern	Augmentation	Size	Dice	Precision	Recall	Specificity
1-μm	excluded	256×256	0.761	0.675	0.934	0.962
1-μm	excluded	128×128	0.740	0.638	0.942	0.954
1-μm	excluded	64×64	0.714	0.597	0.960	0.943
1-μm	excluded	32×32	0.697	0.576	0.961	0.937
1-μm	**included**	**256×256**	**0.778**	**0.686**	**0.941**	**0.964**
1-μm	included	128×128	0.740	0.631	0.953	0.951
1-μm	included	64×64	0.693	0.568	0.970	0.935
1-μm	included	32×32	0.715	0.610	0.942	0.948
3-μm	excluded	256×256	0.815	0.749	0.940	0.980
3-μm	excluded	128×128	0.840	0.769	0.941	0.980
3-μm	excluded	64×64	0.809	0.731	0.933	0.975
3-μm	excluded	32×32	0.733	0.618	0.955	0.958
3-μm	**included**	**256×256**	**0.843**	**0.778**	**0.952**	**0.981**
3-μm	included	128×128	0.801	0.707	0.964	0.974
3-μm	included	64×64	0.783	0.683	0.955	0.970
3-μm	included	32×32	0.748	0.633	0.953	0.962

within the prediction at the area of cell borders, the main amount of false positives comes from wrongly segmented unpatterned cells. There are similar results with models on 3 µm data but in general the overall performance is better. A Dice score of 0.84 can be considered as a good result, especially regarding the low amount of data and high amount of variability between the images. A large part of the performance increase is due to a highly increased precision compared to the results on 1 µm data. Therefore, more unpatterned cells are correctly ignored for segmentation and not segmented. This increase compared to 1 µm data could be explained by the nature of the data. While 1 µm patterns are very small and often not easy to detect, 3 µm patterns are fairly large and easier to detect.

Over all models, no general positive effect of data augmentation can be seen. There is a small difference between models on the test set regarding augmentation. Augmentation can slightly increase the performance of both models trained on image size 256×256. The largest difference in 3 µm data due to augmentation is represented in the increase of precision. Still the change in recall and specificity is small. It seems that augmentation cannot or only slightly increase precision and therefore overall performance. This positive effect does not account for models trained on smaller sub-images. In general there is a decline in the Dice score with smaller sub-images. All scores for smaller sub-images than 256×256 pixels are smaller than the best result for each pattern type. This clearly shows a disadvantage of even smaller sub-images. This could be due to the fact that smaller sub-images do not always allow to learn the whole cell structure especially for larger cells. They also produce more artifacts within the prediction resulting in more false positives and reduced precision.

Table 2. Comparison of trained models based on Dice score, precision, recall and specificity.

Pattern	Augmentation	Size	Dice	Precision	Recall	Specificity
1-µm	excluded	256×256	0.787	0.712	0.933	0.969
1-µm	excluded	128×128	0.774	0.688	0.936	0.965
1-µm	excluded	64×64	0.754	0.650	0.952	0.956
1-µm	excluded	32×32	0.738	0.635	0.944	0.953
1-µm	included	256×256	0.791	0.706	0.935	0.968
1-µm	included	128×128	0.757	0.657	0.943	0.957
1-µm	included	64×64	0.714	0.597	0.960	0.944
1-µm	included	32×32	0.749	0.665	0.927	0.961
3-µm	excluded	256×256	0.828	0.772	0.929	0.983
3-µm	excluded	128×128	0.888	0.860	0.929	0.987
3-µm	excluded	64×64	0.865	0.827	0.920	0.983
3-µm	excluded	32×32	0.796	0.710	0.941	0.972
3-µm	included	256×256	0.850	0.793	0.945	0.984
3-µm	included	128×128	0.827	0.747	0.960	0.979
3-µm	included	64×64	0.822	0.749	0.947	0.977
3-µm	included	32×32	0.793	0.704	0.939	0.971

4.4 Post-processing

In Table 2 the final results of the whole workflow tested on the test data set are shown. Post-processing increases the Dice score in all models at least slightly. In general, post-processing have a higher effect on model predictions trained with smaller sub-images. This can be explained by the removal of generated small artifacts of the model within the predicted image. Models trained on smaller sub-images do include a higher amount of small artifacts segmenting single patterns or small parts of cells. With post-processing, these false positive areas are removed, which increases precision and also the Dice score. In general, compared to the prediction of the model itself with post-processing there is almost no change specificity, but therefore a trade-off between a higher increase in precision and therefore a smaller decrease in recall. Besides higher scores, the results over different runs are fairly similar to the Unet prediction result. If primary connected cells are disconnected and the wanted result is reached, it is slightly reflected in the Dice score. Another positive effect is due to size-based filtering. For the best performing segmentation models seen in Table 1 the Dice score changed from 0.778 to 0.79 in 1um images and from 0.843 to 0.85 in 3um images. The best overall performance on 3 µm data could be reached with sub-images of size 128×128 with a score of 0.89. The already high Dice score could be largely increased by post-processing. Because the prediction with models trained on smaller sub-images provides more artifacts. Morphological filtering can improve the result and can separate connected cells from each other while in other images the Unet was already sufficient. Therefore, it is also necessary that the operation does not adapt the prediction too much to keep the prediction of the Unet and preserve the segmented areas. This is also reflected in a consistent or even increasing Dice score. The effect of additional morphological filtering can be seen in Fig. 9.

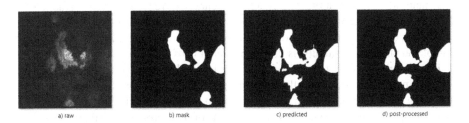

a) raw   b) mask   c) predicted   d) post-processed

Fig. 9. Representative example of the effect of post-processing. The morphological operation removes the connections between the different cells as shown in sub images c and d (Dice score model: 0.714, Dice score post-processing: 0.731.).

5 Conclusion and Outlook

The strategy for segmenting cells for protein-protein interactions on patterned cells used in this research does provide good results and is totally automated. We have showed, depending on the dataset, that there can be a small effect of data augmentation on to the final segmentation accuracy. Post-processing with morphological filtering and size-based filtering has a positive effect onto the performance of the whole workflow. The proposed workflow and the models are integrated into Spottys μ-patterning analysis pipeline. Spotty is a user-friendly software suite that we have developed for simple and extensive studies of fluorescence microscopy images and experiments, with dedicated, generalizable, and reusable algorithms. We have showed the practicability and possibilities of the algorithm and improvements of biomedical image analysis in the context of μ-patterning by improving patterned cell segmentation. With the presented approach and results, we can speed-up and simplify analysis for biologists. The software is already completely functional in its present form, and it has been used effectively in a number of articles [1, 3, 7]. An important step that still had to be performed manually is the cell selection and segmentation. With this work, we are automating this step.

In general dealing with low amounts of data for supervised learning is of high interest in the analysis of biological data and in bioimaging to speed-up and allow ongoing biological experiments. A Dice score of 0.79 and 0.89, respectively, indicate good results considering the high variety of cells and low amount of data. If cells are found they are already good segmented. Proposed post-processing show that the problem of connected cells can be solved by filtering. With the improved prediction on 3 μm images compared to 1 μm images we could increase the accuracy of a part of the workflow. On the other hand, the overall performance is often reduced by segmented cells without a valid pattern generating false positives. One of the problems with the false positive segmented cells is, that cells with a low quality of patterns are often not considered as wanted cells and therefore not in the label. Another limitation is also the separation of connected, cells even if cells can be separated by morphological filtering, overlapping cells with valid patterns or very close cells sharing long borders, without visible intensity differences can still be a problem reducing overall performance by detecting a lower amount of correct cells. More and improved data labels will further improve the segmentation to achieve a higher amount of accuracy to reduce human interaction by adapting the outcome of the segmentation workflow. In the current state also the differentiation between wanted and valid patterned cells and unwanted patterned cells for example due to too low quality, is the main limitation of the current approach.

In the future, we want to improve and expand our solutions for biomedical data analyses and image analysis, especially for the mentioned upcoming projects. Multiple ideas of existing works for example in [2] will be tested for suitability to further improve the shortcomings of the segmentation step. First tests of their proposed method show good results. Similar to that method in the future we expect increased accuracy by integrating the characteristics of the research problem and the data set like using the estimated grid of the gridding step within the network to further increase accuracy by providing additional information especially for the differentiation between wanted patterned and unwanted patterned cells or unpatterned cells. Possible improvements to further enable better possibilities for the model to increase robustness, additional handcrafted features as input channels can be used. Representations could include the grid information as an additional layer. With this information, we expect to provide a possibility to allow distinguishing between unpatterned and patterned cells. To further support the segmentation pipeline a classification model for the detection of single patterns will be used in future. For post-processing also thresholding like the watershed algorithm can be used afterward. Which will lead to higher overall accuracy and therefore for a better fully automatic cell segmentation and use of the model. This shall assure needed efficiency, reproducibility, objectivity, comparability, and accuracy in biomedical data analysis.

Acknowledgements. The work described in this paper is supported by the Center of Excellence for Technical Innovation in Medicine (TIMED, project BIOsens), and the Christian-Doppler Forschungsgesellschaft (Josef Ressel Center for Phytogenic Drug Research). Special thanks to my supervisor Joseph Scharinger.

References

1. Lanzerstorfer, P., Müller, U., Gordiyenko, K., Weghuber, J., Niemeyer, C.: Highly modular protein micropatterning sheds light on the role of Clathrin-mediated endocytosis for the quantitative analysis of protein-protein interactions in live cells. Biomolecules **10**, 540 (2020)
2. Scherr, T.: Cell segmentation and tracking using CNN-based distance predictions and a graph-based matching strategy. PLoS ONE **15**, 1–22 (2020). https://doi.org/10.1371/journal.pone.0243219
3. Hager, R., Müller, U., Ollinger, N., Weghuber, J., Lanzerstorfer, P.: Subcellular dynamic immunopatterning of cytosolic protein complexes on microstructured polymer substrates. ACS Sens. **6**, 4076–4088 (2021)
4. Schurr, J.: Automated Cell Segmentation for Micropatterning Microscopy Images. Paper presented at BIOSTEC 2022 (2021). https://biostec.scitevents.org/Abstracts.aspx
5. Schaller, S., Jacak, J., Borgmann, D., Weghuber, J., Winkler, S.: An image analysis suite for automated spot detection in cellular and nano structures of microscopy images. In: Proceedings of the 20th Annual International Conference on Intelligent Systems For Molecular Biology (ISMB) (2012)
6. Borgmann, D., Weghuber, J., Schaller, S., Jacak, J., Winkler, S.: Identification of patterns in microscopy images of biological samples using evolution strategies. In: Proceedings of the 24th European Modeling And Simulation Symposium, pp. 271–276 (2012)
7. Stadlbauer, V., et al.: Fluorescence microscopy-based quantitation of GLUT4 translocation: high throughput or high content? Int. J. Mol. Sci. **21**, 7964 (2020)
8. Abadi, M., et al.: TensorFlow: large-scale machine learning on heterogeneous systems (2015). https://www.tensorflow.org/. Software available from tensorflow.org
9. Chollet, F.: Keras (2015). https://keras.io
10. Uka, A., Polisi, X., Halili, A., Dollinger, C., Vrana, N.: Analysis of cell behavior on micropatterned surfaces by image processing algorithms. In: IEEE EUROCON 2017–17th International Conference On Smart Technologies, pp. 75–78 (2017)
11. Koohbanani, N., Jahanifar, M., Tajadin, N., Rajpoot, N.: NuClick: a deep learning framework for interactive segmentation of microscopic images. Med. Image Anal. **65**, 101771 (2020)
12. Motsch, V., Brameshuber, M., Baumgart, F., Schütz, G., Sevcsik, E.: A micropatterning platform for quantifying interaction kinetics between the T cell receptor and an intracellular binding protein. Sci. Rep. **9**, 1–10 (2019)
13. Thomas, R., John, J.: A review on cell detection and segmentation in microscopic images. In: 2017 International Conference On Circuit, Power And Computing Technologies (ICCPCT), pp. 1–5 (2017)
14. Ronneberger, O., Fischer, P., Brox, T.: U-net: convolutional networks for biomedical image segmentation. In: International Conference On Medical Image Computing And Computer-Assisted Intervention, pp. 234–241 (2015)

15. Vicar, T., et al.: Cell segmentation methods for label-free contrast microscopy: review and comprehensive comparison. BMC Bioinf. **20**, 1–25 (2019)
16. Xing, F., Yang, L.: Robust nucleus/cell detection and segmentation in digital pathology and microscopy images: a comprehensive review. IEEE Rev. Biomed. Eng. **9**, 234–263 (2016)
17. Jadon, S.: A survey of loss functions for semantic segmentation. In: 2020 IEEE Conference On Computational Intelligence in Bioinformatics and Computational Biology (CIBCB), pp. 1–7 (2020)
18. Buslaev, A., Kalinin, A.: Albumentations: fast and flexible image augmentations. ArXiv E-prints (2018)
19. Diakogiannis, F., Waldner, F., Caccetta, P., Wu, C.: ResUNet-a: a deep learning framework for semantic segmentation of remotely sensed data. ISPRS J. Photogrammetry Remote Sens. **162**, 94–114 (2020)
20. Iakubovskii, P.: Segmentation Models Pytorch. GitHub Repository (2019). https://github.com/qubvel/segmentation_models.pytorch
21. Radosavovic, I., Kosaraju, R., Girshick, R., He, K., Dollár, P.: Designing Network Design Spaces (2020)
22. Nalepa, J., Marcinkiewicz, M., Kawulok, M.: Data augmentation for brain-tumor segmentation: a review. Front. Comput. Neurosci. **13**, 83 (2019)
23. Ali, M., et al.: Evaluating very deep convolutional neural networks for nucleus segmentation from brightfield cell microscopy images. SLAS DISCOVERY: Adv. Sci. Drug Disc. **26**, 1125–1137 (2021)

Automated Data Adaptation
for the Segmentation of Blood Vessels

Andreas Haghofer[1,4(✉)], Thomas Ebner[2], Philipp Kainz[2], Michael Weißensteiner[2],
Nassim Ghaffari-Tabrizi-Wizsy[3], Isra Hatab[3], Josef Scharinger[5],
and Stephan Winkler[1,4]

[1] Bioinformatics Reasearch Group, University of Applied Sciences Upper Austria,
Softwarepark 11-13, Hagenberg, Austria
[2] KML Vision GmbH, Nikolaiplatz 4/2, Graz, Austria
[3] Otto Loewi Research Center, Immunology and Pathophysiology, Medical University of Graz,
Heinrichstraße 31, Graz, Austria
[4] Department of Computer Science, Johannes Kepler University, Altenberger Strae 69,
Linz, Austria
Andreas.Haghofer@fh-hagenberg.at
[5] Institute of Computational Perception, Johannes Kepler University, Altenberger Straße 69,
Linz, Austria
https://bioinformatics.fh-hagenberg.at/,
https://www.kmlvision.com/

Abstract. In the field of image analysis used for diagnostic processes, domain shifts constitute a significant obstacle. Domain shifts lead to an incompatibility of an otherwise well-performing AI model for image segmentation. Accordingly, if two different machines image the same tissue, the model may provide better results for one of the two images depending on the similarity of the image data compared to the training data for generating the AI model. In this paper, we analyzed how the input images of a neural network have to be adapted to provide better segmentation results for images which are previously not compatible with the used model. Therefore, we developed two approaches to increase a model's segmentation quality for a dataset with initially poor results. The first approach is based on heuristic optimization and creates a set of image processing algorithms for the data adaptation. Our algorithm selects the best combination of algorithms and generates the most suitable parameters for them regarding the resulting segmentation quality. The second approach uses an additional neural network for learning the incompatible dataset's recoloring based on the resulting segmentation quality. Both methods increase the segmentation quality significantly without the need for changes to the segmentation model itself.

Keywords: Heuristic optimization · Machine learning · Image processing

1 Introduction

The affordability of high-performing computers and the fast-growing number of use cases increased the adaption of image segmentation algorithms using neural networks

A. C. A. Roque et al. (Eds.): BIOSTEC 2022, CCIS 1814, pp. 53–72, 2023.
https://doi.org/10.1007/978-3-031-38854-5_4

in medical applications. Popular neural networks such as the Unet [3] and its constantly improving variations represent the state-of-the-art segmentation models in medical imaging. To be able to provide the demanded segmentation quality, all these algorithms rely on labeled data for the so-called training process where the network learns which parts of the provided images are relevant.

Using data augmentation [4] techniques such as rotation, cropping, and color manipulation to artificially increase the number of learning samples, models like Unet [3] could be trained on just a few sample images. Nevertheless, for a newly arrived dataset it's sometimes not possible to achieve the same segmentation quality as during the training and also testing. Due to changes in the imaging setup, different image parameters could lead to worse segmentation results, even if the underlying sample might be the same. Even if this lack of generalization can be compensated with data from different imaging setups and varying staining concentrations, it is often not affordable to cover all possible variations during the modeling process.

In our case, all the individual datasets of blood vessels provide different properties in terms of their colorization and contrast. The commonly used approach for solving this problem would be an adjustment of the whole model for each of the datasets, which does not represent a suitable solution for our project since the underlying model must stay the same. Due to data limitations and a high variation of the individual data samples, we required a solution that provides an adaptable pre-processing approach to achieve higher compatibility of new datasets with our existing segmentation model. In addition to the already published evolution strategy workflow presented at the Biostec 2022 [1] we also created another pre-processing strategy based on convolutional autoencoders [13] which we will compare to the state-of-the-art method in the results Sect. 3.

Our workflows represent alternatives to the commonly used transfer learning for adapting an existing model for a new dataset. Despite the adaption of the already trained model, we created a pre-processing workflow that can adjust an incompatible dataset to fit the model, which leads to an improved segmentation quality. The main advantage of this approach is that the model itself does not change. Besides a neural network based approach, we also created a heuristic workflow for generating a specialized pre-processing pipeline.

1.1 Problem Description

Using chick embryo models [18] the imaged blood vessels are formed on polymerized collagen through nylon grids. By a magnification of 40x, the individual images were recorded with a resolution between 0.8 and 1.2 µm per pixel. Despite the variations in colorization and contrast, all images provide three color channels with 8 bits per channel. As shown in Fig. 1 our images provide a significant variation in their image properties, especially in their colorization. Dividing the available data, we created two separate datasets, in the following called A and B. Dataset A was created using 150 images with similar image properties like image a in Fig. 1. Dataset B is consists of 27 images with a high variation in image properties as images b, c, d of Fig. 1 indicate.

To be able to focus on the significant pre-processing steps, we needed a measure to identify the differences between two datasets. We wanted to answer the question if the difference is mainly based on the colorization of the blood vessels themselves or within

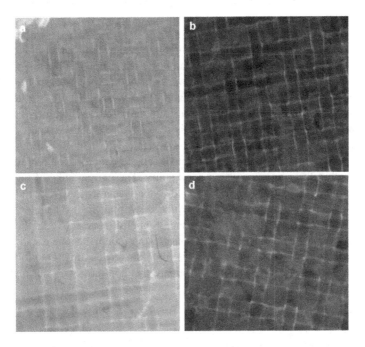

Fig. 1. Examples of blood vessels images formed on polymerized collagen through nylon grids with different properties in terms of colorization and contrast. Source: [1].

the surrounding background. Based on the intensity histograms of each color channel of the individual images, we compared the images using the Hellinger distance built in the OpenCV framework [17].

Based on the exemplary sample shown in Fig. 2, the higher Hellinger Distance between the two backgrounds is significantly higher at 0.61 than the distance of 0.019 between the blood vessel regions. According to these results, we assumed that any change in colorization should result in significant changes to the similarity of two datasets, which also impacts the overall compatibility with a pre-trained segmentation model.

Besides the dataset, we are in the initial position of having an already well-performing neural network model trained on dataset A. The variety of colorization and contrast still inhibits the use of this already trained segmentation neural network on dataset B.

Our workflow aims to increase the segmentation quality on dataset B of the model trained on dataset A. Adding an automated pre-processing workflow preceding the actual application of the segmentation model should improve the segmentation quality without needing to change the model itself. This pre-processing workflow should either be generated by a heuristic-based approach using a selection of image processing algorithms or model-based using a specifically trained neural network.

1.2   State of the Art

The lack of enough training data, representing one major issue for machine learning-based research, could be compensated partially by using transfer learning [2]. Based on the idea that already trained neural networks provide a benefit over training from scratch, this learning technique uses the weights of pre-trained networks instead of random weights during the initialization of the training process. Therefore, the learning algorithm must only adjust the network weights for the new data without learning the whole feature processing from scratch.

Reliable solutions for solving the presented lack of generalization represent a topic of interest within the computer vision community. The current state-of-the-art methods are based on deep learning methods called Cycle-Generative Adversarial Networks [19,20] which can change the staining of images without losing cellular structures, requiring an extensive amount of training data. Some of these networks are also fully self-supervised. They do not need labeled image data to adapt the image staining, which is a significant benefit compared to methods like transfer learning. Due to limitations of the available data, we are not able to compare this approach with our methods and catch up on that in later work.

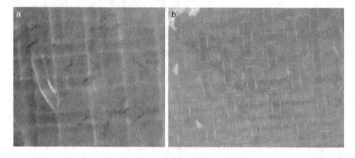

Fig. 2. Sample images of two different datasets representing one example of different image properties. Source: [1].

2   Methods

Besides the algorithmic differences, the amount of needed data represents the main difference between our presented approaches. Our evolution-based approach provides a self-adapting pre-processing pipeline specialized for each new arriving dataset requiring only one labeled image. In contrast, our recoloring networks are comparable with transfer learning in terms of data needed since these networks also have to learn the individual properties of each type of image to achieve an appropriate recoloring result.

A shared requirement between both approaches is the need for an already well-performing segmentation network on similar types of images. In our case, we used an Unet++ [6] based architecture from the segmentation models package for Pytorch [7] with the regnety_120 backbone [5]. Including techniques like data augmentation and image cropping for extending the used dataset A, this model was trained on 82 sample images, validated on 15 samples during the parameter optimization process, and tested on 18 samples that were not used during any of the previous steps. We additionally tested the model on the test samples from the second dataset B, which were also used for our pre-processing approaches.

Our model achieved a Dice Score of 0.6765 on the test samples of dataset A which already provides an impression that the segmentation of these blood vessels is not an easy task, even for these specialized types of neural networks. Based on the low score achieved on Dataset B with a Dice score of only 0.1073, it could be seen that our model was not able to deliver any usable segmentation result on this dataset.

2.1   Heuristic Image Manipulation

Relying on heuristic optimization, our evolution process combines the optimal set of pre-processing algorithms as well as select the appropriate parameters. Instead of testing all possible parameter and algorithm combinations, this type of optimization is based on the idea of natural evolution, where the fittest candidates (sets of parameters and algorithms) build up the parents for the next generation. This fast selection process provides an adaptive pre-processing step for the segmentation of microscopy images of blood vessels based on the resulting segmentation quality of the neural network.

Image Processing Algorithms. The chosen algorithms for the algorithm selection are the following:

- Image blurring
- Contrast adjustment
- Color shift

This pre-selected pool of algorithms was used due to their capability of changing the significant image properties to increase the similarity between two datasets.

As shown in Fig. 3 the significant difference between image a and image b is colorization and contrast beside the visible difference in grid scaling, representing the main problem of a neural network trained on a dataset solely containing images of similar colorization and contrast. Both pictures, image a and image c, provide similar information even if image c is colored differently after applying our pre-processing methods.

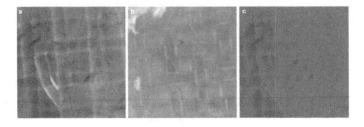

Fig. 3. Pre- and postprocessing images of blood vessels. a: raw image without processing, b: image from training dataset, c: processed image Source: [1].

Despite image c still providing the relevent information about the blood vessels, it is now more similar to the training dataset in terms of colorization and contrast.

This image manipulation is done by the following algorithms, which are parameterized by our algorithm.

Image Blurring. Mostly used for the reduction of image noise, Gaussian blur represents one of the most common image blurring algorithms.

Even if the image on the left shown in Fig. 4 represents a less detailed representation of the raw image due to the application of a Gaussian blur, the required blood vessels are still clearly visible. This algorithm uses a filter kernel of defined size to represent an approximation of the Gaussian curvature [8]. The actual filter step calculates the dot product of each pixel within the filter kernel, until every pixel of the image was part of at least one calculation. The dimension of the kernel matrix, like the one in Fig. 4 is defined by our optimization algorithm.

Contrast Adjustment. An image's contrast can be manipulated by an adjustment of the ratio in the intensity difference between bright and dark areas of image structures.

$$adjustedImage(i, j) = \alpha \cdot image(i, j) + \beta \qquad (1)$$

Using the Eq. 1, each pixel value of each channel is multiplied with a gain α and summed up with a constant β [9].

Highlighting the red blood vessels on the right side of the image the effect of contrast adjustment can be clearly seen in Fig. 5. The values α and β are selected by our algorithm.

Color Shift. Typically used as data augmentation technique, color shifting directly influences the histogram of each color channel by subtracting an offset value, which changes the distribution of the intensities. The used offset values are different for each color channel (oR, oG, oB) as shown in Eq. 2 and are selected by our algorithm.

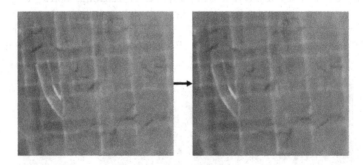

Fig. 4. Example images of blood vessels with and without the application of a 3 × 3 Gaussian blurring kernel. Left: raw image, Right: processed image Source: [1].

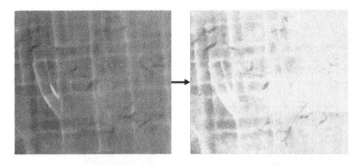

Fig. 5. Example image with applied contrast adjustment compared to a unprocessed image. Left: raw image, Right: contrast adjusted image [1].

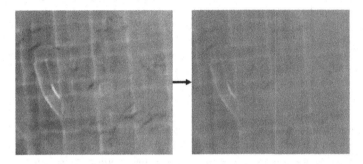

Fig. 6. Example image for the application of a color shift which completely changed the overall blue dominated colorization into a more red dominated one. Left: raw image, Right: processed image [1]. (Color figure online)

$$image(i,j)R = image(i,j)R - oR$$
$$image(i,j)G = image(i,j)G - oG \quad\quad (2)$$
$$image(i,j)B = image(i,j)B - oB$$

Figure 6 shows, that the shift in colors changed the overall blue dominated image to a more red dominated one.

Evolutionary Optimization of Preprocessing Workflows. Acting as an input-manipulation step in front of the actual segmentation model, as visualized in Fig. 7, our evolution strategy-based parameter optimization requires one input image for the optimization. The individual solution candidates (algorithm combination and parameter settings) are generated based on the last iterations candidates with the best fitness or are initially entirely random. Each solution candidate is then used for the pre-processing of the input image. The result of this pre-processing will be fed into the segmentation model, which results in a segmentation mask. This mask, compared to the ground truth label, indicates the quality of the solution candidate. The resulting fitness helps the evolution strategy in selecting the best candidates for the next iteration and adjusts the settings of these candidates to ultimately reach the best solution.

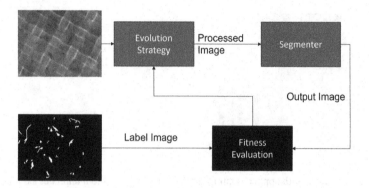

Fig. 7. Representation of our optimization workflow using a labeled image of the new dataset for the optimization by the evolution strategy. Each iteration of the evolution process results in manipulated images segmented by the segmentation model. Based on the segmentation quality, the fitness evaluation indicates the quality of each generated set of algorithms and parameters. This process is repeated until the fitness can no further be improved or a specified amount of iterations are fulfilled. The last iteration's best set of algorithms and parameters represents the best and final result. [1].

Our optimization workflow uses an island-based evolution strategy [10] which requires solution candidates representing the parameter sets to be optimized and the used algorithm combinations. These two parts of the candidates are not optimized in the same way. Whereas the parameters for the algorithms are optimized for each candidate individually, the set and order of the algorithms are selected by using the so-called islands of evolution strategies and never change for one specific solution candidate. This approach significantly reduces the needed processing time by reducing the island during the optimization process.

Solution Candidates. Each solution candidate is therefore built up by the following optimization parameters:

- algorithms used
- order of the algorithms' application
- α -parameter of contrast adjustment
- β -parameter of contrast adjustment
- oR -offset for the red color channel
- oG -offset for the green color channel
- oB -offset for the blue color channel
- kernel size of Gaussian blur

Island Optimization. As the term island indicates, each of them acts as a separate and independent optimization process using its own instance of an evolution strategy. Each instance starts with a randomly generated initial set of parameters for the selected algorithms, which represents a unique combination within the pool of developed islands. This initial represents the parent generation, which is needed to create mutants. These mutants are created by randomly selecting candidates from the parent generation and adding a random number to the parameter values weighted by the evolution parameter σ. Based on their capability to manipulate the input image for the segmentation, so that the final segmentation results improve in quality, each mutant gets a fitness value during the evaluation process. Depending on the quality improvements measured over the whole population of candidates, a reduction in σ transforms the initial random search into a more specific search for the best parameter set. The so-called 1/5 rule realizes this adjustment of σ. Every time 1/5 of the created mutants outperform their parent in the resulting segmentation quality, σ is reduced; otherwise, the σ increases [11]. This process repeats itself until a predefined amount of iterations or a specified threshold value for σ is reached. This process leads to independent evaluations of each set of algorithms, allowing the possibility to compare them using as good parameters as possible after each island's evolution has finished. At the end of this process, the best set of algorithms also uses the best parameters for its algorithms.

Fitness Evaluation. The most important part of each optimization process is evaluating the quality of each possible solution candidate. Representing the only way to distinguish between a good and a bad solution, this function has to be perfectly suitable for solving the problem scenario.

Based on the available labeled images, our workflow includes this ground truth information in the fitness evaluation function. Each evaluation of a mutant starts with applying its set of algorithms using the associated parameters. The segmentation model then processes the resulting image. The resulting binary representation of the segmented blood vessels is compared with the ground truth label using the Dice Coefficient, as shown in Eq. 3 [12].

$$DiceCoefficient = \frac{2 * tp}{2 * tp + fp + fn} \tag{3}$$

Providing an indicator for the similarity between two binary images, this equation represents the perfect measure for our fitness evaluation of the individual solution candidates.

The equation's variable tp represents the true positives, whereas fp represents the falsely as positive predicted pixels. fn represents the resulting falsely as negative predicted pixels.

2.2   Model Based Pre-processing

Following the same concept as the presented evolution strategy pre-processing workflow, our model-based approach also acts as an automated pre-processing step before the actual segmentation model is applied to the images, as shown in Fig. 8.

In the following, we present three different types of artificial neural network based pre-processing, all trained and tested on the same sets of images to be comparable to each other and the results from the heuristic approach. All these models are created using the PyTorch framework [14] as well as Pytorch-lightning [15].

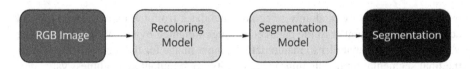

Fig. 8. Visual representation of our model based recoloring workflow where an RGB image is processed by an neural network for a color adaption. Followed by this recoloring, the actual segmentation is done by the segmentation model which results in an segmentation mask.

Convolutional Autoencoder. Representing the baseline for our neural network-based pre-processing workflow, the first model architecture represents a simple convolutional autoencoder structure [13] as shown in Fig. 9. Based on this architecture, we made our proof of concept analysis with different network architectures, which were all based on the simple concept shown in the figure, only varying in the amount and composition of encoding and decoding layers, as well as the size of the input images. All the application results of the following approaches can be found in the result Sect. 3.

The basic idea of this architecture is that the initial image is compressed during several encoding steps of the first network part. The remaining information after this encoding represents the so-called latent space which in theory only contains the significant information needed to reconstruct the image as well as possible. The reconstruction is done by the decoding layers of the network, which result in the reconstructed image. Depending on the number of encoding layers and the convolution and pooling layers, it is possible to significantly reduce the number of parameters from the initial image to the latent space representation, which is one of the use cases for such types of neural networks.

Due to the fact that we only want to recolor the image without the need for compression, we actually increased our initial $512 \times 512 \times 3$ (786 432) parameters of the input

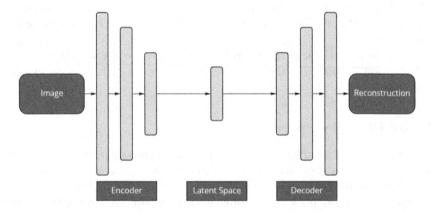

Fig. 9. This conceptual representation of a convolutional autoencoder structure includes three encoding layers, one latent space layer, which represents the encoded information of the initial image, and three decoding layers for the reconstruction of the encoded information. The result should be as similar to the initial image as possible.

image to $256 \times 256 \times 16$ (1.048.576) parameters within the latent space. This prevents detailed information from being lost during the encoding and decoding.

LAB Based Structure Preserving Autoencoder. Based on the same autoencoder concept, the second architecture is created with the theory that we only want the color information to be changed without losing the structural details. This led to the use of the LAB colorspace, which separates the luminance channel (L) from the color information contained in the A and B color channels.

As shown in Fig. 10, we separated the L channel and used an autoencoder structure only for the A and B channels. The L channel was only processed within a kind of parameter extension structure that extends the number of parameters by raising the amount of dimension from the initial $512 \times 512 \times 1$ to $512 \times 512 \times 4$ for the final merging layers which also act as a conversion from the LAB colorspace back to the RGB space. The two channels for A and B are encoded from $512 \times 512 \times 2$ to $256 \times 256 \times 16$, which also extends the number of parameters. The decoder increases the first two dimensions but reduces the third one to a final dimensionality of $512 \times 512 \times 8$, which exactly doubles the number of parameters compared to the latent space. The final merging is needed to reduce the dimensionality from the resulting $512 \times 512 \times 12$ back to the $512 \times 512 \times 3$ of the final RGB image.

Unet. Also based on an encoder/decoder structure, the Unet architecture [3] represents a special type of autoencoders that are commonly used for image segmentation tasks. We also used a variation of this architecture for our segmentation model. Based on the results of the other two approaches, we also used the exact same Unet architecture as we used for the segmentation model itself for the pre-processing. The only difference is that this pre-processing network does not result in binary segmentation but instead outputs RGB images like the other two model architecture presented in this paper.

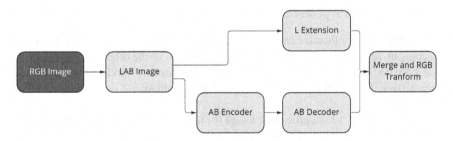

Fig. 10. Conceptual representation of a LAB colorspace-based autoencoder using the luminance channel as a structural preserving channel. Only the A and B channels are encoded, which contain the color information. This combination of an autoencoder structure for the color channels and the structural information in the form of the luminance channel provides a recoloring result without losing the detailed structures.

3   Results

Representing the baseline for all the following results, we also tested the initial segmentation model, which was only trained on one type of blood vessel image and therefore not usable for every new type of image.

As shown in Fig. 11 the resulting binary image after the segmentation (c) does not contain any useful information compared to the ground truth image (b). The lack of generalization should be improved by the presented approaches.

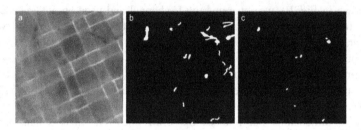

Fig. 11. Segmentation result of the reference model only trained on dataset A. The image on the left (a) represents the raw input image processed by the model. The image in the middle (b) represents the ground truth information. The image on the right (c) represents the segmentation result.

Table 1. List of the heuristic optimization based pre-processing test results using single images of the test partition of dataset B.

Data	Dice score
First test image	0.6168
Second test image	0.5322

3.1   Evolutionary Preprocessing

Representing two application results of our heuristic based pre-processing workflow, the scores in Table 1 are unfortunately not compareable to the other results, due to the use of only one image for the evolution of the pre-processing workflow, and one image for the testing. Despite this limitation, this results still prove the usability as described in the following.

As shown in Fig. 12 the processed image (b) led to a way better segmentation result (e) compared to the raw segmentation result (d) of the unprocessed image (a). The combination of contrast adjustment, image blurring, and color shift improved the initial Dice score achieved on this image from 0.2353 to 0.6168. The used parameters for this generated pre-processing pipeline are the following:

- Algorithm order: contrast, blur, color shift
- α: 1.5498
- β: 1
- μ: red: 0, green: 0, blue: 213
- Gaussian kernel size: 3×3

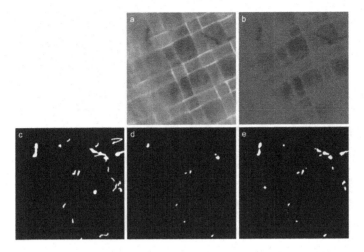

Fig. 12. Segmentation result of an image (a) out of the same dataset as the image used for the optimization process. The processed image (b) with the corresponding segmentation result (e) provides significantly more information of the ground truth (c) compared to the raw segmentation result (d).

The parameters show that our algorithm only applied a color shift on the blue channel of the image, which makes sense due to the overall blue-dominated colorization of the raw image.

This result shows that it is possible to create a pre-processing workflow which is able to change the image properties in a way that the segmentation quality can be increased. The success of this approach relies on the similarity within the dataset the pre-processing pipeline is generated for.

As shown in Fig. 13 image a and image b are colored in a similar way which may indicate that it could be possible to use the same pre-processing workflow for both images. Even if the segmentation quality of image b could be improved with the pro-

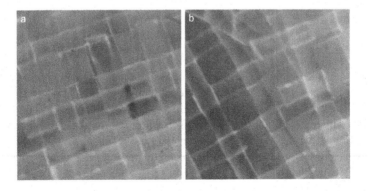

Fig. 13. Example images of blood vessels with similar colorization.

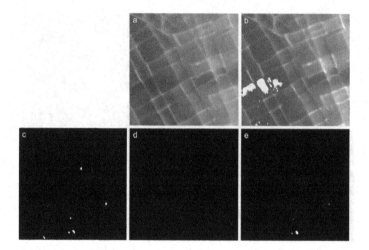

Fig. 14. Segmentation result of an image a with a similar colorization as the image used for the opimization process. The processed image b provides clearly visible artifacts. The segmentation result (e) still provides more information of the ground truth(c) compared to the raw segmentation result (d).

cessing pipeline of image A as shown in Fig. 14. Major artifacts were generated due to an over-saturation within the left part of the image.

Despite the drawback of these artifacts it was still possible to improve the segmentation quality on this image from a Dice score of 0.0 to 0.5322 which might be to little information to be usable for most applications.

Based on these results, we also created an extended version of our evolution strategy workflow, which allows the inclusion of more than one image for the optimization. This test provides insights if this workflow can also provide a general pre-processing pipeline that could be used to prepare every new image for an existing segmentation model.

Figure 15 visualizes the expected result of this test. Linear transformations are not suitable for a generalized workflow which lead to completely useless segmentation results.

3.2 Transfer Learning and Retraining

Exactly this generalization should be provided by the second type of pre-processing we described in this paper based on artificial neural networks. In contrast to linear transformations as used for the heuristic approach, these networks are able to perform non-linear transformations. Despite the comparison with the original segmentation model, we also included two additional baseline tests in the results. The first represents the commonly used transfer learning, and the second represents a completely new trained network only using dataset B.

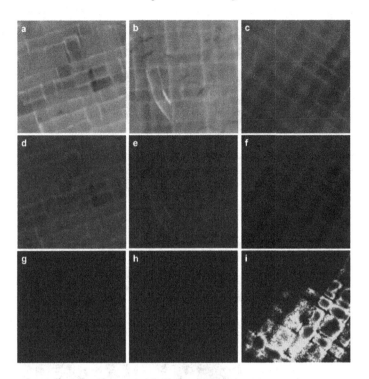

Fig. 15. Segmentation results using the same generated pre-processing workflow generated by using several images of different colorization. The two images a and b are used for the optimization. Image c was not used. The raw images a, b, c are providing a more vivid colorization compared to the processed images d, e, f. However, the processed images are still colored more similar to their raw counterparts compared to the other processed images. This lack of color adjustment result in completely useless segmentation results shown in the images g, h, i. Source: [1]

Table 2. List of the neural networks' test results using the test partition of dataset B. All models were tested on the same test partition.

Method	Dice score
Original model	0.1073
Transfer learned model	0.5022
Newly trained model	0.4990
RGB Autoencoder	0.2547
LAB Autoencoder	0.3730
Unet++	0.5301

As shown in Fig. 16, the transfer learning approach is able to adjust the initial model well enough to provide a way better segmentation result than the model the training was based on. The overall Dice score on the test data was improved from 0.1073 of the original model to 0.5022.

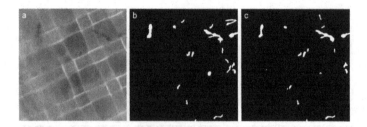

Fig. 16. Segmentation result of a model trained using transfer learning. The image on the left (a) represents the input image. The image in the middle (b) illustrates the ground truth. The image on the right (c) represents the output of the segmentation model.

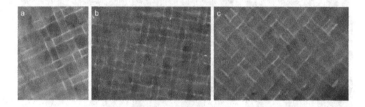

Fig. 17. Example images out of the test partition of dataset B. They provide an impression of the variety in colorization and contrast.

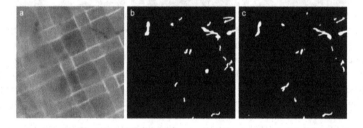

Fig. 18. Segmentation result of a newly trained model only on dataset B which leads to the segmentation results represented by the image on the right (c) using the input image on the left (a) with the corresponding ground truth in the middle (b).

Even if this is still significantly lower than the score of the original model on dataset A, the main benefit of this approach is that this score is achieved on different types of images within dataset B as indicated by the examples out of the test data shown in Fig. 17

Besides the transfer learning approach, we also trained a new Unet only on dataset B containing different types of blood vessel images. As seen in Fig. 18 the resulting segmentation (c) could still not provide nearly all blood vessels seen in the ground truth image. This is reflected in the overall Dice score on the test data of 0.4990, which is actually lower than the transfer learning-based model. Based on these results, it was not possible with these approaches to achieve similar performance on dataset B as the original model could achieve on dataset A.

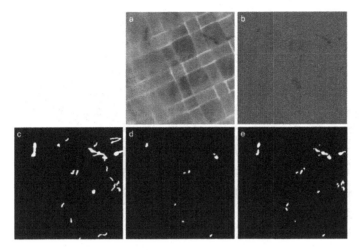

Fig. 19. Baseline result for a recoloring neural network based on an encoder/decoder structure. The input image (a) was processed by the autoencoder resulting in the recolored version (b), which led to the segmentation result (e). Image d represents the segmentation result of the raw image (a). Image c represents the ground truth.

3.3   Recoloring Neural Network

Representing an overview of the model neural networks' test results, Table 2 shows the Dice scores of the different approaches on the test partition of dataset B. A detailed explanation of these results is presented in the following sub-sections. Regarding the transfer learning approach results, the following three results of the recoloring neural networks should be mainly considered in their capability of improving the initial segmentation performance. The primary purpose of the presented workflows was not to outperform transfer learning but instead to provide an alternative.

Autoencoder. Representing the baseline for our recoloring workflow, the resulting Dice score on the test data of 0.2547 doubled, compared to the initial score of 0.1073. But realistically, it is still not even close to representing an alternative to transfer learning. As shown in Fig. 19, the network seems to focus on highlighting the blood vessels by increasing the contrast to the background. If this kind of pre-segmentation was the goal, it could also be seen why it does not work properly due to the fact that not all blood vessels were highlighted, as seen in the segmentation image (c).

LAB-Autoencoder. Although the LAB-based recoloring network could outperform the RGB autoencoder significantly by increasing the Dice score to 0.3730, the most exciting part of this result is that the network created a recolored image where the background and the blood vessels are recolored in complementary colors [16] of a greenish background and more reddish blood vessels as shown in image b of Fig. 20. This behavior seems to be better compatible with the segmentation network than the RGB recoloring, which lead to a better result.

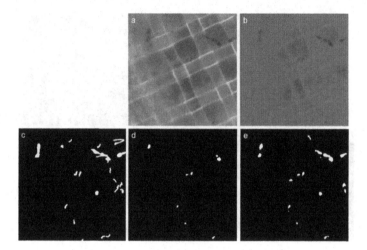

Fig. 20. Segmentation result of the LAB colorspace-based recoloring network. Image a represents the raw image, whereas image b is generated by the recoloring network using image a as input. Image e represents the segmentation result by using image b as input, whereas image d is generated by using image a as input. Image c is used as ground truth.

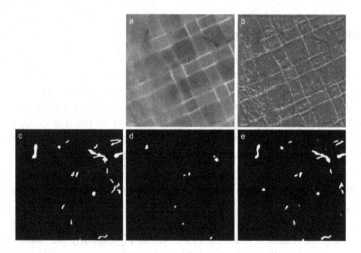

Fig. 21. Segmentation result of an Unet as a recoloring network. Image a represents the raw image, image b the recolored version of image a. The segmentation result of using image b as input is represented by image e, whereas the segmentation result using image a as input is represented by image d. Image c is used as ground truth.

Unet. Using an Unet as recoloring network even outperforms the transfer learning model, providing the best Dice score of 0.5301. As shown in Fig. 21 this pre-processing network seems to follow a comparable approach to the RGB autoencoder where it provides a kind of pre-segmentation. As seen in image b, all the blood vessels are highlighted in pink compared to the greyish background. Even if this still does not come close to the segmentation result of the original model on dataset A, this result proves that our recoloring workflow could be considered as an alternative to transfer learning for our use case.

4   Conclusion

Regarding the presented results, we can say that the two presented approaches of pre-processing images to increase the compatibility with an already existing segmentation neural network are not quite compareable considering their use-cases. Despite the lack of a general pre-processing workflow for all new arriving images, our evolution strategy-based workflow offered a suitable pre-processing for new datasets that share similar image properties. If this similarity is given, this approach could provide an alternative to transfer learning. When a general pre-processing workflow is needed, the use of transfer learning seems still to be the easiest way to go by the fact that no extra network is required. For use-cases where the actual segmentation network can not be changed, an Unet-based architecture as a generic pre-processing network seems to be a suitable solution which, in our case, even worked better than transfer learning. In our future work, we will improve the comparability of our evolution strategy based on results with the other methods, including the mentioned state-of-the-art method cycle gans. Especially the extension of our database should enable these extended test runs, which will provide additional insight into our approaches' usability and the possible use cases compared to the state-of-the-art methods.

Acknowledgements. The work described in this paper was supported by the Center of Excellence for Technical Innovation in Medicine (TIMED), the Dissertation Programme of the University of Applied Sciences Upper Austria, and the Austrian Research Promotion Agency (FFG, project no. 881547).

References

1. Haghofer, A.: Heuristic domain shift adaptation for the analysis of blood vessel images. Paper presented at BIOSTEC 2022. https://www.insticc.org/node/TechnicalProgram/biostec/2022/presentationDetails/110288
2. Weiss, K., Khoshgoftaar, T.M., Wang, D.D.: A survey of transfer learning. J. Big Data 3(1), 1–40 (2016). https://doi.org/10.1186/s40537-016-0043-6
3. Ronneberger, O., Fischer, P., Brox, T.: U-Net: convolutional networks for biomedical image segmentation. In: Navab, N., Hornegger, J., Wells, W.M., Frangi, A.F. (eds.) MICCAI 2015. LNCS, vol. 9351, pp. 234–241. Springer, Cham (2015). https://doi.org/10.1007/978-3-319-24574-4_28
4. Shorten, C., Khoshgoftaar, T.M.: A survey on image data augmentation for deep learning. J. Big Data 6(1), 1–48 (2019). https://doi.org/10.1186/s40537-019-0197-0
5. Radosavovic, I., Kosaraju, R., Girshick, R., He, K., Dollár, P.: Designing network design spaces. In: Proceedings of the IEEE Computer Society Conference On Computer Vision And Pattern Recognition (2020)
6. Zhou, Z., Rahman Siddiquee, M.M., Tajbakhsh, N., Liang, J.: UNet++: a nested U-Net architecture for medical image segmentation. In: Stoyanov, D., et al. (eds.) DLMIA/ML-CDS - 2018. LNCS, vol. 11045, pp. 3–11. Springer, Cham (2018). https://doi.org/10.1007/978-3-030-00889-5_1

7. Iakubovskii, P.: Segmentation Models Pytorch. GitHub Repository (2019). https://github. com/qubvel/segmentation_models.pytorch
8. Getreuer, P.: A Survey of Gaussian Convolution Algorithms. Image Processing On Line (2013)
9. Szeliski, R.: Computer vision: algorithms and applications. Choice Reviews Online (2011)
10. Haghofer, A., Dorl, S., Oszwald, A., Breuss, J., Jacak, J., Winkler, S.M.: Evolutionary optimization of image processing for cell detection in microscopy images. Soft Comput. **24**(23), 17847–17862 (2020). https://doi.org/10.1007/s00500-020-05033-0
11. Rechenberg, I.: Evolutionsstrategie 94. Frommann-Holzboog (1994)
12. Dice, L.: Measures of the amount of ecologic association between species. Ecology (1945)
13. Turchenko, V., Chalmers, E., Luczak, A.: A Deep Convolutional Auto-Encoder with Pooling - Unpooling Layers in Caffe (2017)
14. Paszke, A., et al.: PyTorch: an imperative style, high-performance deep learning library. Adv. Neural Inf. Process. Syst. **32**, 8024–8035 (2019). http://papers.neurips.cc/paper/9015-pytorch-an-imperative-style-high-performance-deep-learning-library.pdf
15. Falcon, W., et al.: Pytorch lightning. GitHub, vol. 3 (2019). https://github.com/pytorchlightning/pytorch-lightning
16. Green-Armytage, P.: Complementary Colors. Encyclopedia Of Color Science And Technology, pp. 523–535 (2016). https://doi.org/10.1007/978-1-4419-8071-7_264
17. OpenCV Open Source Computer Vision Library (2015)
18. Deryugina, E., Quigley, J.: Chapter 2 Chick Embryo chorioallantoic membrane models to quantify angiogenesis induced by inflammatory and tumor cells or purified effector molecules. Methods Enzymol. **444**, 21–41 (2008)
19. Mahapatra, D., Bozorgtabar, B., Thiran, J.-P., Shao, L.: Structure preserving stain normalization of histopathology images using self supervised semantic guidance. In: Martel, A.L., et al. (eds.) MICCAI 2020. LNCS, vol. 12265, pp. 309–319. Springer, Cham (2020). https://doi.org/10.1007/978-3-030-59722-1_30
20. Roy, G., et al.: Robust Mitosis Detection Using a Cascade Mask-RCNN Approach With Domain-Specific Residual Cycle-GAN Data Augmentation (2021)

Security Analysis of the Internet of Medical Things (IoMT): Case Study of the Pacemaker Ecosystem

Guillaume Bour[1]([✉])(iD), Anniken Wium Lie[2], Jakob Stenersen Kok[3],
Bendik Markussen[4], Marie Elisabeth Gaup Moe[5](iD), and Ravishankar Borgaonkar[1](iD)

[1] SINTEF Digital, Strindvegen 4, Trondheim, Norway
{guillaume.bour,ravi.borgaonkar}@sintef.no
[2] Norwegian Police IT Services, Oslo, Norway
[3] Techfolk, Oslo, Norway
[4] Bekk, Oslo, Norway
[5] Norwegian University of Science and Technology, Trondheim, Norway
marie.moe@ntnu.no

Abstract. During the pandemic, the Internet of Medical Things (IoMT) has played a key role in reducing unnecessary hospital visits and the burden on health care systems by providing home-based hospital services and ambulatory nursing services. As IoMT devices handle patient data and are connected over the Internet to the complex hospital Information and Communication Technology (ICT) infrastructure, their role in the transformation of healthcare services will introduce a range of new potential risks. Over the past years, several demonstrated attacks in the healthcare domain have indicated cyber security challenges for integrating IoMT devices.

In this paper, we experimentally evaluate the potential risks that accompany the integration of a given IoMT device, here a connected pacemaker, from a hardware and network security perspective. We take a black box testing approach to the pacemaker ecosystem and find key shortcomings that enable several practical and low-cost attacks that impact a patient's safety and privacy. In particular, we demonstrate the ability to gain control over the home monitoring device and to perform man-in-the-middle attacks. We find that it is possible to bypass hardware security protection mechanisms, to perform remote denial of service attacks, and other attacks. Lastly, we discuss the potential trade-offs in security protection choices and mitigation techniques.

Keywords: IoMT · IoT security · Pacemaker · Medical device · Cyber security

1 Introduction

Hospital-at-Home is expected to become the new norm in the coming decade. Technology has made major changes to the way healthcare is provided, and thanks to the fourth

This work was funded by Reinforcing the Health Data Infrastructure in Mobility and Assurance through Data Democratization, a five-year project (grant number 28885) under the Norwegian IKTPLUSS-IKT and Digital Innovation programme.

industrial revolution, humans will live longer and healthier lives. Consultations will take place over video, and IoMT sensors will take care of monitoring vital in real time, issuing alerts if anything appears abnormal. More intrusive devices such as Implantable Medical Devices (IMD) will also become increasingly connected.

Connecting patients' homes means expanding the attack surface of the system. Patients' safety has always been a key priority in medical devices. Pacemakers, for instance, are built with "fail-safe" modes which they will switch to in case something goes wrong with their programming; this keeps the pacemaker generating a constant pulse until a pacemaker technician can re-progam the device for the patient. Cyber security of medical devices, on the other hand, has not been paid much attention by researchers, nor has it been publicly debated until the last decade. The healthcare domain is, however, not spared by cyber criminals, and attacks like the WannaCry ransomware that struck the world in May 2017 have shown that hospitals and medical devices are at risk for being infected via collateral damage even if the attack was not specifically targeted towards them. A cyber attack can have a real impact on human lives. A poor implementation of cyber security in the edge systems of the Home Hospital could have catastrophic consequences not only for the patients' privacy but also for their safety. Having secure connected medical devices is thus a must-have in order to pave the way to future home-care. Connected pacemakers constitute some of the most life critical medical devices and were among the first to be "connected". As such, they can provide us with evidence of the evolution of cyber security in medical devices over time.

Connected IMD in the form of modern pacemakers are not a new medical innovation but the evolution of technology from the fifties and sixties. In the seventies "on-demand" pacemakers were developed that would sense the patient's cardiac activity and adjust the pacing accordingly. These pacemakers could be remotely programmed through a radio-frequency telemetry link. The first pacemakers driven by microprocessors appeared in the nineties. These devices were able to detect cardiac events and could adapt their internal pacing based on the patient's needs. The first *connected* pacemakers appeared in the early 2000s, with the addition of an external device that would connect wirelessly to the pacemaker and upload its data to a remote server via the Internet, thus reducing the need for patients to go to the clinic for a check-up. Today, this remote connectivity is becoming more and more popular in use. An external device, sometimes called a "bedside monitor", which we in this paper will refer to as the Home Monitoring Unit (HMU), is used to gather the pacemaker's data and upload it to a remote server accessible to the clinician through a web interface.

Over the past three years, we have been analyzing the security of the pacemaker ecosystem of one of the main vendors on the market today. We looked at three different generations of HMU devices and compared their security to document the state-of-the-art and to see how security implementation in these devices has evolved over time.

Our main results, presented in a previous paper [3], suggest that even if the overall security of the devices has improved, the medical device manufacturers are still lagging behind and have failed to implement common security practices. In this paper, we highlight the methodologies used to test the devices from both a hardware and a network perspective. In particular, we present new results obtained through the fuzzing of the generic modem used by the pacemaker HMU. We have implemented a fuzzing framework using a GSM network test bed. The equipment (software defined radio) needed for fuzzing infrastructure is inexpensive and readily available. We followed ethical response procedures and reported our attacks based on identified vulnerabilities to the concerned manufacturers.

The paper is organized as follows. Section 2 provides the background of our work, including a description of the principle of the pacemaker and its ecosystem, along with the interactions between its different components. Here we also review the relevant related work and the threat model used in our research. In Sect. 3 we outline the methodology used along with the different setups used to perform the security analysis. Section 4 presents our main findings, from a hardware, firmware, communication and infrastructure perspective. Those findings are not pacemaker-specific and can be considered for all connected medical devices that present similar architecture. Potential attack scenarios are also presented. Section 5 provides a discussion of the results along with mitigations. Section 6 concludes the paper.

2 Background

2.1 The Pacemaker Ecosystem

Pacemakers and Implantable Cardioverter Defibrillators (ICD) are active implantable medical devices, which are defined in the Norwegian regulatory framework [15] as "*Any active medical device which is intended to be totally or partially introduced, surgically or medically, into the human body or by medical intervention into a natural orifice, and which is intended to remain after the procedure.*" Both pacemakers and ICDs are battery-powered devices surgically implanted in a patient to treat a heart related condition. They differ in the conditions they are treating, as ICDs are not only capable of continuous monitoring the heart rhythm and pacing the heart with electrical pulses, but also of delivering an electrical shock to the heart if required. In this paper, because both ICDs and pacemakers are similar devices from the cyber security point of view, they will both be referred to as pacemakers.

Pacemakers are constructed to last for around 10 years varying on their usage, before having to be replaced due to the battery running out. The devices are able to deliver pacing when required and in a way that is adapted to each patient. This means that the clinician needs a way to program the device in a non-invasive way for the patient. As previously mentioned, an RF-telemetry link was introduced to the devices in the 70s to program some parameters in the pacemaker. Since then, pacemakers have evolved into complex embedded devices, driven by a microcontroller. Once implanted, they are not standalone devices which are left there for ten years waiting to be replaced, but take place in an ecosystem that allows for monitoring the devices and also the patients' condition.

The Home Monitoring Unit is an example of a communication device that enables this remote regular monitoring by connecting wirelessly to the pacemaker, reading and transmitting data from it. Figure 1 presents the pacemaker ecosystem.

The Pacemaker. Implanted in the patient's body, this is the main device of the ecosystem. As already explained, it generates an electric impulse that helps regulate the heart rhythm.

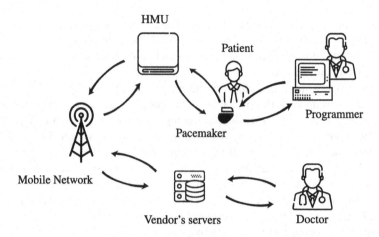

Fig. 1. Diagram of the vendor's pacemaker ecosystem [4].

The Programmer. The programmer is an external computer used by a clinician to program the pacemaker. Programming the pacemaker is achieved wirelessly by placing the programming head of the programmer in close proximity of the pacemaker. While old pacemakers used to communicate with the programmer over the 175 kHz band, newer ones tend to use 402–405 MHz Medical Implant Communications (MICS) band [25]. The communication of the pacemaker with the programmer is triggered by applying a magnetic field on the implant, causing a magnetic switch inside it to close [12]. This magnetic field is emitted by the programming head. It should be noted that pacemakers from different vendors require different programmers due to differences in communication protocols, and that a programmer of a specific vendor usually supports several pacemakers/ICD devices from the same vendor.

The HMU. The HMU is a router-like device in charge of collecting telemetry data from the implant and transmitting it. The device is paired with a pacemaker, placed in the patient's home and receives the data sent by the pacemaker at a pre-configured time (for instance every night at 2:00). The HMU also communicates with the pacemaker over the 402–405 MICS band, which allows for longer range communications than the 175 kHz band. This data is then sent to a backend server, usually owned by the pacemaker manufacturers. Similar to the programmer, pacemakers from different manufacturers require different HMUs. Some newer pacemakers communicate over Bluetooth Low Energy with an app installed on the patient's smartphone, eliminating the need for an external HMU device.

The Operator's Network. In order to transmit the data to the backend server, the HMU needs connectivity. To achieve that without having to rely on patients' internet connection and also for ease of use, manufacturers usually have contracts with Telecom operators. That way, the HMUs are shipped with a SIM card to access the Global System for Mobile Communication (GSM) or 3G networks, or with access to the internet through telephone lines for older versions. The HMU either connects directly to the server which is exposed on the public Internet or connects to a Virtual Private Mobile Network (VPMN) which gives it access to the server. This implementation varies with vendors.

Vendor's Backend Infrastructure. This infrastructure is used to receive data sent by the HMU, process it and make it accessible to the clinician through an online platform. Alerts may also be triggered if something looks irregular, for instance, if no data has been uploaded in a while for a given HMU, or if there is a problem with the patient's condition. This allows the clinician to call in the patient for a follow-up checkup if necessary.

2.2 Related Research

While wireless communication technology has been a feature of pacemakers since the seventies, security researchers have only been taking an interest in this topic for around 15 years. In 2008, Halperin et al. published the first research paper describing a security attack against a commercial pacemaker [12]. Their research targeted the communication between the pacemaker and its programmer. Using Software Defined Radio (SDR), they partially reversed engineered the communication protocol in use and, with that knowledge, were able not only to eavesdrop and decode the communication, but also to perform data replay attacks. They were able to interrogate the pacemaker to reveal the patient's data containing personal information such as patient's name, diagnosis, etc. They were also able to change parameters of the pacemaker, such as the patient's name, implantation date, or even therapies (that includes turning off all therapies). Finally, and more frightening, they were able to trigger a shock on the ICD, which could have fatal consequences on a real patient if delivered at an inappropriate time. They thus highlighted the severity of the lack of security mechanisms for implantable medical devices.

In more recent research from 2016, Marin et al. carried out similar research on the latest generation of pacemakers [19]. Their research highlights several weaknesses in the communication protocol and shows that a weak adversary can perform attacks even with low capabilities. Three kinds of attacks were performed. First, the researchers managed to access private patient information from the telemetry information, even though some obfuscation technique has been done by the manufacturer. Secondly, they performed Denial-of-Service attacks. By keeping the device in "interrogation" mode, they were able to send messages to the device over a long-range communication channel and thus drastically reduce the implant battery life. Finally, they found that there is no mechanism against replay attacks and that an adversary without any knowledge of the protocol could simply replay captured messages and spoof the programmer.

A report exposing vulnerabilities in the pacemakers and HMUs manufactured by St. Jude (now Abbot) was published by Muddy Waters Capital LLC in 2016 [2]. Amongst the vulnerabilities that were presented was a way to perform a battery-draining attack on the pacemakers or forcing them to pace at a rhythm that would be potentially fatal for the patient. These attacks were carried out by first compromising the HMU, which was then used to attack the pacemaker. Even if no attack has been publicly reported exploiting these vulnerabilities, the disclosure of this report had a potentially severe impact on the 260 000 HMUs deployed in patients' homes at the time. As a result, the vendor issued a firmware update at the beginning of 2017 to mitigate the vulnerabilities.

In 2017, Rios and Butts evaluated the security of the pacemaker ecosystems of the four major vendors [23]. They presented several weaknesses, in the programmers, the pacemaker implants, and the HMUs. Weaknesses include vulnerable third-party software, lack of authentication between devices, unencrypted filesystems and firmware, removable hard-drives, and unsigned firmware. The conclusion is that the whole industry is quite immature in terms of cyber security. They highlight that this is not only the case for one unique vendor but that all vendors are impacted.

Attacking the mobile network interface of embedded device is not new either: in 2011 Mulliner et al. published their research on the possibility of launching large scale attacks against phones by exploiting vulnerabilities in the Short Message Service (SMS)-client software [11,20]. In particular, they developed a platform-agnostic testing framework which allows fuzzing SMS messages over a software-based GSM network. They concluded that an attacker can send malformed SMSs resulting in the receiver's phone being disconnected from the network forcing the user to reboot it. Similar work was conducted by Weinmann who focused on the whole cellular basebands from different manufacturers rather than on the SMS-interface only [27]. They combined Mulliner et al.'s approach with reverse engineering of different stacks to identify flaws. In today's devices, the baseband's stacks and applications commonly run on a separate co-processor or chip with their own operating system and memory. Despite this separation, their work demonstrated the ability for an attacker to fully compromise a device by compromising the baseband's processor.

2.3   Threat Model

In this paper, we aim at understanding the evolution of the security measures in the pacemaker ecosystem and to evaluate its current maturity when it comes to cyber security. In our research, we have considered two classes of adversaries:

With Physical Access to an HMU. It is possible to buy HMU devices online, sometimes at the low price range of $20–$50. Since these are much easier to obtain compared to a pacemaker or a pacemaker programmer, one can afford to experiment with them without the fear of breaking an expensive device.

Capable of Setting up a Fake Base Station (FBS). Such an attacker has access to Software Defined Radio equipment, which is also affordable. The HackRF One[1] manufactured by Great Scott Gadgets costs around $350. In order to perform fuzzing of the devices' modems, an attacker might also want to acquire the modems separately as this will allow for easier debugging (for instance by using it together with a RaspberryPi instead of the real device).

The two main facets that we want to look at in this research are the safety and privacy of the patient. To do this, we study the impact of different attacks on the patient's treatment and how it could be interfered with, directly or indirectly. Home monitoring has proven to save lives and as such, any attacks allowing an attacker to disrupt the service is also considered [10]. Regarding the patient's privacy, we look at what attacks would enable an attacker to access any kind of private data about the patient.

As mentioned in the introduction of this paper, motivations to attack the pacemaker ecosystem vary. Attacks against the patient's privacy are mostly driven by financial

---

[1] See https://greatscottgadgets.com/hackrf/.

motives, in order to monetize the medical data on the black market. These attacks can have a great impact if they can be leveraged on a large scale. Safety related attacks could also be motivated by financial profit, for example we can imagine that an adversary could leverage a vulnerability in an extortion attempt by threatening a patient or maybe even a medical device manufacturer asking for a ransom. Targeted attacks against a single individual in order to harm or kill are less likely, except if it is a person of high interest. In both cases, one can imagine that we are facing organized crime or a nation-state threat actor. However, we cannot exclude single opportunistic attackers.

3   Methodology

3.1   Targets

Medical devices either speak to a gateway (the HMU in the case of the pacemaker) or are powerful enough to communicate with a network infrastructure directly. As such, the HMU is a good case study for security testing, and this is why we decided to look more into it. More specifically, we focused on two main attack vectors: *physical* and *network*. In both cases, a black box testing methodology was followed, as the tested components were proprietary hardware and software of which we had very little knowledge. In order to be as close to a real-world scenario as possible, we used commercial off-the-shelf (COTS) equipment whenever possible, and tried to keep the cost of an attack as low as possible.

The targeted devices from our lab were acquired second hand and are all BIOTRONIK's devices. This manufacturer was chosen because no prior security research had been published for this particular pacemaker brand, and no known vulnerabilities had previously been disclosed for its devices. Devices in our research project include three different generations of the HMU:

V1: From 2000 to 2010, one of the first HMUs on the market, using the GSM network for connectivity. This version is not used anymore.
V2: From the 2010s, in two models: one using the standard land line service for its connectivity, the other one using the GSM network. This version is not commercially available anymore, but is still in use.
V3: From 2016, using the 3G network for connectivity. This is the current commercially available version. It is worth noting this version is "mobile" and thus not necessarily only accessible in the patient's home.

3.2   Black Box Testing

Definition. The Black Box Testing methodology is a way to assess a software, a device or more generally a system from the outside while having very little knowledge about its internals. The attacker analyzes the outputs of the box obtained by sending some inputs or just by passively listening, and then tries to deduce the internals of the target. Having made some guesses, the attacker can adjust her inputs to confirm her thoughts or to exploit the target (see Fig. 2).

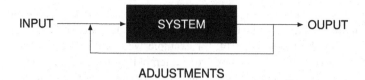

ADJUSTMENTS

Fig. 2. High Level Diagram of the Black Box Testing Methodology [4].

This methodology has several advantages compared to others that can be used to assess a system. Indeed, its primary objective is to test a system under real conditions, to emulate a real attack scenario. This means that such a test might catch errors made during the deployment of the system such as default passwords, misconfigurations in general or even the lack of security trainings of operators (weak passwords). This methodology also presents a low false positive ratio as the security expert can assess the risks associated with a vulnerability directly, i.e., if the vulnerability can be exploited or not. Black Box Testing also has some drawbacks. By definition, the attacker has very little information about the target and might miss some vulnerabilities that would have been detected by code and/or configuration review. Despite this, it remains an excellent way to assess how a system stands against attacks and to get an idea of the path an attacker would take to compromise the solution, thus giving indications on how to tackle potential low hanging fruits. It can be later be completed by a deeper assessment following a grey or white box approach if applicable.

Ordinarily, the ecosystems for connected medical devices are for the most part proprietary. They usually rely on commercially available components and communicate using standardized frequency bands (such as MICS) but the rest (communication protocol with the gateway or with the backend infrastructure) is custom-made. The Black Box Testing methodology thus fits well not only for our research on the pacemaker ecosystem, but for security research on any connected medical devices. This is valid for the three approaches presented in the next subsections.

3.3 Hardware Testing Methodology and Setup

Methodology. Our process can be split into five different tasks (see Fig. 3). The first is the *Hardware Analysis*. Once we acquire a device, we start analyzing its components, which means knowing what the exposed interfaces are, debug interfaces, but also the chips that are on the board. To know that, opening the device to access the Printed Circuit Board (PCB) and analyze it is often required.

Knowing the components and available interfaces, we can then start looking for *documentation* such as datasheets, Request for Comments (RFC) or any other relevant information about the device. The goal of that second step is to understand the overall system and come up with some first hypotheses about it.

From those hypotheses, we then come with *testing* scenarios to be performed on the device and that will have two possible outcomes: either a success or a failure. However, the success or the failure of a testing scenario is determined by the expected result, which means in reality that even failure brings us information about the system.

Indeed, the results of a specific scenario need to be interpreted. This interpretation will be called a *finding*. Those findings are then used to look for new documentation and/or infer new hypotheses about the device. For example, if the hypothesis is "the device has debug ports exposed on the Universal Asynchronous Receiver Transmitter (UART) pins and is providing the attacker with a shell when connected to it", then the testing of that particular scenario will lead to either a confirmation or a rejection of the hypothesis. The interpretation is here quite easy as it is the hypothesis itself. This finding can then be reinjected in the documentation phase to infer new testing hypotheses like "the attacker is given a root shell when connecting to the UART console" or "the attacker can access the filesystem when connecting to the UART console".

Those findings are finally gathered to be *reported*. The reporting step is the one where the device is considered back in its whole ecosystem. That means the findings are interpreted again, but then with regard to different metrics. In the case of the above example, one can wonder what is the impact of the attacker having access to the filesystem on a medical device. The interpretation will be different when linked to other findings such as "The users' data are stored in cleartext on the device" or "The users' data are not stored on the device". Mitigation measures are also included in the reporting step.

Those steps can be mapped with the Open Source Security Testing Methodology Manual (OSSTMM) which is widely used to assess ITs' systems' security [14]. Indeed, the first two steps (*hardware analysis* and *documentation*) correspond to the *information gathering* (or approach) phase in the OSSTMM. The *contact* phase is then used followed by the *exploitation* phase, which are here mapped with the testing and findings phases. In the OSSTMM, the information gathered during the first phase along with the information gathered directly by the *contact* phase is then use to exploit the system and gain access. In our process, the information required to exploit, and gain access comes from previous testings. Finally comes the *reporting phase*, including mitigation. In the OSSTMM, one more phase is sometimes used depending on the engagement: the persistence one. In our case, persistence is studied as a hypothesis which is then tested and reported as any other findings.

Our methodology also follows the OWASP Firmware Security Testing Methodology [1]. While this methodology is more targeted towards more complex systems (running a Linux-based Operating System for instance), it remains applicable for simpler firmware. The hardware testing presented in this paper covers all 9 stages to some extent (considering that there are no file systems in the extracted firmware).

Testing Setup. We used a combination of several COTS equipment to perform hardware testing on the devices. This equipment varied, depending on the stage we were at. *The shikra* was used to interface with low-level data interfaces via USB (it proved to be more reliable than a standard USB-to-TTL adapter). We used a *logic analyzer* to detect non standard baud rates and the *JTAGulator* to identify the pinout of the JTAG interface when it was not labelled. The latter does so by trying all possible permutations. Once the pins were known, we used a *Raspberry Pi zero* as our UART/JTAG/SPI connector. Having one Raspberry Pi Zero configured with all the required tools allowed us to gain time to collect the content of the different Integrated Circuits (IC) on the PCB.

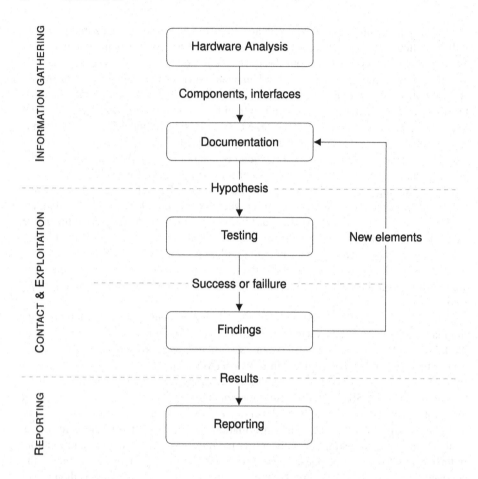

Fig. 3. Black Box Methodology iterative cycles used for our research [4].

3.4 Network Testing Setup

From a network perspective, we used two different setups, to match the two kinds of network interfaces available on the different devices and used to send data to the back-end server:

- We developed a *modem emulator* to interact with the device using a telephone line (HMU (V2)).
- We setup a *Fake Base Station* (based on OpenBTS) to interact with the GSM (V2) and 3G (V3) versions of the HMUs. In addition, a network jammer was used to prevent the HMU from connecting via the 3G network, forcing a so-called downgrade attack. A virtual machine was set up to emulate the backend server of the manufacturer (as shown in Fig. 4) [4, 18].

These two setups allowed us to interact with the devices not only at the mobile network level, but also to directly capture the proprietary protocol used to exchange patient's data and the device's logs.

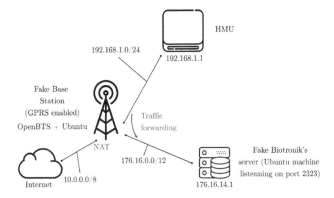

Fig. 4. Network diagram of the emulated network [4].

3.5 Modem Fuzzing Setup

The OWASP Foundation defines Fuzzing as "*a Black Box software testing technique, which basically consists in finding implementation bugs using malformed/semi-malformed data injection in an automated fashion.*"

We developed a custom fuzzing framework to fuzz the modem of the latest version of the HMU. Our framework is inspired by the initial work of Mulliner et al. [20] and built on top of the network testing setup from Lie [18]. Our fuzzing framework has the following components and characteristics:

- An infrastructure to send malformed SMS to the device. Achieving this required us to re-introduce the *testcall* feature in OpenBTS.
- A payload generator. This is not performed randomly, but rather in a context aware way: we used the Python package *smspdu* together with the *Intruder Payloads* from BurpSuite to generate our SMS PDU payloads.
- A monitoring service. When fuzzing, it is necessary to detect when a given payload triggers a bug or a vulnerability in the fuzzed device. This also allows for reproduceability. Traffic monitoring using *tcpdump* was used for this.

Figure 5 shows the overall Architecture of the Fuzzing Framework. Details on its development and capabilities can be found in [16].

3.6 Ethical Considerations

Given that the devices available in our lab have been acquired on the second-hand market, and that some of them were not new, they could have contained potentially sensitive data. This data has been systematically redacted from this paper and from previous publications. The Norwegian Centre for Research Data (NSD) was notified at the beginning of our project, and approved our patient data protection plan.

As the vulnerabilities discovered in the pacemaker ecosystem during our research could have had a potential impact on patients' safety and security, our findings were kept under embargo for one year. During this time, the research findings were shared with

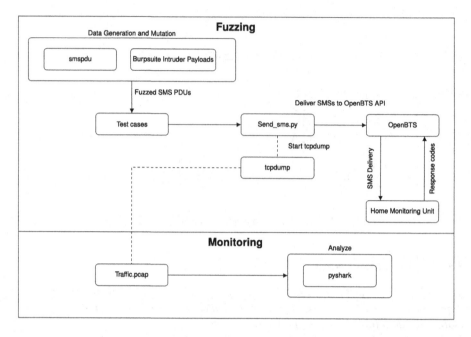

Fig. 5. Architecture of the Fuzzing Framework [16].

the vendor (BIOTRONIK) in the form of a vulnerability report. The vendor cooperated according to a coordinated vulnerability disclosure process and appropriately analyzed and validated our report. They then shared their responses to each reported vulnerability, and we discussed each point in detail. During these discussions, they also provided sufficient information to confirm that patient harm arising from the vulnerabilities is very unlikely. BIOTRONIK recommends that healthcare providers and patients continue to use the investigated devices as intended and follow device labelling. The coordinated vulnerability disclosure process also involved the German Federal Office for Information Security (BSI), the German Federal Office for Medical Devices (BfArM), the US Cyber Security and Infrastructure Agency (CISA) and the US Food and Drug Administration (FDA). As a result of this process, CISA issued an advisory [6].

The vulnerabilities discovered as part of the modem fuzzing not only impact the vendor's devices, but also all devices using that specific modem (and potentially all devices using modems from that vendor sharing the same software stack). Additionally, this is why we shared our findings with the modem's manufacturer and kept our results under embargo for two years. The vendor was informed about the vulnerabilities and how to re-produce attack-scenarios documentations.

4   Security Analysis

In this section, we present the findings from our security analysis on the different versions of the HMU. We first cover raw findings, split into four categories: Hardware,

Firmware, Communication and Infrastructure. Then, we detail how an attacker can chain several of the highlighted weaknesses to mount an attack.

4.1 Hardware

Debug Interfaces Available. On all HMU versions analyzed, we were able to discover the UART and JTAG interfaces. On versions 1 and 2 the pins were not labelled, making it harder to determine the JTAG interface. On the latest version, however, pins were labelled. On all versions, the UART interface seemed disabled, and it was not possible to interact with it. The JTAG interface, on the other hand, was enabled and it is possible to fully control the microcontroller using it. That includes dumping the contents of the Random Access Memory (RAM) as well as the Flash Memory, which gave access to the firmware of the device.

4.2 Firmware

Data Stored Unencrypted on the External Flash. Having physical access to a device, an attacker can use tools such as *flashrom* to dump the content of the external Flash on the PCB, connecting to it directly via SPI. By doing so, we could see that data was stored on it in cleartext.

Firmware not Protected or Obfuscated. Once the firmware was dumped via the JTAG interface, reverse-engineering revealed that it was not encrypted or protected in any way. There was no trace of obfuscation of the code. On the contrary, log strings used by the device were explicit enough to ease the process of reverse engineering. This made it possible to create a script to easily fetch the credentials previously acquired via eavesdropping on the communication channel directly from the firmware, along with other credentials used by the device to connect to the backend server hosted by the manufacturer.

Memory not Protected. The memory was not protected either, meaning that anyone with physical access to the HMU ccould copy it via the JTAG interface and access the data going through the HMU, including the patient's data, if any.

Hard-coded Credentials and Cryptographic Keys. The credentials used by the devices to connect to the network and backend servers were hard-coded and stayed the same for each connection attempt. We observed, however, that they were unique for every device (two different HMUs will use different credentials). On the latest version they were stored on the external flash which is not encrypted and whose content can be read via the Serial Peripheral Interface (SPI). Cryptographic material such as Data Encryption Standard (DES) and Advanced Encryption Standard (AES) keys used in the proprietary protocol were also stored in a similar way.

Broken or Risky Algorithm. In the case of patient data, the proprietary protocol uses AES CBC as the encryption algorithm, however single DES is used in the case of log data going over SMS. DES is a broken algorithm from a security perspective, and log data can thus easily be obtained by an attacker that is able to set up a Fake Base Station in the proximity of the HMU. An attacker having had physical access once to the HMU could also perform the same attack on patient data by getting hold of the DES key. The keys (DES and DES) were, however, random and unique per device.

4.3 Communication

When analyzing the security of the communication link between the HMU and the backend server, we identified several weaknesses in the communication protocol.

Credentials sent in Clear Text to the Modem. When analyzing the version 2 of the HMU, we were able to eavesdrop on the communication between the microcontroller and the modem as the pins of the modem were exposed on the PCB. This allowed us to get access to the credentials used by the device to connect to the manufacturer's VPMN, since these were sent in clear text.

No Mutual Authentication. We were able to spoof the backend server and trick the HMU into sending its data to us, highlighting the lack of mutual authentication between the backend server and the HMU on the first two versions. We did so at two different levels: first at the modem level on the Telephone line version, where we spoofed both the modem and the backend server, and second at the network level, where we used a virtual machine, connected to the same network as our OpenBTS machine, with the proper IP address requested by the HMU, to respond to the TCP request of the HMU (see Fig. 4). The data obtained was encrypted for the most part. However, credentials to connect to the service were sent in cleartext before switching to the encrypted communication.

Usage of a Proprietary Protocol over an Insecure Transport Protocol. Versions 2 and 3 of the HMU use both GPRS and SMS to send data. On both channels, the data is sent using a proprietary communication protocol on top of TCP. Leveraging the hardware vulnerabilities exposed above and the raw network data obtained by interacting with the devices, we were able to reverse engineer the protocol. It packs, compresses (when using GPRS) and encrypts the data. The detailed structure of a data packet is presented in Fig. 6.

Credentials Reuse. The credentials used to connect the VPMN and the backend services are the same and are sent unencrypted in both cases. They are thus very easy to obtain.

Unencrypted Communication with the Pacemaker. Even though we have not done exhaustive research at this interface due to limited access to working compatible pacemakers in our lab, we found that there is no encryption of the data exchanged between the pacemaker and the HMU. That means that attackers who can intercept the radio signal from the pacemaker (the radio band is already known) can also access the patient's data.

Denial of Service of the Modem. Results from the fuzz testing show that an attacker can perform a Denial of Service attack against the modem of the latest version of the HMU (V3) by sending it a specially crafted SMS. This will effectively prevent the HMU from communicating with the backend service before being rebooted.

4.4 Infrastructure

Improper Devices Management. The HMU has two sets of credentials: the first to connect to the network and access the manufacturer VPMN; the second to connect to the service on the backend server. To verify the validity of the credentials, we used them on a phone with the HMU SIM card and manually entered the settings in order to connect to the VPMN. However, when using the version 2 HMU SIM card, we were unable to connect because the SIM card was not valid anymore.

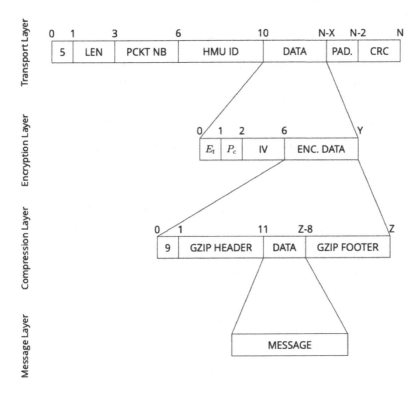

E_t: Encryption type (8 = AES CBC; 7 = 3DES CBC; 6 = DES)

P_c: Padding from the compression layer

Gzip header: 10 bytes starting with 0x1F8B (0x1F: compressed file; 0x8: deflate)

Gzip footer: CRC and length of original data

Fig. 6. Structure of the communication protocol's packet.

It turned out that using a SIM card from an old first version HMU on a newer second version HMU worked: we were able to connect to the VPMN and obtain an IP address inside the VPMN. To ensure we were in the right network, a successful ping request was sent to the server hosting the telemetry collection service. No other testing was performed as this was outside of our research scope and could potentially interfere with the manufacturer's service.

The VPMN is an additional security measure, even though this is not its main purpose. It prevents the patient data telemetry servers from being publicly exposed to the

Internet, something that for instance protects against Denial of Service (DoS) attacks. However, our research showed that this protection can be bypassed by an attacker who acquires an old device with a valid SIM card, highlighting the need for proper decommissioning procedures for old devices.

4.5   General Considerations and Attack Scenarios

By chaining several of the vulnerabilities, we were able to *weaponize* the second version of the HMU. With physical access to the device, an attacker can install a physical device with a wireless communication interface inside of it (the inside of the HMU casing is big enough to add a *RaspberryPi zero*), and that way gain *remote access* to the device. This allows an attacker to not only eavesdrop on all communications between the HMU and the backend server, but also to act as a *Man-in-the-Middle*, the proprietary protocol being known. Such an adversary can also get access to all the data sent by the pacemaker to the HMU. This would enable an attacker to modify the pacemaker telemetry data in order to hide a possible problem, or to create a problem by deleting or modifying pacemaker alerts and warnings that were meant to be sent to the backend server.

In this subsection, we describe three attack scenarios against the HMU and more generally against the whole pacemaker ecosystem. Figures 7, 8 and 9 present the attack trees for these scenarios. Arrows indicate a requirement. An arc between several arrows indicates an "AND" condition while single arrows indicate an "OR" condition.

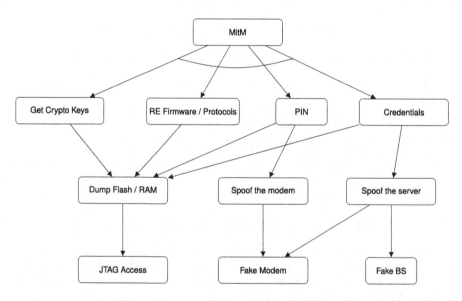

Fig. 7. Attack tree for the "MitM scenario" [3].

The first scenario is the *Man in the Middle* presented in Fig. 7. Given the vulnerabilities described earlier, an attacker can spoof the identity of the HMU for the backend server and vice-versa. This means that an adversary can have full control over the information that is sent between these two entities. In order to target a patient, an attacker could for instance constantly send good reports, suppressing any alerts or warnings from the pacemaker. This could trick a clinician into thinking that the patient is doing great while in reality, the patient might be in urgent need of a check-up, for example, due to the pacemaker battery running out. Having an HMU would thus be more dangerous than having no home monitoring enabled, due to a false sense of security and potentially fewer visits to the clinic.

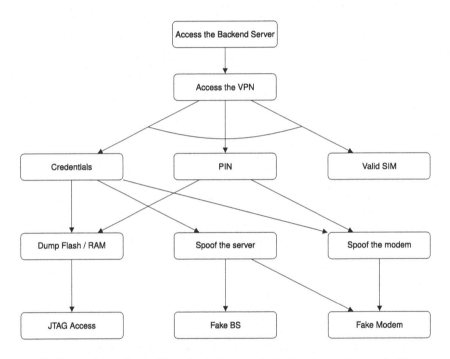

Fig. 8. Attack tree for the "Unauthorized access the backend server" scenario [3].

The second scenario can be described as *Unauthorized access to the backend server* and is presented in Fig. 8. We believe that this is possible with both versions of the HMU, given that the attacker can access credentials that are still valid. The attack tree shows only the GSM attack tree; the attack tree for the T-Line would be similar but easier since it only requires a working telephone line and no valid PIN or SIM. If an attacker can access the Virtual Private Network (VPN) with their computer using the credentials of the HMU, they would have direct access to the backend server (and all machines that reside in the same private network unless proper network segmentation with security monitoring is in place). If any of these machines are compromised, the result could be a significant data leak of personal data. Second-hand HMUs can be bought for a very low price on the internet, some come with their SIM cards still valid as we have demonstrated in our research, thus enabling an attacker to perform such an attack.

The last scenario is a large scale DoS attack on all the HMU devices of the pacemaker ecosystem. Our research has shown that an attacker can make an HMU crash by sending a specially crafted SMS to it. To recover from that crash, the device needs to be rebooted. Performing this attack requires knowledge of the phone number of the targeted device, thus making a large scale attack difficult. Such information could, however, be obtained in case of a data leak from the manufacturer or from the network provider. It could also come from an internal source. The attack tree for this attack is presented in Fig. 9.

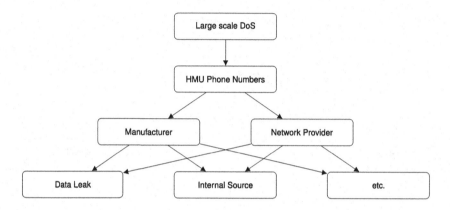

Fig. 9. Attack tree for the "Large scale DoS" scenario.

5   Discussion

5.1   Results

Our research confirms what was highlighted by Rios and Butts: the industry is overall still quite immature when it comes to cybersecurity [23]. Indeed, from a hardware point of view, an attacker with physical access to a device can easily get access to patients' data with no need for extensive knowledge or expensive equipment. From our observations, best security practices were not applied when it comes to hardware security given our findings of vulnerabilities that can all be described as commonly found in embedded devices. From a network perspective, several weaknesses have been identified in the protocol that is used by the HMU to communicate with the backend server, such as the credentials sent in clear text over TCP, the usage of a weak cipher to send data using SMS or the lack of mutual authentication in the second version of the HMU.

To be fair, it is also important to highlight that there is a notable evolution in terms of security between the versions. The latest version of the HMU seems to implement mutual authentication and stronger cryptographic ciphers than the previous versions. We can also point out that even though the second version has been found to have several weaknesses and vulnerabilities, the telemetry data was already encrypted using AES CBC with the keys being randomly generated and unique per device.

5.2 Trade-Offs in the Medical Industry

When designing IMDs, there are several security objectives to keep in mind. These are the regular six following properties: Confidentiality, Integrity, Availability, Non-repudiation, Authorization and Authentication. One also needs to consider the two modes under which these security properties have to be respected: *normal operation mode* and *emergency mode*. In the normal operation mode, the patient is in a state where it is reasonable to assume strict control of which devices can interact with the IMD, and it is feasible to implement strong access control, through the mean of cryptographic protocols for instance. Camara et al. explain that ideally, the device should not be detectable by unauthorized parties in this mode, and should "*ignore data requests or device reprogramming commands*" [5]. In emergency mode, even though the previously mentioned security objectives are important, it is vital that the device be accessible, for example if the patient is to undergo an emergency procedure for which the pacemaker must be deactivated.

It is thus a challenge for manufacturers to develop devices that fulfill all these characteristics. Zheng et al. highlight the trade-offs that come with the pacemaker ecosystem [30]. The first one is related to the emergency mode: *security vs accessibility*. Indeed, the purpose of the pacemaker is to save the patient's life and should not be an obstacle during an emergency surgery. The second trade-off is, *emergency access vs secure checkup access*. Securing the regular access while having an emergency access, which is almost like a security backdoor, is a challenge, especially when one must also take into account the battery life of the device. This leads to the third trade-off which is *limited resources vs strong cryptography*. Indeed, to secure the device, one needs to implement strong cryptography which requires intense processing power, this conflicts with the with low power capabilities and the long battery life time required by the implanted devices. This can even be abused by an attacker that launches Denial of Service (DoS) attacks in the form of constant wireless communication requests to drain the device battery, leading to a premature pacemaker battery depletion which requires surgery and thus setting the patient's life at higher risk from complications.

5.3 Device Management and Credentials Invalidation

As shown in our research, hospitals and device manufacturers already have challenges when it comes to asset management of devices through their entire lifecycle. One example of this is the lack of de-commissioning of old HMU devices containing SIM cards that still had valid credentials for connecting to the manufacturer's back end systems. Asset management might become an even greater challenge when it comes to managing the future "hospital at home". Getting rid of hardcoded credentials, deprecating certificates and expired cryptographic keys and also the detection of potential rogue devices joining the network will have to be implemented to mitigate the risk.

5.4 Mitigation and Defense

As mentioned in the previous section, building safe and secure medical devices means facing several trade-offs. Several solutions have been proposed to solve the problem of having a secure access to the device while allowing access in emergency situations. Zheng et al. wrote a review [28] of the different mechanisms that could be used:

External Proxy-based Solutions. This idea was first proposed by Denning et al., and consists, as the name indicates, in having an external device called the Communication Cloakers to protect the implant [7]. This external device is carried by the patient and protects the implant from attacks in everyday life. In an emergency situation, when the clinician does not have access to the distributed key, she can simply remove the proxy. However, this also means that if patients forget or lose their proxy device, their implant becomes vulnerable to attacks again.

Biometric-based Access Control. This type of solution uses patients' biometric features in order to provide access. For instance, the Heart-to-Heart (H2H) scheme [24] makes sure that the pacemaker can only be accessed by a programmer in physical contact with the patient by using ECG signals to generate the crypto material to establish a secure wireless communication. Other solutions might use different biometric features, such as fingerprints, iris or even voice [29].

Proximity-based Security Schemes. In these schemes, the proximity of the device is used to determine whether or not a functionality is available. For instance, changing the device settings, which is a critical operation, requires close proximity (a few centimeters) while home monitoring is allowed up to 10m. If some authentication scheme such as Ultrasonic-AC [22] combine proximity and security credentials, others can be based on magnetic fields or short-range communication protocol. This is in fact what is currently used to secure pacemakers. Proximity-based security schemes have however been proven to be vulnerable if the attacker uses strong magnetic fields or simply use powerful and sensitive transceivers and high gain antennas [19].

Key Distribution Supporting Emergency Access. These schemes rely on cryptography to achieve secure access in normal situations while also keeping an emergency access. This includes symmetric cryptography, in which the key is distributed to authorized devices. For emergency situations, it is proposed that the key is carried by the patient, either with a smart card, on a bracelet or simply tattooed on the skin (with UV ink for instance) [26]. Public key cryptography can also be used. However, in the case of an emergency situation, the programmer needs to contact a trusted party to obtain the certificate that can be used to derive a symmetric key, and this requires access to the Internet. In addition, public key cryptography is not compatible with the low energy requirements of the pacemakers. Finally, it is possible to use biometric features to generate keys, as already explained for biometric-based solutions.

In their review, Zheng et al. also suggest possible solutions to address the resource constraints of IMDs [28].

Lightweight Cryptography. In order to preserve the implant energy, manufacturers need to use lightweight cryptography protocols. Marin et al. propose a key agreement protocol that is an alternative to the proposal of Halperin et al., that was to add a standard symmetric key authentication and encryption between the ICD and the programmer, thus requiring the key to be safely stored on the programmer and opening the door to it being leaked. Marin et al. propose a semi-offline protocol: the IMD is in charge of computing a new key for the new period. To do so, the programmers need to contact the vendor to obtain the key for the period. That way, if the programmer is lost, or not in use anymore, it will not receive any updated key, and thus the ecosystem goes back to a secure state when the key is changed. Even though the new key computation is expensive for the IMD, this is a rare event and is thus not a problem.

Energy Harvesting. Another way to protect medical devices is through energy harvesting. Halperin et al. propose zero-power defenses for IMDs. These defenses include detection of attacks, prevention of attacks and a key exchange mechanism. As a detection mechanism, they propose to add a way to make the patient aware that there is something out of the ordinary happening, by for instance playing a "beep" if the security is disabled on the implant. The zero-power idea is to use a piezo-element driven by wireless communication (thus alerting a patient that wireless communication is taking place).

Separate Security Unit. Last but not least, the usage of a separate security unit that would be in charge of the security can mitigate the impact on the battery of the implant. This is for instance something that can be pushed to the external proxy device proposed above.

Moving away from the communication channel, another area that needs improvements is the software security. Li et al. propose a way to improve the trustworthiness of medical device software with formal verification methods [17]. They applied their approach to the firmware of a pacemaker and "demonstrated its ability to detect a range of software vulnerabilities that compromise security and safety." The idea behind formal verification is not only to check for common vulnerabilities such as buffer overflows, use after free, etc. but also to go from the device specifications to verifiable properties. This can be, for example, the voltage of the pacing for a pacemaker in a given configuration. This approach allows the verification of real-world properties.

The healthcare domain has recently been plagued with cyber attacks in the form of ransomware attacks, where the intrusion often comes as a result of poor practices related to software patching and software inventory management. One mitigation that might help IT staff in deciding which software security updates need to be applied for securing medical devices is the introduction of a *Software Bill of Materials (SBOM)*, where the manufacturer declares all software components in a device. In 2018, the FDA published a Medical Device Safety Action Plan where one of the proposed actions was to require medical device manufacturers to include an SBOM as part of their premarket submissions.

Securing devices to which an attacker might have physical access is difficult. As mentioned in the Microsoft's Ten immutable Laws of Security, *"If a bad guy has unrestricted physical access to your computer, it's not your computer anymore."* This is even more true for embedded medical devices, which usually do not come with as strong security defense mechanisms as computers. Indeed, adding strong hardware security to medical devices such as the Home Monitoring Unit also has a cost, and manufacturers might have to make a choice between security and costs, given that the money that is invested in the security of an HMU is not being used for developing treatment functionality, which saves lives. In addition to this, there is also the race to market and the strict certification process that does not allow easily making changes to an already approved design.

Fuzzing is a powerful methodology which can be used by both attackers and developers to discover bugs and potential vulnerabilities. Fuzzing might, however, not catch all issues, and manufacturers should ensure their devices are resilient to events such as crashes of external components (a modem for instance).

The industry is unfortunately not yet at the point where we can expect very strong cyber security in medical devices. As demonstrated by our research, basic security practices remain to be applied. A first step towards a more secure pacemaker ecosystem is the implementation of well-known best practices for hardware security, which, even if they do not protect against all attackers, can surely raise the cost of an attack, and simply discourage many attackers. Guides such the Secure Design Best Practice Guide by the IoT Security Foundation [13] provide a checklist of security measures to be adapted to a product, already during the design phase. When it comes to securing the firmware, the OWASP foundation offers a project for Embedded Application Security [21] that should be taken into account.

5.5   New Regulations

The European Union (EU) currently has two regulations medical devices manufacturers have to comply with: REGULATION (EU) 2017/745 (MDR) and REGULATION (EU) 2017/746 (IVDR) which apply from the 26th of May 2021 and 2022 respectively. These two new regulations replace older EU directives and aim at creating a regulatory framework for medical devices, to improve safety, quality and reliability.

In particular, the new regulation is paving the way for more testing of medical devices and should ease the work for manufacturers when it comes to fixing software (for instance, no need to re-certify for every minor change). This should also benefits security researchers as it will ease the responsible disclosure process.

Unfortunately, while great on paper, putting the regulation in practice comes with challenges. There are currently few devices certified with the new scheme as medical devices tend to have a long life. It will thus be hard to make legacy devices compliant with the new regulations, and this for quite some time still due to the also slow roll out of new devices.

6   Conclusion

Security of IoMT is a hot topic today, especially in the healthcare domain due to the need for patient safety and protection of critical data. In this paper, we evaluated the security aspects of the pacemaker ecosystem with a focus on hardware and network security architecture.

We have shown how the security protection features of several components in the pacemaker ecosystem are flawed. Leveraging physical access to the device and following a reverse engineering approach, we demonstrated that an attacker can expose the patient's data. Fuzzing the wireless communication chip of the device revealed vulnerabilities allowing an attacker to remotely trigger a DoS attack on the device.

Our focus was on the impacts of insecurity of the pacemaker ecosystem on patient safety. However, our results also imply that integrating such IoMT devices with major shortcomings into the complex hospital infrastructure could open the door to attacks with impacts that are potentially as devastating as a ransomware attack on hospital services [8,9].

Acknowledgments. We very much appreciate the contributions of Éireann Leverett that did some of the initial hardware testing to discover the HMU debug interfaces. Finally, we are grateful to Snorre Aunet and Ingulf Helland from NTNU who took time to help us solder a connector on the HMU.

This work was funded by Reinforcing the Health Data Infrastructure in Mobility and Assurance through Data Democratization, a five-year project (grant number 28885) under the Norwegian IKTPLUSS-IKT and Digital Innovation programme. The authors gratefully acknowledge the financial support from the Research Council of Norway.

References

1. OWASP firmware security testing methodology. https://scriptingxss.gitbook.io/firmware-security-testing-methodology/
2. Block, C.C.: Muddy waters report - St. Jude Medical, Inc. Technical report, Muddy Waters Capital LLC (2016). http://www.muddywatersresearch.com/research/stj/mw-is-short-stj/
3. Bour, G., Moe, M.E.G., Borgaonkar, R.: Experimental security analysis of connected pacemakers. In: Roque, A.C.A., Fred, A.L.N., Gamboa, H. (eds.) Proceedings of the 15th International Joint Conference on Biomedical Engineering Systems and Technologies, BIOSTEC 2022, Volume 1: BIODEVICES, Online Streaming, 9–11 February 2022, pp. 35–45. SCITEPRESS (2022). https://doi.org/10.5220/0010816900003123
4. Bour, G.N.: Security analysis of the pacemaker home monitoring unit: a blackbox approach. Master's thesis, NTNU (2019)
5. Camara, C., Peris-Lopez, P., Tapiador, J.E.: Security and privacy issues in implantable medical devices: a comprehensive survey. J. Biomed. Inform. **55**, 272–289 (2015)
6. CISA: ICS Medical Advisory (ICSMA-20-170-05) (2020). https://us-cert.cisa.gov/ics/advisories/icsma-20-170-05. Accessed 30 Sept 2021
7. Denning, T., Fu, K., Kohno, T.: Absence makes the heart grow fonder: new directions for implantable medical device security. In: HotSec (2008)
8. Digital, N.: A clear and present danger (2022). https://digital.nhs.uk/features/a-real-and-present-danger
9. Europol: Covid-19 sparks upward trend in cybercrime (2022). https://www.europol.europa.eu/media-press/newsroom/news/covid-19-sparks-upward-trend-in-cybercrime
10. Færestrand, S.: Telekardiologi for jernmonitorering av pacemaker og icd (2010). https://www.legeforeningen.no/contentassets/4896657d08894a6886de725113d89de4/hjerteforum3-2010web08telemedisin.pdf
11. Golde, N., Feldmann, A.: SMS vulnerability analysis on feature phones. Master's thesis (2011)
12. Halperin, D., et al.: Pacemakers and implantable cardiac defibrillators: software radio attacks and zero-power defenses. In: 2008 IEEE Symposium on Security and Privacy (SP 2008), pp. 129–142. IEEE (2008)
13. Secure design best practice guide (2020). https://www.iotsecurityfoundation.org/wp-content/uploads/2019/03/Best-Practice-Guides-Release-1.2.1.pdf
14. ISECOM: OSSTMM. https://www.isecom.org/OSSTMM.3.pdf
15. Justis- og beredskapsdepartementet, Helse- og omsorgsdepartementet: Forskrift om medisinsk utstyr (2005). https://lovdata.no/dokument/SF/forskrift/2005-12-15-1690/%2FT1%2Ftextsection1-5#/T1/textsection1-5

16. Kok, J.S., Markussen, B.A.: Fuzzing the pacemaker home monitoring unit. Master's thesis, NTNU (2020)
17. Li, C., Raghunathan, A., Jha, N.K.: Improving the trustworthiness of medical device software with formal verification methods. IEEE Embed. Syst. Lett. **5**(3), 50–53 (2013)
18. Lie, A.W.: Security analysis of wireless home monitoring units in the pacemaker ecosystem. Master's thesis, NTNU (2019)
19. Marin, E., Singelée, D., Garcia, F.D., Chothia, T., Willems, R., Preneel, B.: On the (in) security of the latest generation implantable cardiac defibrillators and how to secure them. In: Proceedings of the 32nd Annual Conference on Computer Security Applications, pp. 226–236 (2016)
20. Mulliner, C., Golde, N., Seifert, J.P.: SMS of death: from analyzing to attacking mobile phones on a large scale (2011). https://www.usenix.org/conference/usenix-security-11/sms-death-analyzing-attacking-mobile-phones-large-scale
21. OWASP embedded application security (2020). https://owasp.org/www-project-embedded-application-security/
22. Rasmussen, K.B., Castelluccia, C., Heydt-Benjamin, T.S., Capkun, S.: Proximity-based access control for implantable medical devices. In: Proceedings of the 16th ACM Conference on Computer and Communications Security, pp. 410–419 (2009)
23. Rios, B., Butts, J.: Security evaluation of the implantable cardiac device ecosystem architecture and implementation interdependencies (2017)
24. Rostami, M., Juels, A., Koushanfar, F.: Heart-to-heart (H2H) authentication for implanted medical devices. In: Proceedings of the 2013 ACM SIGSAC Conference on Computer & Communications Security, pp. 1099–1112 (2013)
25. Savci, H.S., Sula, A., Wang, Z., Dogan, N.S., Arvas, E.: Mics transceivers: regulatory standards and applications [medical implant communications service]. In: Proceedings of the IEEE SoutheastCon, pp. 179–182. IEEE (2005)
26. Schechter, S.: Security that is meant to be skin deep using ultraviolet micropigmentation to store emergency-access keys for implantable medical devices (2010)
27. Weinmann, R.P.: Baseband attacks: remote exploitation of memory corruptions in cellular protocol stacks. In: WOOT, pp. 12–21 (2012)
28. Zheng, G., Shankaran, R., Orgun, M.A., Qiao, L., Saleem, K.: Ideas and challenges for securing wireless implantable medical devices: a review. IEEE Sens. J. **17**(3), 562–576 (2016)
29. Zheng, G., et al.: Finger-to-heart (F2H): authentication for wireless implantable medical devices. IEEE J. Biomed. Health Inform. **23**(4), 1546–1557 (2018)
30. Zheng, G., Zhang, G., Yang, W., Valli, C., Shankaran, R., Orgun, M.A.: From WannaCry to WannaDie: security trade-offs and design for implantable medical devices. In: 2017 17th International Symposium on Communications and Information Technologies (ISCIT), pp. 1–5. IEEE (2017)

Parallel Lossy Compression for Large FASTQ Files

Veronica Guerrini[1]([✉])[ID], Felipe A. Louza[2][ID], and Giovanna Rosone[1][ID]

[1] Department of Computer Science, University of Pisa, Pisa, Italy
{`veronica.guerrini,giovanna.rosone`}`@unipi.it`
[2] Faculty of Electrical Engineering, Federal University of Uberlândia,
Uberlândia, Brazil
`louza@ufu.br`

Abstract. In this paper we present a parallel version for the algorithm BFQzip, we introduced in [Guerrini et al., BIOSTEC – BIOINFORMATICS 2022], that modifies the bases and quality scores components taking into account both information at the same time, while preserving variant calling. The resulting FASTQ file achieves better compression than the original data. Here, we introduce a strategy that splits the FASTQ file into t blocks and processes them in parallel independently by using the BFQzip algorithm. The resulting blocks with the modified bases and smoothed qualities are merged (in order) and compressed. We show that our strategy can improve the compression ratio of large FASTQ files by taking advantage of the redundancy of reads. When splitting into blocks, the reads belonging to the same portion of the genome could end up in different blocks. Therefore, we analyze how reordering reads before splitting the input FASTQ can improve the compression ratio as the number of threads increases. We also propose a paired-end mode that allows to exploit the paired-end information by processing blocks of FASTQ files in pairs.

Availability: The software is freely available at https://github.com/veronicaguerrini/BFQzip

Keywords: FASTQ compression · EBWT · Positional clustering · Reordering reads

1 Introduction

Next-generation sequencing (NGS) technology has transformed almost every research field in biology. NGS has made large-scale whole-genome sequencing (WGS) accessible to a larger number of researchers, and has allowed to gain insights and to explore applications as never possible before. DNA sequence data generated by the NGS technology are usually stored using the standard FASTQ file format.

An earlier version of this contribution appeared in the Proceedings of the 15th International Joint Conference on Biomedical Engineering Systems and Technologies: Bioinformatics [26].

A FASTQ file stores sequences of nucleotides with quality scores sequences that encode the probabilities of sequencing errors for each base. More in details, for each sequencing data (called *read*), the FASTQ file format comprises three main components: (i) read identifier with information related to the sequencing process (*header*), (ii) nucleotides sequence with the DNA fragment (*bases*), and (iii) qualities sequence, with the estimation of base calling confidence (*quality scores*). The last two components are divided by a "separator" line, which is generally discarded by compressors as it contains only a "+" symbol optionally followed by the same header.

In particular, each component of a FASTQ file has the following features: The *headers* generally consist of multiple fields encoding information such as the sequence ID or the instrument ID; thus, the information can be redundant as the per-field encoding is similar between different reads. The *bases* (nucleotides sequences) may be repetitive according to the sequencing depth; indeed, a high-coverage dataset contains more reads that cover the same genome position than a low-coverage dataset. The *quality scores* sequences encode the integer values representing the estimated error probability. If P is the probability that the base is incorrect, its Phred quality score is $Q = -10 \log(P)$. They are represented by printable ASCII characters (*e.g.* using the phred+33 encoding), whose range of values can vary depending on the sequencing machine.

The majority of the state-of-the-art compressors for FASTQ files focus on compressing one of the two main components, (ii) *bases* or (ii) *quality scores*, and apply known techniques or other tools to the other one.

The approaches for the *bases* compression are lossless, that is they do not perform modifications or information loss, but exploit the inherent redundancy of DNA sequences to compress them [13,18]. Some of them allow to lose the original order of reads to place sequences from close regions of the genome next to each others to improve compression, *e.g.* [13,27,49].

Differently, the *quality score* component is generally compressed lossy: some modifications are applied to improve compression at the cost of a little distortion effect. These compressors can be divided into two groups according to whether the biological information is exploited (*i.e.* read-based) or not. Many read-based approaches provide or need to compute a corpus based on a known reference or other external information (besides the FASTQ file itself), *e.g.* [24,51,53]. On the other hand, reference-free strategies generally do not use any biological information: they compress the *quality scores* either read by read independently (*e.g.* Illumina 8-level binning), or computing some statistics on them, *e.g.* SCALCE [27]. Among the reference-free strategies that evaluate the related biological information of the *bases* component are BEETL [29] and LEON [5].

Burrows-Wheeler Transform (BWT). The BWT was introduced by M. Burrows and D. Wheeler in the 1990s s [10] as a reversible transformation on texts to improve data compression [50]. Almost 10 years later, the BWT has been used as the building block for compact text indexing [22].

Therefore, the BWT has become the unifying tool for textual compression and text indexing, becoming an extremely useful tool in various applications, as for comparing DNA sequence collections by direct comparison of compressed text indexes [17], metagenomic classification [25], sequence alignment [40], DNA mapping [32] and genome assembly [52].

The greatest advantage of the BWT is that its output generally has a good local similarity (occurrences of a given symbol tend to occur in blocks) and then turns out to be highly compressible. This property, known as *clustering effect*, is a consequence of the fact that the BWT builds a list containing the cyclic rotations (resp. suffixes) of the input string in lexicographic order, and this sort tends to move the rotations (or suffixes) prefixed by the same substring close together in the sorted list, leading to runs of identical symbols in the concatenation of the last (or the preceding) symbol of each element of the sorted list. An interested reader can find relevant works about the clustering effect in [35,38,41,42,48] and references there in.

In this work, we use the extended BWT (EBWT) for string collections [37], and we consider the construction algorithm introduced in [4] that works in semi-external memory and it is particularly fast for short reads, at the cost of making the set of input strings ordered, since it requires appending a (distinct) end-marker to each string (related works and different implementations can be found in [20,21,31,33,34]). We point to [8] for a thorough study about sorting conjugates and suffixes in a string collection, and to [12] for a recent analysis of several BWT variants for string collections.

Reordering of Reads. Some studies have shown that reordering the reads in the FASTQ file allows to obtain a higher compression at the expense of losing information about the original order of the reads (unless it is not saved).

The authors in [16] observed that it is possible to reorder strings within an input collection while building their EBWT – by means of the algorithm introduced in [4] – in order to reduce the number of runs of equal symbols in the resulting EBWT string. The main underlying idea is that one can reorder the symbols within particular blocks of the EBWT, called 'same-as-previous' intervals, that are associated with suffixes that are equal up to the end-markers. Indeed, the order of symbols in these intervals only depends on the relative ordering of the end-markers, and changing their order determines a different ordering in the input collection. The same authors introduce two heuristics: in the first heuristic (named SAP-order) the symbols are grouped into as few runs as possible and in the second, the symbols are permuted in according to the Reverse Lexicographic Order (named RLO). Experiments showed that both RLO and SAP-order improve the overall compression.

Recently, the authors in [6, Section 5] provided a linear time algorithm that reorders the end-markers (and, thus, it reorders input strings) so that the number of runs of equal symbols in the EBWT string is minimized. Another work on the re-ordering of the strings in a collection related on the BWT can be found in [11].

Nevertheless, the problem of reordering short-reads in a FASTQ file for data compression purposes was also addressed independently by the BWT. It has been explored with SCALCE [27] a reorganization of the reads based on Locally

Consistent Parsing as a 'boosting' scheme for compressing them. Further, the tool HARC [14] has been designed for reordering reads approximately according to their genome position and then for encoding them as to remove the redundancy between consecutive reads and to achieve a better compression. In [13], the authors of HARC contributed to introducing SPRING that includes significant improvements on HARC and supports variable-length reads.

Our Contribution. In this paper, we introduce a strategy suitable for the compression of large FASTQ files by extending and parallelizing the algorithm BFQzIP described in [26].

BFQzIP is a read-based, reference- and assembly-free lossy compression approach based on the EBWT, which by careful modifications on data, reduces noise from the *bases* and modifies the *quality scores* taking into account both information at the same time, while preserving variant calling.

The basic idea is that each *base* in a read can with high probability be predicted by its context, and its *quality score* can be smoothed without distortion effects on downstream analysis. In our strategy, we use contexts of variable-order thanks to the EBWT positional clustering [46].

Our parallel strategy splits the input FASTQ file into t blocks and processes them all together in parallel with BFQzIP, the resulting blocks with the modified bases and smoothed qualities are merged (in order) and then compressed with the PPMd or BSC. We show that our strategy can improve the compression ratio of large FASTQ files by taking advantage of the redundancy of reads. When splitting into blocks, the reads belonging to the same portion of the genome could end up in different blocks. Therefore, we analyze how reordering reads before splitting the input FASTQ can improve the compression ratio as the number of threads increases. Indeed, processing highly related reads together improves the compression ratio and mitigates the loss in compression ratio when the number of threads increases.

We evaluated RLO and SPRING reordering methods. We performed the RLO by ordering all the reads lexicographically from right to left, that has been shown to reduce the number of runs in the EBWT and has improved the compressibility especially for short reads [16]. We also tested the SPRING reordering implemented as a stand-alone tool for placing reads approximately according to their genome position.

Finally, we implemented a paired-end mode for our parallel BFQzIP tool that allows to exploit the paired-end information by processing blocks of reads in pairs.

2   Background

Let S be a string (also called sequence) of length n on the alphabet Σ. We denote the i-th symbol of S by $S[i]$. A *substring* of any S is denoted as $S[i,j] = S[i] \cdots S[j]$, with $S[1,j]$ being called a *prefix* and $S[i,n]$ a *suffix* of S.

Let $\mathcal{S} = \{S_1, S_2, \ldots, S_m\}$ be a collection of m strings on the alphabet Σ. We assume that each string $S_i \in \mathcal{S}$ has length $n_i + 1$, since we append a special end-marker symbol $\$_i$ to each S_i, *i.e.* $S_i[n_i + 1] = \$_i$, such that each $\$_i$ does not belong to Σ and it is lexicographically smaller than any other symbol in Σ.

Data Structures. The Burrows-Wheeler Transform (BWT) [10] of a text T (and the EBWT of a string collection $\mathcal{S}$ [4,37]) is a reversible transformation that permutes the symbols of T (and of $\mathcal{S}$) so that symbols preceding similar contexts are carried in clusters.

For our target application, we focus on the EBWT of a collection of m strings $\mathcal{S}$, as described in [4]. Let N be the sum of the lengths of all strings in $\mathcal{S}$, *i.e.* $N = \sum_{i=1}^{m}(n_i + 1)$. The output of the EBWT is a string $\mathsf{ebwt}(\mathcal{S})$ of length N such that, for $1 \leq i \leq N$, $\mathsf{ebwt}(\mathcal{S})[i]$ is the symbol that circularly precedes the i-th suffix of the lexicographic sorted list of suffixes of all strings in $\mathcal{S}$. In particular, let $S_j[k, n_j + 1]$ be the i-th suffix of the lexicographic sorted list, for some $1 \leq j \leq m$ and $1 \leq k \leq n_j + 1$, it holds $\mathsf{ebwt}(\mathcal{S})[i] = S_j[k - 1]$, if $k > 1$, and $\mathsf{ebwt}(\mathcal{S})[i] = \$_j$, if $k = 1$. Note that the implementations can use a single symbol $\$$ as end-marker for all strings, and consider the end-markers from different strings implicitly sorted on the basis of their index in the input collection, *i.e.* $\$_i < \$_j$, if $i < j$. See Table 1 for an example. We say the suffix $S_j[k, n_j + 1]$ is the *context* associated with position i in $\mathsf{ebwt}(\mathcal{S})$.

The *LF-mapping* is a fundamental property of the EBWT (and BWT), which states that the i-th occurrence of symbol x on the string $\mathsf{ebwt}(\mathcal{S})$ and the first symbol of the i-th lexicographically-smallest suffix that starts with x correspond to the same position in the input string collection. The *LF-mapping* allows us to reconstruct $\mathcal{S}$ in linear time, and to perform the so-called backward search to find range of suffixes prefixed by a given substring that plays a key role in text indexing (see [3,22] for more details).

A data structure that is often used combined with the EBWT is the *longest common prefix* (LCP) array [36]. The LCP array of $\mathcal{S}$, $\mathsf{lcp}(\mathcal{S})$, is an array of length $N + 1$ such that $\mathsf{lcp}(\mathcal{S})[1] = \mathsf{lcp}(\mathcal{S})[N + 1] = 0$ and, for any $2 \leq i \leq N$, $\mathsf{lcp}(\mathcal{S})[i]$ is the length of the longest common prefix between the two contexts associated with the positions i and $i - 1$ in $\mathsf{ebwt}(\mathcal{S})$. The LCP-intervals, introduced in [2], of LCP-value k are maximal intervals $[i, j]$ that satisfy: $\mathsf{lcp}(\mathcal{S})[r] \geq k$, for all $i < r \leq j$, and there exists x, $i < x \leq j$ such that $\mathsf{lcp}(\mathcal{S})[x] = k$. Thus, the contexts of an LCP-interval of LCP-value k share the first k symbols.

Dealing with FASTQ files, for each sequence of bases, we have a sequence of corresponding quality scores. Thus, we associate the EBWT output string of the bases, $\mathsf{ebwt}(\mathcal{S})$, with the string $\mathsf{qs}(\mathcal{S})$ obtained by concatenating the quality scores permuted in the same way as bases symbols. In this way, for each position i in the EBWT, we know the base symbol $\mathsf{ebwt}(\mathcal{S})[i]$ and its associated quality score $\mathsf{qs}(\mathcal{S})[i]$. Note that a dummy symbol in $\mathsf{qs}(\mathcal{S})$ is associated with each end-marker in $\mathsf{ebwt}(\mathcal{S})$. See Table 1 for an example of the qs string (a space is used as dummy symbol).

Positional Clustering. The positional clustering framework [44,46] detects blocks of EBWT symbols whose associated contexts approximately cover the same genome position.

Table 1. Extended Burrows-Wheeler Transform (EBWT), LCP-array, and the string qs for the set $\mathcal{S} = \{$AACGTATTG, ACGAGTACGACT, TTAACGTATT$\}$ with associated quality scores {!#! <:<;: @,? > @AAA=JJGIJ,BABHH#!!8;}.

i	lcp	B_{min}	B_{thr}	ebwt	qs	Sorted suffixes	i	lcp	B_{min}	B_{thr}	ebwt	qs	Sorted suffixes
1	0	0	0	G	@	$	18	1	0	0	A	G	CT$
2	0	0	0	T	J	$	19	0	1	0	T	:	G$
3	0	0	0	T	;	$	20	1	0	0	C	J	GACT$
4	0	0	0	**T**	A	AACGTATT$	21	2	0	1	**C**	>	GAGTACGACT$
5	8	0	1	**$**		AACGTATTG$	22	1	1	0	**A**	A	GTACGACT$
6	1	1	0	**T**	A	ACGACT$	23	3	0	1	**C**	H	GTATT$
7	4	0	1	**$**		ACGAGTACGACT$	24	5	0	1	**C**	!	GTATTG$
8	3	1	1	**A**	B	ACGTATT$	25	0	1	0	C	I	T$
9	7	0	1	**A**	!	ACGTATTG$	26	1	0	0	T	8	T$
10	2	0	1	**G**	J	ACT$	27	1	0	0	**T**	B	TAACGTATT$
11	1	1	0	**G**	@	AGTACGACT$	28	2	0	1	**G**	A	TACGACT$
12	1	0	0	T	!	ATT$	29	2	0	1	**G**	#	TATT$
13	3	0	1	**T**	:	ATTG$	30	4	0	1	**G**	<	TATTG$
14	0	1	0	A	=	CGACT$	31	1	1	0	**T**	;	TG$
15	3	0	1	**A**	?	CGAGTACGACT$	32	1	0	0	A	!	TT$
16	2	1	1	**A**	H	CGTATT$	33	2	0	1	**$**		TTAACGTATT$
17	6	0	1	**A**	#	CGTATTG$	34	2	0	1	**A**	<	TTG$

It has been inspired by the well-known property of the EBWT that symbols associated with equal contexts are contiguous in the ebwt string, thus forming substrings that are commonly called clusters. For instance, clusters associated with maximal intervals $[i,j]$ such that $\mathsf{lcp}[r] \geq k$, for all $i < r \leq j$, are known to share a right context w of length at least k characters. Nevertheless, the length of the common context w is at least k, and it could be longer for some sub-intervals. Moreover, those clusters are detected by fixing the length k a-priori.

In order to overcome the limitation of LCP-intervals-like strategies, the authors of [46] introduced the positional clustering framework that allows to detect clusters without fixing a value for the length k, but exploiting "local minima" of the LCP-array that mark context changes in the EBWT. We remark that, in this strategy, clusters do not depend on the choice of k, rather they are automatically detected, in a data-driven way, so that the length of the common right context w is of variable order.

Then, a positional cluster can be defined by using two binary vectors: B_{min} and B_{thr}, where $B_{min} = 1$ if and only if it holds $\mathsf{lcp}[i-1] > \mathsf{lcp}[i] \leq \mathsf{lcp}[i+1]$, for all $1 < i \geq N$, i.e. $\mathsf{lcp}[i]$ is a local minimum, and $B_{thr}[i] = 1$ if and only if $\mathsf{lcp}[i] \geq k_m$, for some k_m. The parameter k_m is a threshold that helps to trim clusters corresponding to short random contexts, that are statistically not significant.

An *EBWT positional cluster* PosCluster $[i,j]$ is a maximal substring ebwt$[i,j]$ where $B_{thr}[r] = 1$, for all $i < r \leq j$, and $B_{min}[r] = 0$, for all $i < r \leq j$. See, for instance, Table 1, in which positional clusters for $k_m = 2$ are in bold and delimited by lines.

By definition, we have that any two EBWT positional clusters, $\mathsf{PosCluster}[i,j]$ and $\mathsf{PosCluster}[i',j']$, such that $i \neq i'$ are disjoint, *i.e.* either $j < i'$ or $j' < i$. Moreover, if we set $k_m = k$, any EBWT positional cluster may be a proper sub-interval of a maximal cluster $\mathsf{ebwt}[i,j]$ such that $\mathsf{lcp}[r] \geq k$, for all $i < r \leq j$. In addition, any maximal cluster $\mathsf{ebwt}[i,j]$ when chopped at the local minima of $\mathsf{lcp}[i,j]$ originates multiple consecutive EBWT positional clusters. For instance, in Table 1, the LCP-interval $[6,10]$ of value $k = 2$ is split in two positional clusters $[6,7]$ and $[8,10]$.

3   Noise Reduction of DNA Sequences and Smoothing Quality Scores

In this section we present the main phases of BFQZIP, a EBWT-based lossy compression method, first introduced in [26].

Data Structures Building. Let $\mathcal{S}$ be the collection of bases sequences stored in a given input FASTQ file. The first phase computes the EBWT of $\mathcal{S}$, obtaining together with $\mathsf{ebwt}(\mathcal{S})$ the associated string of permuted quality scores, $\mathsf{qs}(\mathcal{S})$.

Then, in the following phases, by using $\mathsf{ebwt}(\mathcal{S})$ and $\mathsf{qs}(\mathcal{S})$, we handle and modify the information related to both the permuted bases and their associated quality scores in order to build a new FASTQ file to be compressed.

In order to exploit the biological information contained in the FASTQ file, we employ the notion of positional clustering based on the crucial clustering property of the EBWT.

Positional Cluster Detecting. We recall the aim of positional clustering is to detect blocks of characters in $\mathsf{ebwt}(\mathcal{S})$ sharing a common context, and approximately covering the same genome position, without a fixed context length. The authors in [44,46] showed that those blocks can be detected between local minima of the LCP-array (see Sect. 2).

Thus, according to the positional clustering, we detect blocks in $\mathsf{ebwt}(\mathcal{S})$, and thus in $\mathsf{qs}(\mathcal{S})$. Yet, in order to filter out clusters corresponding to short random contexts, a minimum threshold value k_m for that length is required.

As in [44], BFQZIP computes all the EBWT positional clusters by representing and navigating the $\mathsf{ebwt}(\mathcal{S})$ through the compressed suffix tree described in [45] (see also [47] for more details). In fact, the authors of [44] do not have the LCP-array calculated explicitly, but they compute the bitvectors B_{min} and B_{thr} that define EBWT positional clusters by navigating the indexed $\mathsf{ebwt}(\mathcal{S})$ and by storing only entries of the LCP-array that are local minima in B_{min} and those larger than the threshold value k_m in B_{thr}. Such a strategy comes as a modification[1] of the method first introduced in [45].

---

[1] By using the code/library at https://github.com/nicolaprezza/bwt2lcp.

Alternatively, BFQzip can work in external memory without navigating the compressed suffix tree of the ebwt($\mathcal{S}$). In this case, we need to build also the lcp($\mathcal{S}$), and by reading it in a sequential way, we can compute all the EBWT clusters.

Noise Reduction. Let PosCluster$[i, j]$ be a EBWT positional cluster (abbreviated as cluster). BFQzip analyzes the base symbols in PosCluster$[i, j]$ and may change some of them according to their quality scores and which symbols appear in it.

We call *frequent symbol* of PosCluster$[i, j]$ any symbol that occurs over a threshold percentage in PosCluster$[i, j]$. The basic idea is to change bases symbols that are different from the frequent symbols of their clusters, as to reduce the noise of that cluster while preserving the variant calls. For this reason, we take into account only clusters that have no more than two frequent symbols (for example, by setting the threshold percentage to 40%).

The bases symbols that are candidates to be changed are called *noisy bases.* Formally, a base symbol b in PosCluster$[i, j]$ is a noisy base, if it is different from the most frequent symbols of PosCluster$[i, j]$ and none occurrence of b in PosCluster$[i, j]$ has a high quality score. In other words, any occurrence of a noisy base b of PosCluster$[i, j]$ is associated with a low quality value in qs$[i, j]$. Recalling that symbols in any cluster usually correspond to the same genome location [46], any base symbol different from the most frequent symbols and having a low quality score (which indicates a high error probability) is likely to be noise.

In order to replace noisy bases of PosCluster$[i, j]$, we need to distinguish mainly two cases: (i) one frequent symbol, or (ii) more frequent symbols.

In case (i), we have that PosCluster$[i, j]$ contains a unique frequent symbol c, and we replace any occurrence of the noisy base b by c.

In case (ii), we analyze the case in which there are two different frequent symbols c and d in PosCluster$[i, j]$ (no more than two frequent symbols are allowed in our setting). Then, for each occurrence of c and d, we compute a context of length ℓ that in the corresponding read precedes it (*i.e. left context* of the considered symbol). We take advantage of the backward search applied to ebwt($\mathcal{S}$) to compute left contexts (for example, we set $\ell = 1$ in our experiments). We also compute the left context of the noisy base, and if it coincides with the left contexts of all the occurrences either of c or of d, then we substitute b either with c or with d. Nonetheless, if the left contexts preceding c and d are the same, no base replacement is performed.

Quality Score Smoothing. While analyzing clusters for noise reduction, we perform a smoothing on qs($\mathcal{S}$) by replacing the quality scores associated with symbols within clusters.

For any PosCluster$[i, j]$, we denote by Q the score used to smooth quality scores in qs$[i, j]$. We defined Q by using different strategies[2]:

---

[2] Note that the value Q does not depend on the cluster analyzed only in strategy (a).

(a) Q is a default value;
(b) Q is the quality score corresponding to the mean probability error in $\mathsf{qs}[i,j]$;
(c) Q is the maximum quality score appearing in $\mathsf{qs}[i,j]$;
(d) Q is the average of the quality scores in $\mathsf{qs}[i,j]$.

The smoothing process consists in substituting Q for any value $\mathsf{qs}[r]$, $i \leq r \leq j$, if and only if $\mathsf{qs}[r]$ is greater than Q or $\mathsf{ebwt}[r]$ is an occurrence of a frequent symbol (regardless of its quality score).

Indeed, quality scores of bases that can be predicted by their context add little information, and thus they can be smoothed. In general, the average of the quality score appearing in a cluster does not coincide with the quality score associated with the mean error probability, which is obtained by transforming each quality score within the cluster into its corresponding error probability.

Another additional feature of BFQZIP to compress further quality scores is the possibility of reducing the number of the alphabet symbols appearing in $\mathsf{qs}(\mathcal{S})$. This is a well-known and standard technique used in the literature by other compressors. In particular, the additional smoothing strategy implemented in BFQZIP is the alphabet reduction to only 8 different symbols from the Illumina 8-level binning.

4   Parallel Strategy and Paired-End Mode

Our parallel strategy splits the input FASTQ file into t blocks $B_1, B_2, \ldots, B_t$ of nearly equal sizes (except for the last one), where t is the number of threads. Each block B_i is processed independently from the others in a parallel way by using BFQZIP to perform *noise reduction* and *quality score smoothing* locally to reads within the block. Then, by using the LF-mapping on the EBWT related to each B_i, we retrieve the order of symbols in B_i and build a new FASTQ block having each component (*i.e.*, both the sequences of bases and the sequences of quality scores) modified as described in the previous section.

The resulting FASTQ blocks with the modified information are merged in the original order $B_1, B_2, \ldots, B_t$ into a new (modified) FASTQ file, which is given as input to be compressed with PPMd or BSC. Figure 1 shows the overall strategy performed by BFQZIP: in particular, Fig. 1a shows the strategy used in [26], and Fig. 1b its parallel version.

This strategy can reduce the compression ratio of large FASTQ files as BFQZIP cannot take fully advantage of redundancies that traverse blocks boundaries. In the next section we show that reordering the reads before the split of the input FASTQ can improve the compression ratio as the number of threads t increases.

Figure 1b shows the additional feature of first reordering the reads and then splitting the input FASTQ file into t blocks. Indeed, under the hypothesis that the reads in the same block are related to their mapping (similar) positions on the genome, an increasing number of blocks splitting the FASTQ file may not affect the compression ratio achieved.

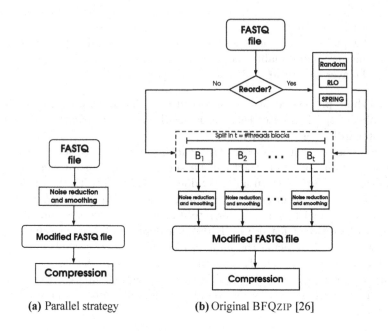

Fig. 1. Original BFQzip vs Parallel BFQzip (this paper)

Furthermore, in our parallel strategy, we introduce the possibility to process paired-end reads together, so that the pairing information is exploited to perform modifications to both bases and quality scores. In particular, we designed a paired-end mode so that each block B_i contains reads that are in pairs. Note that if a reordering is applied to the dataset to process, we need to check that the pairing in files is preserved.

Finally, in our compression scheme, the header component of a FASTQ file comprising of read titles can be either omitted (inserting just the '@' as header) or kept as it is in the original file.

5   Experiments

In this section we assess our parallel framework based on BFQzip in several aspects, evaluating it on Whole Genome Sequencing (WGS) data.

Datasets. In order to show the effectiveness of our method, we selected two datasets, described in Table 2, of paired-end reads with the same length but with diverse composition[3]. The two mates are stored in distinct files (_1 and _2). More in details, we use the *Caenorhabditis Elegans* dataset (SRR065390) comprising 33, 808, 546 paired-end reads of length 100 (33.6× a coverage of the genome) that

---

[3] We recall that a paired-end read is a pair consisting of two reads (or mates), such that the second read occurs in the genome at a known distance after the first one.

has been previously studied by the *Sequence Squeeze* [28] entrants and in [4]. We also considered a larger dataset from the *Homo Sapiens* individual NA12878 (ERR174324) comprising 223,571,196 paired-end reads of length 100–102, which corresponds to a 15×-coverage WGS dataset.

Table 2. The WGS paired-end datasets used for our evaluation. Each dataset comprises two files (_1 and _2), whose number of reads and read length are given in columns 3 and 4. We report the sizes in bytes of original FASTQ files (raw data) and FASTQ files with all headers removed (*i.e.*, replaced by '@').

Dataset	Name	N. reads	Len.	FASTQ size (in bytes)	
				with headers	without headers
Illumina WGS	SRR065390_1	33,808,546	100	11,282,985,734	6,964,560,476
of *C. Elegans*	SRR065390_2	33,808,546	100	11,282,985,734	6,964,560,476
Illumina WGS	ERR174324_1	223,571,196	100	72,676,271,264	46,055,666,376
of *H. Sapiens*	ERR174324_2	223,571,196	102	73,570,556,048	46,949,951,160

Reordering of Reads. We choose to evaluate the RLO and SPRING reorderings, and to preprocess the FASTQ file by using direct tools that build the reordered FASTQ file[4]. We also build a dataset obtained by shuffling the reads randomly for a negative control.

Table 3 shows the compression ratio of the original FASTQ files without headers by using two well-known compressors, PPMd [15,39] and BSC[5], when the different reorderings are used. The ratio is defined as compressed size over the original size, where original file sizes are reported in Table 2. The best results are highlighted in bold.

Table 3. Compression ratios of the original FASTQ files by using PPMd and BSC, and different reorderings: OO = Original order, RO = Random order, RLO = Reverse Lexicographic order, SO = SPRING order.

Dataset	Ratio (OO)		Ratio (RO)		Ratio (RLO)		Ratio (SO)	
	PPMd	BSC	PPMd	BSC	PPMd	BSC	PPMd	BSC
SRR065390_1	0.2234	0.2141	0.2094	0.2029	**0.2009**	**0.1468**	0.2243	0.2148
SRR065390_2	0.2279	0.2184	0.2144	0.2082	**0.2072**	**0.1553**	0.2288	0.2191
ERR174324_1	0.2535	0.2423	0.2538	0.2425	**0.2348**	0.2322	0.2427	**0.2026**
ERR174324_2	0.2639	0.2523	0.2643	0.2526	**0.2459**	0.2427	0.2544	**0.2167**

---

[4] https://github.com/shubhamchandak94/Spring/tree/reorder-only.
[5] http://libbsc.com/.

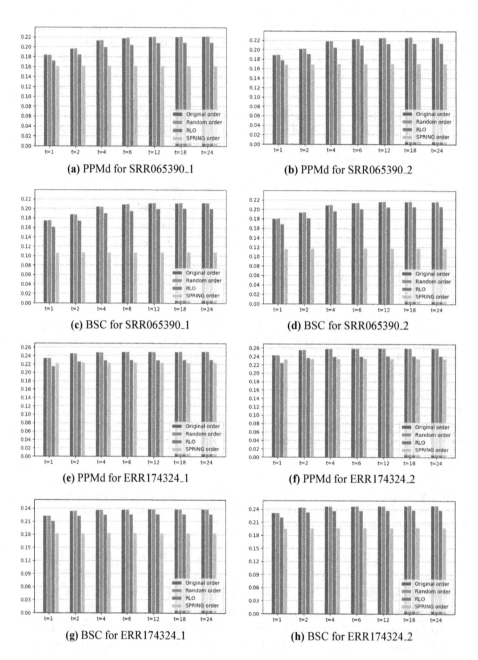

Fig. 2. Compression ratio by using PPMd and BSC when paired-end reads of SRR065390 and ERR174324 datasets are processed separately.

Experiments Goals. We compare the compression ratio of the resulting modified FASTQ file produced by the parallel BFQzip to the original FASTQ file (showed in Table 3).

For our experiments, we use the same parameter setting as that evaluated in [26], considering FASTQ files with headers replaced by '@'.

We recall that we split the input file into t blocks containing approximately the same number of reads, and reads belonging to the same portion of the genome could end up in distinct blocks analyzed by different threads. Thus, in this analysis, we study the reordering effect of the reads before splitting the input collection.

Moreover, since t corresponds to the number of threads, we study how the ratio compression and the resource usage vary in our heuristic when t changes. Clearly, the output of original (sequential) BFQzip could differ from that obtained by varying the number of threads, due to the fact that the information processed by BFQzip in parallel is limited to the thread block. For this reason, we expect the best compression occurs when the whole information contained in the dataset is processed, or when the information is "well-distributed" among the blocks.

Another analysis of our pipeline concerns the compression effect when the pairing information is exploited. We observe that when one reorders paired-end files, one must keep the same order of reads in both files. In fact, the SPRING reordering tool when working in paired-end mode outputs files that have paired reads in corresponding position. Or, when shuffling reads, we keep the same random permutation on both files. Conversely, in the case of the RLO strategy, we could only sort one of the two paired-end files, and apply the same read order to the second file (without actually using the RLO on it).

Reordering Effect in Parallel Pipeline. Figure 2 shows the reordering effect by using PPMd or BSC when each FASTQ file is individually processed (*i.e.* without using the paired-end information). As expected, when the number of threads increases, the compression ratio worsens for the original and random ordering for both datasets. The same effect happens mainly when RLO is used for dataset SRR065390. Nevertheless, if the SPRING reordering is used, the compression ratio holds for all the number of threads considered for both datasets.

We can also see that the reordering of the reads is generally useful for compression (cf. Table 3), and for our pipeline, the SPRING reordering allows to obtain a better compression ratio when the number of threads increases. We believe this depends on the fact that SPRING sorts the reads approximately to their genome position by taking into account the overlap of prefix/suffix of reads (up to a Hamming distance).

Paired-End Mode. Figure 3 shows that compression ratios are improved not only by reordering reads, but also by using the pairing information. In fact, when the information of both files is used to perform modifications, we gain in compression ratio for both files (_1 and _2).

We remark that if the RLO is used, only one file obtains a greater improvement in compression ratio (*i.e.* file _1). We believe this is due to the fact that the other file is reordered according to the first one. A similar behavior could be noted for the SPRING reordering. However, also in the paired-end mode, the SPRING reordering holds the compression ratio as the number of threads increases.

Effect on the Number of Runs. The analysis of the number of runs in the EBWT string is important because several studies [1,23,38,41] consider this value as a measure of repetitiveness of the input collection.

Figure 4 shows the number of runs in the EBWT string obtained from the FASTQ file output of our parallel BFQzip considering the different reordering strategies and different number of threads. We can see that when BFQzip is applied we reduce the number of runs of the original file, not only if a reordering is applied. However, the number of runs increases as a greater number of threads is used, similarly to what happens in the compression ratio analysis. Nevertheless, differently from the results on compression ratio, the number of runs for RLO is much smaller than the number of runs achieved by SPRING reordering, which indicates that not only the number of runs determines a good compression ratio when PPMd or BSC are used.

Finally, Fig. 5 shows similar results for the analysis on the number of runs in the EBWT string of each modified FASTQ obtained by BFQzip in paired-end mode.

Time and Memory Usage. In our experiments, we build the data structures during the pre-processing phase by using gsufsort [33]. Nevertheless, the EBWT construction can be performed with any tool, *e.g.* [4,7,9,20,33] according to the resources available (which is a good feature).

Figure 6 shows separately the running time and the memory usage of the pre-processing performed by gsufsort and the following phases for obtaining a new modified FASTQ (with both noise reduction and quality scores smoothing) in the case of the larger dataset ERR174324_1. These experiments were done on a machine with Intel Xeon E5-2630 v3 20M Cache 2.40 GHz, 386 GB of RAM and a 13 TB SATA storage. The operating system was Debian GNU/Linux 8 (kernel 3.16.0-4) 64 bits.

We remark that the time and memory consumption in these two steps is the same for all the reordering strategies tested.

The time improvement when the number of threads increases is significant. Comparing with the sequential algorithm (1 thread), BFQzip was 14 times faster when using 24 threads (a similar time improvement also holds for the smaller dataset). Whereas the internal memory usage remains approximately the same for all threads numbers. That is due to the fact that the memory mainly depends on the size of the EBWT, *i.e.* the number of bases in the input FASTQ, which is equal to the number of quality scores (*e.g.* it is about 21 GB for ERR174324_1). Nevertheless, the peak memory is registered during the pre-processing phase (gsufsort), while the following phases use a much smaller amount of memory.

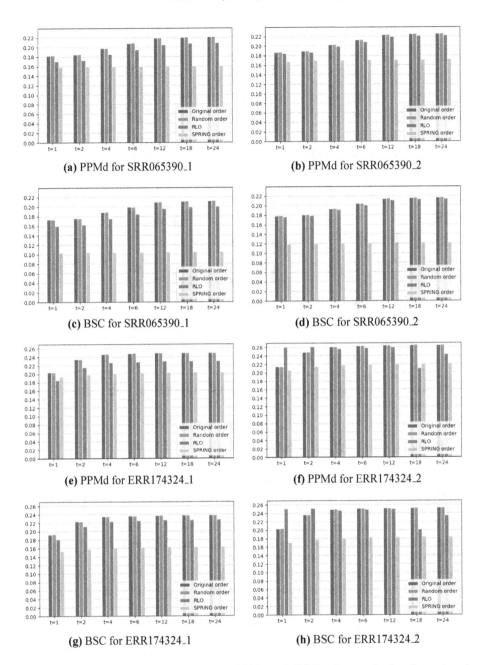

Fig. 3. Compression ratio by using PPMd and BSC when paired-end reads of SRR065390 and ERR174324 datasets are processed in paired-end mode.

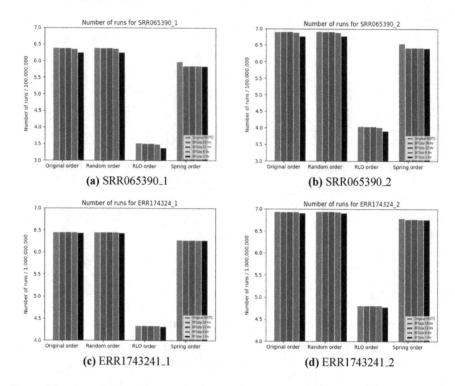

Fig. 4. Number of runs when paired-end reads of SRR065390 and ERR174324 datasets are processed independently.

6   Effects on Variant Calling

Whenever we use a lossy compression scheme, the impact of modified data on downstream analysis should be evaluated. In this section, we show that our lossy parallel strategy preserves the genotyping accuracy.

We designed the validation by using BWA-MEM [30] to align sequences to the reference (in our case, the latest build of the human reference genome, GRCh38/hg38) and GATK-HaplotypeCaller [19] to call variants. Then, we compare the set of variants retrieved (called) from a modified FASTQ with the set of variant from a baseline by using the function `rtg vcfeval` from the RTG Tools[6].

The function evaluates agreement between called and baseline variants using the following performance metrics. True positive (TP) are variants matching between baseline and query (the set of called variants); false positives (FP) are variants mismatching, *i.e.* variants in the called set but not in the baseline; false negatives (FN) are baseline variants missing in the set of called variants.

According to these metrics, we compute precision (PREC) to measure the proportion of true called variants, and sensitivity (SEN) to measure the pro-

---

[6] https://www.realtimegenomics.com/products/rtg-tools.

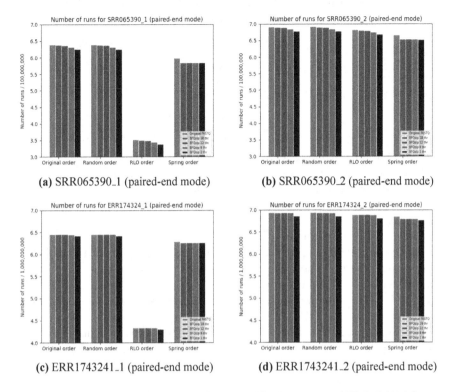

(a) SRR065390_1 (paired-end mode)

(b) SRR065390_2 (paired-end mode)

(c) ERR1743241_1 (paired-end mode)

(d) ERR1743241_2 (paired-end mode)

Fig. 5. Number of runs when paired-end reads of SRR065390 and ERR174324 datasets are processed in paired-end mode.

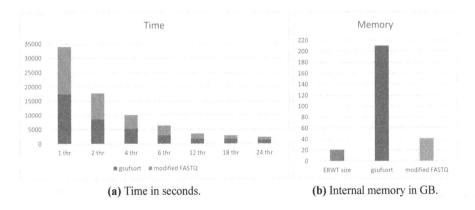

(a) Time in seconds.

(b) Internal memory in GB.

Fig. 6. Time (in seconds) and memory usage (in GB) of BFQZIP parallel strategy for the human dataset ERR174324_1 with original read order.

portion of called variants among those in the baseline. We also compute the harmonic mean between sensitivity and precision (known as F-score):

$$\text{PREC} = \frac{TP}{TP + FP} \tag{1}$$

$$\text{SEN} = \frac{TP}{TP + FN} \tag{2}$$

$$\text{F-score} = \frac{2 \cdot SEN \cdot PREC}{SEN + PREC} \tag{3}$$

For evaluation purposes, we used the Whole Genome *C. Elegans* dataset SRR065390 and, similarly to other studies [43], we extracted chromosomes 1 and 20 from the real human dataset ERR174324. In this section, we not only tested our strategy, but also other lossy compressors that have been shown to preserve called variants.

Recall that BFQzIP combines DNA bases and quality score information both to apply a noise reduction and to smooth the quality scores, and to the best of our knowledge, there are no other existing tools designed for that.

Nevertheless, for comparison purposes, we consider the tools BEETL[7] [29] and LEON[8] [5] as done in [26], as they are both reference-free and read-based lossy compressors, alike BFQzIP. They smooth only the quality scores component according to the biological information in the bases component, yet without modifying the bases themselves.

BEETL is based on the EBWT and takes as input about the same data structures as BFQzIP. BEETL smooths to a constant value the quality scores corresponding to runs of the same symbol that are associated with LCP-values greater than a threshold value c. Whereas LEON is based on a probabilistic *de Bruijn graph* built from the set of reads that is used to perform a lossy transformation of the quality scores. It could be considered assembly-based [5].

Note that both BEETL and LEON have been tested on the same *C. Elegans* dataset SRR065390. Thus, for BEETL we used the parameter setting described in [29] (*i.e.* `-c 5 -s 10 -r 62`), and for LEON we used default parameters (see [5]). We also tested another reference-free compressor, SCALCE[9] [27], which modifies the reads ordering and allows to smooth the quality scores on the basis of statistics on the whole quality scores component. Analogously, SCALCE was run with the same parameter setting as [27] for quality scores smoothing (*i.e.* `-p 30`).

Table 4 and 5 report the evaluation results obtained by `rtg vcfeval` when comparing the variants retrieved from a modified FASTQ (produced by any tool) to the set of variants from the original (unsmoothed) FASTQ used as baseline.

We can observe that our method provides the highest precision and F-score for all the number of threads tested (1, 6, 12 threads are reported). Thus, with

---

[7] https://github.com/BEETL/BEETL/blob/RELEASE_1_1_0/scripts/lcp/
applyLcpCutoff.pl.

[8] http://gatb.inria.fr/software/leon/.

[9] http://sfu-compbio.github.io/scalce/.

Table 4. Evaluation by means of `rtg vcfeval` of the called variants for dataset SRR065390: comparison between raw variants from a modified FASTQ and raw variants from the original FASTQ used as baseline.

	BFQzip			BEETL	LEON	SCALCE
	1 thr	6 thr	12 thr			
PREC (%)	94.83	97.85	**98.20**	92.15	92.52	87.43
SEN (%)	95.87	97.73	**97.89**	90.70	96.54	85.89
F-score (%)	95.35	97.79	**98.04**	91.42	94.49	86.65

Table 5. Evaluation by means of `rtg vcfeval` of the called variants for chromosomes 1 and 20 from the human dataset ERR174324: comparison between SNPs from a modified FASTQ and SNPs from the original FASTQ used as baseline.

	CHR 1						CHR 20					
	BFQzip			BEETL	LEON	SCALCE	BFQzip			BEETL	LEON	SCALCE
	1 thr	6 thr	12 thr				1 thr	6 thr	12 thr			
PREC (%)	99.84	99.89	**99.91**	99.39	99.35	99.60	99.79	99.90	**99.90**	99.28	99.28	99.21
SEN (%)	99.87	99.93	**99.94**	99.51	99.41	99.49	99.68	99.87	**99.92**	99.39	98.85	98.93
F-score (%)	99.86	99.91	**99.93**	99.45	99.38	99.55	99.73	99.89	**99.91**	99.34	99.07	99.07

respect to the original FASTQ file, we preserve a higher number of variants (TP) and introduce the lowest number of new ones (FP). Then, we may conclude that we preserve information of the original FASTQ more than the other tools (see also Table 5, where SNPs calling is evaluated for the human dataset[10]).

We also analyzed the effect on variant calling when the paired-end mode is used on the *C. Elegans* dataset SRR065390, and we obtained results comparable to those in Table 4.

7   Conclusions and Discussion

In this paper, we presented a parallel framework based on the lossy reference-free and assembly-free compression approach for FASTQ files named BFQzip, first introduced in [26], that allows to exploit the paired-end information FASTQ files in pairs.

The introduced parallel strategy splits the FASTQ file into t blocks and processes them in parallel with BFQzip, the resulting blocks with the modified bases and smoothed qualities are merged (in order) and then compressed with the compressor tools PPMd or BSC.

---

[10] SNPs calling pipeline available at https://github.com/veronicaguerrini/BFQzip/blob/main/variant_calling/pipeline_SNPsCall.sh.

In this paper, we focused our attention on how the compression obtained by our parallel pipeline is affected by the splitting of the blocks, by the reordering of reads in the input collection and by the using of the paired-end information. We showed that SPRING reordering holds the compression ratio as the number of threads (*i.e.* split blocks) increases and it is better than when using the RLO reordering strategy. We also showed that RLO allows us to obtain the least number of runs in the modified base component when the EBWT is applied to it, which indicates that the compression ratio achieved by PPMd or BSC do not depend directly on the number of runs of the given transformed string.

We also showed that the splitting of the input FASTQ file guarantees the preservation of the variant calling with respect to the original file. Our parallel version slightly reduces the compression ratio and preserves performance on variants calling showing a better resource usage compared to the version introduced in [26].

In the preliminary version [26], we showed that the resulting FASTQ file with the modified bases achieves better compression than the original data, and that is also confirmed by experiments in this paper. As in the preliminary version [26], our tool, in terms of variant calling, keeps the same accuracy as the original FASTQ data and preserves the variant calls of the original FASTQ file better than BEETL and LEON. We also tested the compressor SCALCE, which also exploits an its own reordering of the reads, showing our tool preserves the variant calls of the original FASTQ file better than it. We believe the detrimental effect in validation of our competitors is due to the fact that they compress the quality score component a lot (they do not modify the bases component) obtaining a better compression ratio than BFQzIP, but a worse validation. So, the comparison is not completely fair. For instance, the ratio compression of LEON and SCALCE applied to *C. Elegans* dataset SRR065390_1 is respectively 0.1447 and 0.1314 by using PPMd, and 0.1085 and 0.1232 by using BSC. Indeed, we recall that LEON truncates all quality values greater than '@' and SCALCE provides a lossy transformation scheme to reduce the alphabet size of the quality scores component by reducing the variability among the quality scores. While BEETL achieves a compression ratio comparable to BFQzIP (0.1838 by using PPMd and 0.1760 by using BSC).

Regarding our used resources, we can affirm that our tool suffers in two particular steps: the pre-processing phase for the construction of the data structures and the reconstruction of the FASTQ file after we have modified of the bases and quality scores components. However, we believe that these two steps can be overcome in the future, given that new strategies for these purposes continue to be introduced in the literature. A further strength of our tool is the fact that it is independent of both the construction algorithms of the data structures and the compressor used in the last step.

Acknowledgments. The authors thank Prof. Nalvo Almeida (UFMS, Brazil) for granting access to the computer used in the experiments.

Funding. Work partially supported by MIUR, the Italian Ministry of Education, University and Research, under PRIN Project n. 20174LF3T8 AHeAD ("Efficient Algorithms for HArnessing Networked Data"). and by PNRR - M4C2 - Investimento 1.5, Ecosistema dell'Innovazione ECS00000017 - "THE - Tuscany Health Ecosystem" - Spoke 6 "Precision medicine & personalized healthcare", funded by the European Commission under the NextGeneration EU programme.

F.A.L. acknowledges the financial support of CNPq (grant number 406418/2021-7) and FAPEMIG (grant number APQ-01217-22).

References

1. Sensitivity of string compressors and repetitiveness measures (2023). https://doi.org/10.1016/j.ic.2022.104999
2. Abouelhoda, M.I., Kurtz, S., Ohlebusch, E.: Replacing suffix trees with enhanced suffix arrays. J. Discrete Algorithms **2**(1), 53–86 (2004). https://doi.org/10.1016/S1570-8667(03)00065-0
3. Adjeroh, D., Bell, T., Mukherjee, A.: The Burrows-Wheeler Transform: Data Compression, Suffix Arrays, and Pattern Matching. Springer, New York (2008). https://doi.org/10.1007/978-0-387-78909-5
4. Bauer, M., Cox, A., Rosone, G.: Lightweight algorithms for constructing and inverting the BWT of string collections. Theor. Comput. Sci. **483**, 134–148 (2013). https://doi.org/10.1016/j.tcs.2012.02.002
5. Benoit, G., et al.: Reference-free compression of high throughput sequencing data with a probabilistic de Bruijn graph. BMC Bioinform. **16**, 1–14 (2015). https://doi.org/10.1186/s12859-015-0709-7
6. Bentley, J.W., Gibney, D., Thankachan, S.V.: On the complexity of BWT-runs minimization via alphabet reordering. In: ESA. LIPIcs, vol. 173, pp. 15:1–15:13. Schloss Dagstuhl-Leibniz-Zentrum für Informatik, Dagstuhl, Germany (2020). https://doi.org/10.4230/LIPIcs.ESA.2020.15
7. Bonizzoni, P., Della Vedova, G., Pirola, Y., Previtali, M., Rizzi, R.: Multithread multistring Burrows-Wheeler transform and longest common prefix array. J. Comput. Biol. **26**(9), 948–961 (2019). https://doi.org/10.1089/cmb.2018.0230
8. Bonomo, S., Mantaci, S., Restivo, A., Rosone, G., Sciortino, M.: Sorting conjugates and suffixes of words in a multiset. Int. J. Found. Comput. Sci. **25**(08), 1161–1175 (2014)
9. Boucher, C., Cenzato, D., Lipták, Z., Rossi, M., Sciortino, M.: Computing the original eBWT faster, simpler, and with less memory. In: Lecroq, T., Touzet, H. (eds.) SPIRE 2021. LNCS, vol. 12944, pp. 129–142. Springer, Cham (2021). https://doi.org/10.1007/978-3-030-86692-1_11
10. Burrows, M., Wheeler, D.: A Block Sorting data Compression Algorithm. Technical report DIGITAL System Research Center (1994)
11. Cazaux, B., Rivals, E.: Linking BWT and XBW via Aho-Corasick automaton: applications to run-length encoding. In: CPM. LIPIcs, vol. 128, pp. 24:1–24:20. Schloss Dagstuhl-Leibniz-Zentrum fuer Informatik, Dagstuhl, Germany (2019). https://doi.org/10.4230/LIPIcs.CPM.2019.24
12. Cenzato, D., Lipták, Z.: A theoretical and experimental analysis of BWT variants for string collections. In: Bannai, H., Holub, J. (eds.) 33rd Annual Symposium on Combinatorial Pattern Matching (CPM 2022). Leibniz International Proceedings in Informatics (LIPIcs), vol. 223, pp. 25:1–25:18. Schloss Dagstuhl - Leibniz-Zentrum für Informatik (2022). https://doi.org/10.4230/LIPIcs.CPM.2022.25

13. Chandak, S., Tatwawadi, K., Ochoa, I., Hernaez, M., Weissman, T.: SPRING: a next-generation compressor for FASTQ data. Bioinformatics **35**(15), 2674–2676 (2018)
14. Chandak, S., Tatwawadi, K., Weissman, T.: Compression of genomic sequencing reads via hash-based reordering: algorithm and analysis. Bioinformatics **34**(4), 558–567 (2017). https://doi.org/10.1093/bioinformatics/btx639
15. Cleary, J., Witten, I.: Data compression using adaptive coding and partial string matching. IEEE Trans. Commun. **32**(4), 396–402 (1984). https://doi.org/10.1109/TCOM.1984.1096090
16. Cox, A., Bauer, M., Jakobi, T., Rosone, G.: Large-scale compression of genomic sequence databases with the Burrows-Wheeler transform. Bioinformatics **28**(11), 1415–1419 (2012). https://doi.org/10.1093/bioinformatics/bts173
17. Cox, A.J., Jakobi, T., Rosone, G., Schulz-Trieglaff, O.B.: Comparing DNA sequence collections by direct comparison of compressed text indexes. In: Raphael, B., Tang, J. (eds.) WABI 2012. LNCS, vol. 7534, pp. 214–224. Springer, Heidelberg (2012). https://doi.org/10.1007/978-3-642-33122-0_17
18. Deorowicz, S.: Fqsqueezer: k-mer-based compression of sequencing data. Sci. Rep. **10**(1), 1–9 (2020)
19. DePristo, M.A., et al.: A framework for variation discovery and genotyping using next-generation DNA sequencing data. Nat. Genet. **43**(5), 491–498 (2011). https://doi.org/10.1038/ng.806
20. Egidi, L., Louza, F.A., Manzini, G., Telles, G.P.: External memory BWT and LCP computation for sequence collections with applications. Algorithms Mol. Biol. **14**(1), 6:1–6:15 (2019). https://doi.org/10.1186/s13015-019-0140-0
21. Egidi, L., Manzini, G.: Lightweight BWT and LCP merging via the gap algorithm. In: Fici, G., Sciortino, M., Venturini, R. (eds.) SPIRE 2017. LNCS, vol. 10508, pp. 176–190. Springer, Cham (2017). https://doi.org/10.1007/978-3-319-67428-5_15
22. Ferragina, P., Manzini, G.: Opportunistic data structures with applications. In: FOCS, pp. 390–398. IEEE Computer Society (2000). https://doi.org/10.1109/SFCS.2000.892127
23. Giuliani, S., Inenaga, S., Lipták, Z., Prezza, N., Sciortino, M., Toffanello, A.: Novel results on the number of runs of the Burrows-Wheeler-transform. In: Bureš, T., et al. (eds.) SOFSEM 2021. LNCS, vol. 12607, pp. 249–262. Springer, Cham (2021). https://doi.org/10.1007/978-3-030-67731-2_18
24. Greenfield, D.L., Stegle, O., Rrustemi, A.: GeneCodeq: quality score compression and improved genotyping using a Bayesian framework. Bioinformatics **32**(20), 3124–3132 (2016). https://doi.org/10.1093/bioinformatics/btw385
25. Guerrini, V., Louza, F., Rosone, G.: Metagenomic analysis through the extended Burrows-Wheeler transform. BMC Bioinform. **21**, 21–25 (2020). https://doi.org/10.1186/s12859-020-03628-w
26. Guerrini., V., Louza., F., Rosone., G.: Lossy compressor preserving variant calling through extended BWT. In: Proceedings of the 15th International Joint Conference on Biomedical Engineering Systems and Technologies - BIOINFORMATICS, pp. 38–48. INSTICC, SciTePress (2022). https://doi.org/10.5220/0010834100003123
27. Hach, F., Numanagić, I., Alkan, C., Sahinalp, S.C.: SCALCE: boosting sequence compression algorithms using locally consistent encoding. Bioinformatics **28**(23), 3051–3057 (2012). https://doi.org/10.1093/bioinformatics/bts593
28. Holland, R.C., Lynch, N.: Sequence squeeze: an open contest for sequence compression. GigaScience **2**(1), 2047–217X (2013). https://doi.org/10.1186/2047-217X-2-5

29. Janin, L., Rosone, G., Cox, A.J.: Adaptive reference-free compression of sequence quality scores. Bioinformatics **30**(1), 24–30 (2014). https://doi.org/10.1093/bioinformatics/btt257
30. Li, H.: Aligning sequence reads, clone sequences and assembly contigs with BWA-MEM. arXiv:1303.3997 (2013)
31. Li, H.: Fast construction of FM-index for long sequence reads. Bioinformatics **30**(22), 3274–3275 (2014). https://doi.org/10.1093/bioinformatics/btu541, source code: https://github.com/lh3/ropebwt2
32. Li, H., Durbin, R.: Fast and accurate short read alignment with Burrows-Wheeler transform. Bioinform. **25**(14), 1754–1760 (2009). https://doi.org/10.1093/bioinformatics/btp324
33. Louza, F.A., Telles, G.P., Gog, S., Prezza, N., Rosone, G.: gsufsort: constructing suffix arrays, LCP arrays and BWTs for string collections. Algorithms Mol. Biol. **15**, 1–5 (2020)
34. Louza, F.A., Gog, S., Telles, G.P.: Inducing enhanced suffix arrays for string collections. Theor. Comput. Sci. **678**, 22–39 (2017). https://doi.org/10.1016/j.tcs.2017.03.039
35. Mäkinen, V., Navarro, G., Sirén, J., Välimäki, N.: Storage and retrieval of highly repetitive sequence collections. J. Comput. Biol. **17**(3), 281–308 (2010)
36. Manber, U., Myers, G.: Suffix arrays: a new method for on-line string searches. In: ACM-SIAM SODA, pp. 319–327 (1990)
37. Mantaci, S., Restivo, A., Rosone, G., Sciortino, M.: An extension of the Burrows-Wheeler Transform. Theoret. Comput. Sci. **387**(3), 298–312 (2007)
38. Mantaci, S., Restivo, A., Rosone, G., Sciortino, M., Versari, L.: Measuring the clustering effect of BWT via RLE. Theor. Comput. Sci. **698**, 79–87 (2017). https://doi.org/10.1016/j.tcs.2017.07.015
39. Moffat, A.: Implementing the PPM data compression scheme. IEEE Trans. Commun. **38**(11), 1917–1921 (1990). https://doi.org/10.1109/26.61469
40. Na, J.C., et al.: FM-index of alignment with gaps. Theor. Comput. Sci. **710**, 148–157 (2018)
41. Navarro, G.: Indexing highly repetitive string collections, part I: repetitiveness measures. ACM Comput. Surv. **54**(2), 29:1–29:31 (2021)
42. Navarro, G.: Indexing highly repetitive string collections, part II: compressed indexes. ACM Comput. Surv. **54**(2), 26:1–26:32 (2021)
43. Ochoa, I., Hernaez, M., Goldfeder, R., Weissman, T., Ashley, E.: Effect of lossy compression of quality scores on variant calling. Brief. Bioinform. **18**(2), 183–194 (2016). https://doi.org/10.1093/bib/bbw011
44. Prezza, N., Pisanti, N., Sciortino, M., Rosone, G.: Variable-order reference-free variant discovery with the Burrows-Wheeler transform. BMC Bioinform. **21**, 1–20 (2020). https://doi.org/10.1186/s12859-020-03586-3
45. Prezza, N., Rosone, G.: Space-efficient computation of the LCP array from the Burrows-Wheeler transform. In: Annual Symposium on Combinatorial Pattern Matching (CPM). vol. 128. Schloss Dagstuhl- Leibniz-Zentrum fur Informatik GmbH, Dagstuhl Publishing (2019). https://doi.org/10.4230/LIPIcs.CPM.2019.7
46. Prezza, N., Pisanti, N., Sciortino, M., Rosone, G.: SNPs detection by eBWT positional clustering. Algorithms Mol. Biol. **14**(1), 3 (2019). https://doi.org/10.1186/s13015-019-0137-8
47. Prezza, N., Rosone, G.: Space-efficient construction of compressed suffix trees. Theoret. Comput. Sci. **852**, 138–156 (2021). https://doi.org/10.1016/j.tcs.2020.11.024

48. Restivo, A., Rosone, G.: Balancing and clustering of words in the Burrows-Wheeler transform. Theor. Comput. Sci. **412**(27), 3019–3032 (2011). https://doi.org/10. 1016/j.tcs.2010.11.040
49. Roguski, L., Ochoa, I., Hernaez, M., Deorowicz, S.: FaStore: a space-saving solution for raw sequencing data. Bioinformatics **34**(16), 2748–2756 (2018)
50. Rosone, G., Sciortino, M.: The Burrows-Wheeler transform between data compression and combinatorics on words. In: Bonizzoni, P., Brattka, V., Löwe, B. (eds.) CiE 2013. LNCS, vol. 7921, pp. 353–364. Springer, Heidelberg (2013). https://doi. org/10.1007/978-3-642-39053-1_42
51. Shibuya, Y., Comin, M.: Better quality score compression through sequence-based quality smoothing. BMC Bioinform. **20-S**(9), 302:1–302:11 (2019). https://doi. org/10.1186/s12859-019-2883-5
52. Simpson, J.T., Durbin, R.: Efficient construction of an assembly string graph using the FM-index. Bioinformatics **26**(12), 367–373 (2010)
53. Yu, Y.W., Yorukoglu, D., Peng, J., Berger, B.: Quality score compression improves genotyping accuracy. Nat. Biotechnol. **33**(3), 240–243 (2015). https://doi.org/10. 1038/nbt.3170

Comparing Different Dictionary-Based Classifiers for the Classification of Volatile Compounds Measured with an E-nose

Rita Alves[1,2,3], Joao Rodrigues[1(✉)], Efthymia Ramou[2,3], Susana I. C. J. Palma[2,3], Ana C. A. Roque[2,3], and Hugo Gamboa[1]

[1] LIBPhys (Laboratory for Instrumentation, Biomedical Engineering and Radiation Physics), Faculdade de Ciencias e Tecnologia, Universidade Nova de Lisboa, Caparica, Portugal
`jmd.rodrigues@campus.fct.unl.pt`
[2] Associate Laboratory i4HB- Institute for Health and Bioeconomy, School of Science and Technology, NOVA University Lisbon, 2829-516 Caparica, Portugal
[3] UCIBIO - Applied Molecular Biosciences Unit, Department of Chemistry, School of Science and Technology, NOVA University Lisbon, 2829-516 Caparica, Portugal

Abstract. Electronic noses (e-noses) are devices that mimic the biological sense of olfaction to recognize gaseous samples in a very fast and accurate manner, being applicable in a multitude of scenarios. E-noses are composed of an array of gas sensors, a signal acquisition unit and a pattern recognition unit including automatic classifiers based on machine learning. In a previous work, a text-based approach was developed to classify volatile organic compounds (VOCs) using as input signals from an in-house developed e-nose. This text-based algorithm was compared with a 1-nearest neighbor classifier with euclidean distance (1-NN ED). In this work we studied other text-based approaches that relied in the Bag of Words model and compared it with the previous approach that relied in the term frequency-inverse document frequency (TF-IDF) model and other traditional text-mining classifiers, namely the naive bayes and linear Support Vector Machines (SVM). The results show that the TF-IDF model is more robust overall when compared with the Bag of Words (BoW) model. An average F1-score of 0.84 and 0.70 was achieved for the TF-IDF model with a linear SVM for two distinct gas sensor formulations (5CB and 8CB, respectively), while an F1-score of 0.66 and 0.71 was achieved for the BoW model for the same formulations. The text-based approaches appeared to be less reliable than the traditional 1-NN ED method.

Keywords: Electronic nose · Volatile organic compounds · Euclidean distance · Morphology · Classification · Bag of words · TFIDF

1 Introduction

Volatile biomarkers are found to be related with specific diseases. These volatiles can be found in body fluids from a patient and their detection is a possible source of information to diagnose a specific disease. There are several methods to detect the presence of volatiles, being electronic noses (e-noses) one of the possible options.

© The Author(s), under exclusive license to Springer Nature Switzerland AG 2023
A. C. A. Roque et al. (Eds.): BIOSTEC 2022, CCIS 1814, pp. 121–140, 2023.
https://doi.org/10.1007/978-3-031-38854-5_7

Odors are the perception the brain develops when recognizing a gas, being it a single VOC or a VOC mixture. The singularity of e-noses is that, unlike analytical chemistry laboratorial equipment, e-noses do not identify individual VOCs present in a gas sample. Instead, they recognise the odor or the "fingerprint" formed by the specific mixture of VOCs present in the gas to identify the nature of the sample. E-noses mimic the biological olfaction process by combining arrays of gas sensors, dedicated signal processing, and pattern recognition algorithms. Due to their portability, fast response and non-invasive operation, they gained importance as a potential non-invasive diagnostics tool. E-noses were first mentioned and developed by Persaud and Dodd [37] in 1982. With further developments in electrical, optical and computational technology, e-noses started to be equipped with machine learning, and were widely used for VOC' pattern recognition [3]. These devices provide an electrical response to the presence of individual VOCs or VOC mixtures, which represent the identity of the sample and can be used to train machine learning models for future automatic recognition. Undeniably so, many promising applications were designed for odours recognition in a broad range of fields, such as environment monitoring [6,29,52], medical diagnostics [4,8,10,16,20,21,36,42], public security affairs [22], agricultural production [7,25], and food industry [6,7,29,45].

In the previous work we tested two classifiers for the classification of VOCs with two different gas sensor formulations in the same in-house developed e-nose prototype. The first was a standard 1-NN ED method, while the second was a novel text-based based method that relied in a transformation of the signals into a set of sentences based on the signal's dynamics and used a text-mining method to perform the classification stage. The propose method was a dictionary-based classification method that uses the Synthatic Search on Time Series (SSTS) [41] tool to perform a sentence-based representation of the signal. From this, the sentences are analyzed as pure text with standard strategies in text-mining. In this particular case, we used the TF-IDF model with a linear SVM [2], which was recommended in the literature. Following this previous work we experimented other text-mining approaches with different combinations, namely the usage of the BoW model and TF-IDF model with different classifiers. These methods fall in the category of dictionary-based methods and rely on the signals' morphology described by a set of ordered patterns. The performance of each combination will be compared to understand which is more appropriate for the VOC classification.

The main objective of this work are a) to evaluate the performance of a set of new gel-like optical gas sensors [23] to correctly label a series of individual VOCs, and b) to compare the performance of new text-based classification methods with the previously suggested best approach that uses a TF-IDF model with a linear SVM classifier. We observed that the other text-based classifiers that relied in BoW models are not as reliable as the previously identified TF-IDF model and standard 1-NN ED classifier. However, the usage of dictionary-based methods show room for improvement.

2 Related Work

2.1 E-nose for Disease Diagnosis

Humans can recognize odours because the human brain learns to recognize smells associated with distinct odorant samples (e.g. objects, animals, food, environment, etc.). This concept is the base for the development of e-noses, starting with the works of Persaud and Dodd [37]. With further technological developments, it was soon understood that these systems could be used for medical purposes. Patients often release VOCs that provide relevant indicators regarding their health condition [31]. However, current strategies for the recognition of these VOCs is limited, due to being expensive and complex to use [40]. Considering this, e-noses started to be considered for these purposes [25] and several commercially available electronic noses can be found, such as: Aeonose from The eNose Company [27]; Cyrano Sciences' Cyranose 320 from Sensigent, Intelligent Sensing Solutions [13]; Bloodhound BH-114 [28]; AirSense Portable Electronic Nose from AirSense Analytics [34], among others.

Novel research is also found for e-nose development. For instance, Liang et al. [30] were able to detect the presence of *Eschericia Coli, Staphylococcus aureus*, and *Pseudomonas aeruginosa* in *in-vitro* cultures of the individual strains or of mixtures of strains. To do that, an electronic nose with 24 MOS and 6 electrochemical sensors array and PCA and SVM methods were used. In 2012, Qinghua He et al. [19] developed a classification algorithm to detect wounds infections. A method based on particle swarm optimization was used to find the optimal SVM model parameters. Features were extracted through wavelet transform. In this study, the performance of radial basis function and SVM algorithm were compared, concluding the last achieved the best performance. Additionally, electronic noses have been widely used in diagnosing respiratory diseases through exhaled breath [11]. Examples of such applications can be found in works of Fens et al. [16] for the distinction between asthma and COPD. Dragonieri et al. [12] followed the same methodology and were able to distinguish asthma patients with different disease severities. Vries et al. [51] also used an e-nose to distinguish asthmatic patients from healthy individuals. Other works are also found for cancer detection [1,9,10,39,43,53,54], tuberculosis [4,8,36,48], pneumonia [20,21,49] and chronic kidney disease [42]. Other e-noses were also developed to study urine samples with many purposes [5,24,38].

Recently, a new class of gas sensors was proposed and is being explored for classification of individual VOC in an in-house built e-nose [14,17,23]. In this particular case, the signal is generated by chemical changes that occur in the sensor when exposed to a VOC, and the resulting response of that change is converted to an electrical signal. The resulting signal from the interaction of the sensor with the VOC is produced using unique sensing materials that change their optical properties according to the VOC they are exposed to [44]. This sensing materials are a new class of hybrid gels that contain Liquid Crystal (LC) and Ionic Liquid (IL), forming LC-IL droplets. When exposed to a VOC, the configuration of LC inside the droplets change and creates different optical patterns that can be measured [14,23,44]. The e-nose used in this work to record the VOC samples employs this gas sensing technology.

2.2 Signal Classification

The response generated by e-noses are signals (time series). In the literature, an exhaustive list of methods are available for the purpose of time series classification. These methods are divided into shaped-based and structure-based methods [26]. Shape-based methods perform local comparisons between time series, being the most well-known and reference methods for comparison of time series the Euclidean distance (ED) and the Dynamic Time Warping (DTW) distances [33]. Both methods have been extensively used in this problematic, performing specially well in short time series. ED and DTW are usually combined with a k-Nearest Neighbour (NN) classifier [46].

Structure-based methods rely on broader characteristics of time series, such as the presence of specific morphological structures or patterns, being more adequate for longer signals [46]. A subcategory of such methods are dictionary-based methods, which use relevant segments of the time series and compile them as a dictionary of patterns [55] or words [32,46,47]. These methods have showed good performances in benchmarks evaluations [46]. Dictionary-based methods, such as the Bag of Patterns (BoP), rely on a transformation of the time series into a sequence of symbols by means of methods such as the *Symbolic Aggregate approXimation* (SAX) [32]. This method was inspired by the Bag of Words model from the text mining scenario, using SAX as the symbolic transformer [33]. Further, proposed methods were conceptually inspired on the *BoP*, using the same reasoning. Other techniques are found, such as *Bag of SFA Symbols* (BOSS) and Word ExtrAction for time SEries cLassification (WEASEL) [46,47].

3 Acquisition Setup and Dataset

In this work, an in-house built optical e-nose was used to record the response of hybrid gel sensors to a set of different VOCs [14,23,44]. The optical e-nose explores the optical properties of the hybrid gel sensors. The e-nose's schematic and system used in this work are presented in Fig. 1. The system is built with a delivery and detection system, which are controlled by an arduino system. The delivery system is responsible for leading the gas sample towards the sensor array. It has two air pumps, two relays, and the chamber where the sample is placed. The exposure pump pushes environmental air through the headspace of the liquid VOC sample, to carry the VOCs into the sensors chamber. The recovery pump pushes environmental air to the sensors's chamber to reestablish the initial conditions. This alternation between both pumps generates the VOC exposure/recovery cycles [35].

Each sensor will have a response that can vary in morphology according to the VOC that is inserted into the sensor chamber. This variation is a benefit for its identification. In this work, an optical e-nose is used with two hybrid gel sensor formulations to test the ability of two classifiers to correctly label the VOC to which the e-nose is exposed. Multiple experiments have been acquired for both gel sensors, as the purpose is to label a VOC based on a classifier trained with a database of past experiments.

The data set comprises signals from 11 known VOCs (acetone, acetonitrile, chloroform, dichloromethane, diethyl ether, ethanol, ethyl acetate, heptane, hexane, methanol, and toluene) acquired with sensing gels with two different formulations.

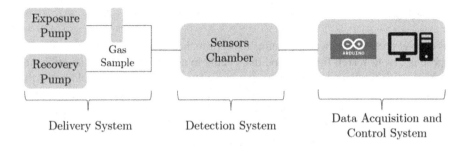

Fig. 1. Schematic of the e-nose and its systems. Image from [2].

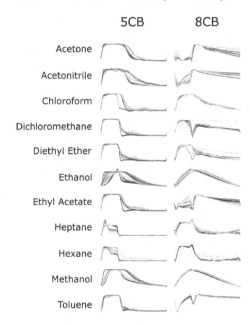

Fig. 2. Representation of overlapped cycles obtained with the optical sensing gels containing bovine gelatin with the IL [BMIM][DCA] and LC 8CB, and the IL [BMIM][DCA] and the LC 5CB for all VOC. Figure from [2].

The gels are composed of a polymer (the bovine gelatin) and molecules of LC and IL. The sensor formulations that were tested contain bovine gelatin and are tagged as: (1) the IL [BMIM][DCA] and the LC 8CB; and (2) the IL [BMIM][DCA] and the LC 5CB. The first formulation was used in 3 experiments, resulting in 444 analyzed cycles (=$\tilde{3}$7 cycles/VOC), while the second formulation was used in 8 experiments, resulting in 1444 cycles (=$\tilde{1}$20 cycles/VOC). The conditions were the same in all experiments. Examples of the acquired cycles are presented in Fig. 2.

4 Methods

This chapter presents the overall pipeline to perform the analysis and classification. The purpose is first to search for a method that is able to perform the correct identification of a VOC with the knowledge of past experiments. A standard methodology for this type of problems is using a k-nearest neighbor classifier with euclidean distance, which works well with short signals. In addition to the standard euclidean distance method, other dictionary-based methods were tested. In our previous work [2], we employed the usage of a textual representation of the signals to perform its further classification. The method used at the time was the traditional TF-IDF model with an *SVM* classifier. In this case, we extended the experiment by testing other traditional classification methods in text-mining, such as the Bag-of-Words (BoW) model and the Baysian classifier. In that sense, we will compare the results of these methods to understand which is better in this type of problems and with the textual representation used. In addition, these experiments will be compared with the 1-NN euclidean distance classifier.

4.1 Pre-processing

Before the usage of the recorded signals in the mentioned algorithms, a pre-processing stage is needed. This step includes a (1) noise reduction: a median filter with a window size of 1 s is used to ensure high frequency noise and high fluctuations are attenuated; (2) cycle segmentation: a square signal, used to control the pumps of the system, is used to segment the signals from the moment the sensors are exposed to the VOC (exposure phase) to the next exposure phase, dividing it into cycles; and (3) data cleaning: cycles with signal-to-noise ratio higher than 3 and outlier cycles with a high distance to the mean wave are not used in the experiment.

4.2 SSTS for Time Series Text Representation

The proposed methodology is inspired by the reasoning from text data mining for text classification. This pipeline uses the well known *Bag of Words* (BoW) to generate a feature matrix with vectors that represent the frequency of words found for each document, being each vector a vectorized and quantifiable characterization of a text document. The BoW can be used by itself with a simple bayes model or a linear Support Vector Machine (SVM) [18]. It can also be transformed into a term-frequency inverse frequency (*TF-IDF*) matrix, which can be used with the same classifiers. In order to use these text-based methods we need to encode the time series into a symbolic/text representation. There are several methods for symbolic representation of time series, such as SFA or SAX. These resort to a symbolic description rather than a textual one. In this case, we apply SSTS to extract higher level words and convert the signal into several sentences. These higher level words are searched by a query-based approach that has three steps: (1) pre-processing: applies filtering and/or transformation to simplify the signal for the symbolic conversion; (2) connotation: where the symbolic transformation occurs based on specific conversion functions and (3) search: a regular expression pattern is used to search for pre-defined words on the symbolic representation. Each word found is then ordered to form sentences. The overall process is presented in Fig. 3.

4.3   Pattern Search and Sentence Generation

The connotation step is used to encode the signal in a symbolic way. Each step of SSTS can be customized by the user to employ the desired pre-processing methods and search for the most representative patterns in the signal. For example, when searching for moments when the signal is rising, the user selects (1) the pre-processing that best can prepare the signal for this search, (2) the connotation that corresponds to the first derivative, converting each sample of the signal into a character for when it is rising (p), falling (n) or flat (z). From this symbolic transformation, patterns can be converted to words. A sentence can then be built with the ordered words found, which can be as simple as a word representative of the symbol (p - "Rise"), or a combination of symbols (pf - "Rise Fall" - "Peak"). Step one of Fig. 3 shows an example of this process. For this experiment, we used a standard mechanism, converting the signal based on available connotation methods and searching standard words. These are listed in Tables 1 and 2. These patterns were extracted for all signals. The pre-processing was also the same and already mentioned in the previous section. In Table 2, the regular expression patterns are separated into different groups. Each group is used independently to build a sentence, otherwise a sentence would be mixed with ordered patterns that can mix each other and disturb the classification process.

The list of patterns used for this analysis is presented in Table 2.

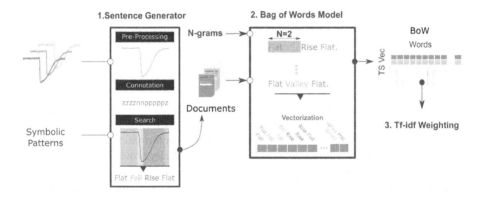

Fig. 3. Sequence of steps used to vectorize the textual representation of the recorded signals. The time series is (1) converted into a set of sentences, which are (2) vectorized into a BoW. The BoW can be (3) converted into a TF-IDF model. From [2].

4.4   Text Vectorization Methods

A sentence can be vectorized by means of a BoW or a TF-IDF model. These methods have the intent of converting text information into a feature vector. To achieve this representation, the BoW model has the number of word/token occurrences in each document. This information is usually stored in a matrix of data with the rows being the documents and the columns are the unique words found. Mathematically, the model calculates the term frequency/raw counts, tf:

Table 1. Connotation (Con) methods and their meaning for each single characters (Char) in which the samples of the time series are translated.

Con	Char	Description
1st Derivative	p	positive slope
	n	negative slope
	z	zero slope
Slope Height	r	positive slope with low increase
	R	positive slope with high increase
	f	negative slope with low increase
	F	negative slope with high increase
Derivative Speed	R	quick positive slope
	r	slow positive slope
	F	quick negative slope
	f	slow negative slope
Amplitude	0	lower than a threshold
	1	higher than a threshold
2nd Derivative	D	Concave
	C	Convex

$$tf_{t,d} = \frac{f_{t,d}}{\sum\limits_{t' \in d} f_{t',d}}, \tag{1}$$

in which t is the term that exists in all documents, d the document, t' the term that belongs to document d. The word/term can also be an N-gram, that is, a junction of two or more words/terms. N-grams provide more contextual information to the model. In this case, the features extracted are purely statistical, but can provide a relevant measure of differences between documents. As a symbolic method is used to create a new representation of time series, this methodology will be used to extract features. The *tf* can give higher relevance to words that occur more frequently, the TF-IDF model tries to balance these more frequently occurring word/terms with how frequently the word appears in all documents. If most of the documents have the that word present, the word might not be relevant. In that sense, TF-IDF maximizes differences between documents by means of including the inverse document frequency term (idf):

$$idf(t, D) = \log \frac{N}{|d \in D : t \in d|}, \tag{2}$$

being D, the set of documents and N the total number of documents. The final equation of the TF-IDF model is:

$$tfidf(t, d, D) = tf(t, d) \cdot idf(t, D) \tag{3}$$

Table 2. The connotation variables, search regular expressions and corresponding words assigned to the pattern searched. The parameter m indicates the size, in samples, of the difference between a peak or a plateau. For this work, m = 20 samples.

Connotation	Search	Word
Derivative	p+	Rising
	n+	Falling
	z+	Flat
Derivative	p+z{,m}n+	Peak
	n+z{,m}p+	Valley
	p+z{m,}n+	posPlateau
	n+z{m,}p+	negPlateau
Slope Height	r+	smallRise
	R+	highRise
	f+	smallFall
	F+	highFall
Slope Height	r+z*F+	smallRisehighFall
	R+z*f+	highRisesmallFall
	f+z*r+	smallFallsmallRise
	F+z*R+	highFallhighRise
	r+z*f+	smallRisesmallFall
	R+z*F+	highRisehighFall
	f+z*R+	smallFallhighRise
	F+z*r+	highFallsmallRise
Derivative Speed	R+	quickRise
	r+	slowRise
	F+	quickFall
	r+	slowFall
	z+	Straight
Ampltiude + Derivative	(0p)+(0z)*(0n)+	lowPeak
	(1p)+(1z)*(1n)+	highPeak
	(0n)+(0z)*(0p)+	lowValley
	(1n)+(1z)*(1p)+	highValley
2nd Derivative + 1st Derivative	(Dp)+	concaveRising
	(Dn)+	concaveFalling
	(Cp)+	convexRising
	(Cn)+	convexFalling

As presented in Fig. 3 (step 2), the BoW is built with an N-gram to have more context about the sequence of words that might describe the shape of the signal. For instance, if the sequence"Flat Rise" is common in one of the classes, it might be a more important feature than the individual counterparts, "Flat" and "Rise". In that sense, an *N-gram* was given to build the BoW. In the example presented, an N-gram of size 2 is used and the final example vector is generated from the sentences of the document. From sentence *"Flat Valley Flat"*, the words "Flat", "Valley", "Flat Valley" and "Valley Flat" are represented. For this work, an *N-gram* value of 10 was used.

In this work, we studied different combinations and methods, namely BoW+NB (Bag of Words with a Naive Bayes Classifier), BoW+SVM (Bag of Words with a Linear SVM classifier) and TF-IDF+SVM (TF-IDF with a Linear SVM classifier). These methods were also compared with the standard k-NN classifier with the euclidean distance (with $k = 3$). The sklearn package from Python was used to perform both vectorization and classification steps, and the k-NN classifier was implemented with the pyts package [15].

Table 3. Results of all methods for the 5CB formulation to classify different VOCs.

VOC	Comb 1			Comb 2			Comb 3			Comb 4			1 NN-ED		
	P	R	F1	P	R	F1	P	R	F1	P	R	F1	P	R	F1
Acetone	0.60	0.63	0.61	0.71	0.70	0.70	0.57	0.38	0.46	0.84	0.78	0.81	0.97	0.82	0.89
Acetonitrile	0.51	0.74	0.61	0.63	0.77	0.69	0.40	0.75	0.52	0.72	0.84	0.79	0.96	0.92	0.94
Chloroform	0.70	0.47	0.56	0.65	0.60	0.62	0.62	0.33	0.43	0.88	0.86	0.86	0.94	0.99	0.96
Dicholoromethane	0.64	0.44	0.52	0.56	0.47	0.51	0.49	0.50	0.50	0.88	0.79	0.83	0.90	0.92	0.91
Diethyl Ether	0.59	0.73	0.65	0.66	0.67	0.66	0.67	0.61	0.64	0.88	0.80	0.83	0.92	1.00	0.95
Ethanol	0.78	0.86	0.82	0.87	0.77	0.82	0.66	0.88	0.75	0.91	0.94	0.92	0.92	0.95	0.93
Ethyl Acetate	0.68	0.68	0.68	0.70	0.71	0.70	0.52	0.64	0.58	0.83	0.84	0.83	0.98	0.91	0.94
Heptane	0.71	0.80	0.75	0.59	0.71	0.65	0.50	0.81	0.62	0.76	0.89	0.82	0.96	0.96	0.96
Hexane	0.65	0.82	0.72	0.68	0.68	0.68	0.61	0.47	0.53	0.88	0.88	0.88	0.96	0.96	0.96
Methanol	0.83	0.61	0.70	0.76	0.80	0.78	0.84	0.44	0.58	0.90	0.88	0.89	0.83	0.92	0.87
Toluene	0.82	0.61	0.70	0.80	0.68	0.74	0.81	0.46	0.58	0.94	0.89	0.92	1.00	0.99	0.99
Total	0.68	0.67	0.66	0.69	0.69	0.69	0.61	0.57	0.56	0.78	0.85	0.84	0.94	0.94	0.94

P - Precision; R - Recall; F1 - f1-score; Comb1: BoW+NB; Comb2: BoW+SVM; Comb3: TF-IDF+NB; Comb4: TF-IDF+SVM; ED: Euclidean Distance.

Table 4. Results of all methods for the 8CB formulation to classify different VOCs.

VOC	Comb 1			Comb 2			Comb 3			Comb 4			1 NN-ED		
	P	R	F	P	R	F	P	R	F	P	R	F	P	R	F
Acetone	1.00	0.90	0.95	0.89	0.78	0.83	1.00	0.84	0.91	0.82	0.90	0.86	0.62	1.00	0.76
Acetonitrile	0.91	0.82	0.86	0.54	0.86	0.66	0.89	0.82	0.85	0.89	0.82	0.85	0.98	0.96	0.97
Chloroform	0.90	1.00	0.95	0.96	1.00	0.98	0.84	1.00	0.91	0.98	0.98	0.98	0.93	1.00	0.96
Dicholoromethane	0.76	0.55	0.64	0.69	0.61	0.65	0.68	0.51	0.58	0.77	0.59	0.67	1.00	0.63	0.77
Diethyl Ether	0.92	0.71	0.80	0.81	0.71	0.76	0.97	0.57	0.72	0.87	0.92	0.89	0.84	0.98	0.91
Ethanol	0.66	0.64	0.65	0.49	0.49	0.49	0.65	0.62	0.64	0.54	0.53	0.53	0.96	0.93	0.94
Ethyl Acetate	0.54	0.62	0.58	0.67	0.35	0.46	0.52	0.58	0.55	0.64	0.56	0.60	1.00	0.75	0.86
Heptane	0.52	0.67	0.59	0.45	0.65	0.54	0.49	0.79	0.60	0.47	0.69	0.56	0.65	0.65	0.65
Hexane	0.40	0.29	0.33	0.43	0.29	0.34	0.21	0.07	0.11	0.43	0.29	0.34	0.69	0.48	0.56
Methanol	0.60	0.65	0.62	0.58	0.45	0.51	0.57	0.65	0.61	0.62	0.51	0.56	0.91	1.00	0.95
Toluene	0.70	0.93	0.80	0.72	0.89	0.79	0.72	1.00	0.84	0.71	0.89	0.79	1.00	1.00	1.00
Total	0.71	0.63	0.71	0.66	0.56	0.63	0.69	0.68	0.66	0.70	0.70	0.70	0.87	0.85	0.85

P - Precision; R - Recall; F1 - f1-score; Comb1: BoW+NB; Comb2: BoW+SVM; Comb3: TF-IDF+NB; Comb4: TF-IDF+SVM; ED: Euclidean Distance.

5   Results and Discussion

5.1   Overall Results

The classification of VOC was performed with both a 1-NN-euclidean classifier and all combinations of text-mining methods. The models were trained with a cross-validation strategy, by selecting one experiment as the testing set of signals and all the other experiments as the training sets. The idea is that a new experiment should be recognized based on previous experiments. The results are presented in Figs. 4 and 5, Tables 3 and 4, respectively. The Tables show the overall precision, recall and F1-score for each VOC, and the Figures show the averaged confusion matrices for both methods.

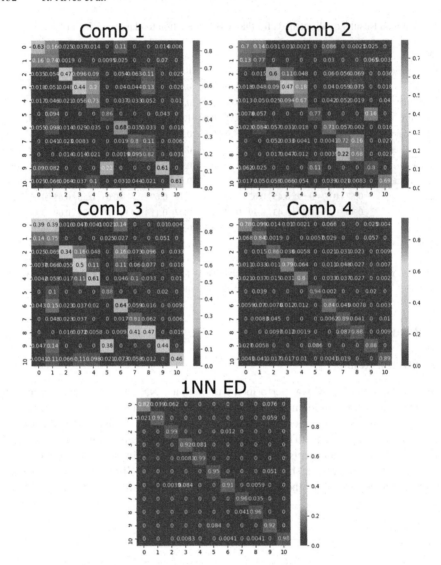

Fig. 4. Confusion matrices of the classification of VOC with the 5CB formulation for all methods. An average f1-score of 0.66 for Comb 1, 0.69 for Comb 2, 0.56 for Comb 3, 0.84 for Comb 4 and 0.94 for the 1-NN ED. The analyzed VOC are labelled from 0 to 10 in the following order: acetone, acetonitrile, chloroform, dichloromethane, diethyl ether, ethanol, ethyl acetate, heptane, hexane, methanol, and toluene.

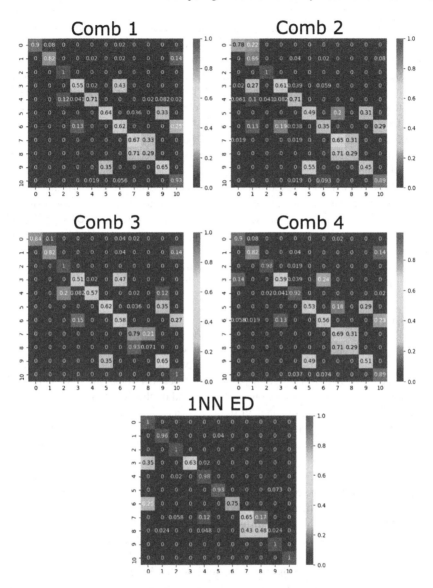

Fig. 5. Confusion matrices of the classification of VOC with the 8CB formulation for all methods. An average f1-score of 0.71 for Comb 1, 0.63 for Comb 2, 0.66 for Comb 3, 0.70 for Comb 4 and 0.85 for the 1-NN ED. The analyzed VOC are labelled from 0 to 10 in the following order: acetone, acetonitrile, chloroform, dichloromethane, diethyl ether, ethanol, ethyl acetate, heptane, hexane, methanol, and toluene.

5.2 Dependence of the Formulation to Classify VOCs

Figures 4 and 5 firstly demonstrate that the simple 1-NN with Euclidean distance is enough to make a correct distinction between different VOCs. This also demonstrates that the response of the e-nose generates signals that are different enough to be differentiated. However, there are noticeable differences between the sensing formulations used. Figure 2 has an illustrative example of the type of cycles generated by the e-nose. Apparently, the shapes seem more distinguishable for the 8CB formulation, but the results indicate the opposite, being the 5CB formulation the one with better results, which suggests that this formulation is more robust to the inherent variability of the sensors from different batches and to the daily conditions that may vary due to slight differences in parameters, as the environmental humidity or temperature. This was not met with the 8CB sensor. In this case, the signals generated are richer in their morphological differences, but a higher variability in the shape of the signal is found between different experiments. More experiments make the classifier better learn the variability in possible electric responses and therefore the signal's shape associated to each VOC. It is also relevant to report that more experiments were recorded with the 5CB formulation, which gives more examples to train the models and probably make better assessments.

Overall, the 5CB formulation was able to provide better results than 8CB with all classification methods.

5.3   Performances of Text-Mining Methods

Different text-mining combinations were used to classify the VOCs. The results show that the combination of TF-IDF with a Linear SVM classifier had a better performance. Between the BoW and the TF-IDF, with the same linear SVM classifier, the latter had a better performance. This result follows what is found on the literature and enhances the fact that weighting words based on their frequency in each document gives a better evaluation of how much relevant is the word to show differences between text-documents. In addition, the naive bayes classifier, in combination with the BoW model, had a similar performance to the BoW with the SVM classifier. The differences in performances are seen in different VOCs, which suggests that the BoW model has information that can be used to separate the classes, and several classifiers could be combined and used to complement the classification with this model. In a future work, the differences in the classification process of these different combinations should be better understood so that methods can be used together to make a correct prediction.

As understood in our previous work [2], the TF-IDF model shows a better promise than other text-mining methods. It is able to describe the morphology of time series based on a higher-leveled sequence of ordered text-based patterns. This method was able to mostly correctly classify each VOC, with an average f1-score of 84% for the 5CB formulation and 72% for the 8CB formulation.

Several mistakes were made by the text-based method, having more difficulties in classifying VOC that had very similar morphology. For instance, the 8CB sensor exhibited a very similar response to Ethanol and Methanol, as well as to Heptane and Hexane (Fig. 2). In that sense, more mistakes are made between these compounds, which is also verified with the euclidean method but with less impact in the overall performance. Overall, the 1-NN-euclidean method achieved a better performance, with an average f1-score of 94.0% and 81.4% for the 5CB and 8CB formulations, respectively.

It is also noticeable that similar shaped VOC responses are more difficult to separate. Considering that the text-based methods rely in higher structural information, having to distinguish shapes with a similar behavior is more difficult. It is a characteristic of dictionary-based methods. This is very well expressed between Methanol and Ethanol for formulation 8CB, the shape is exactly the same, but differences in how the signal rises and falls are what enable the distinction made by the euclidean method. This might be an indication that the text-based method should be applied in longer time series, where there are distinctive ordered patterns that characterize the signal. In addition, other textual patterns should be considered for shorter length time series, to reflect smaller different nuances between signals. Moreover, a grid search over the variables of the method should be performed to optimize the performance, namely for the n-gram value and peak size (m parameter in Table 2).

6 Conclusion and Future Work

In this work we studied two sensing gel formulations to use in an e-nose for the classification of VOCs. The main reasoning was to train a model with previous databases acquired with the same e-nose formulations and recognize the VOC in a new experiment. For this, several models were studied to be trained with the available datasets. We studied both dictionary-based methods (proposed text-based methods) as well as a shape-based method (1-NN ED method).

The results show that the 5CB formulation produces signals that are more easily recognized by the strategies used as well as more reproducible between different experiments, considering the variability inherent to sensor production and daily environmental conditions. The 8CB formulation produces signals that seem more distinguishable visually, and more experiments should be recorded to contemplate the variations in shape that occur between different experiments.

The methods also had different outcomes. The 1-NN ED method was the most successful in performing the classification of the VOC samples compared with the proposed text-based strategy. This means that the standard euclidean distance is a robust, quick and simple candidate to be used in this context. The text-based methods proposed were not as good as the euclidean distance, but showed promising results, considering that it is a method that relies in higher-leveled features. The combination of a TF-IDF model with a Linear SVM classifier was the most reliable in these experiments and should be considered over other combinations, such as BoW with a naive bayes method or a Linear SVM classifier as well. Another relevant conclusion is that using a combination of the BoW model and TF-IDF model can give complementary information, but further research should be made in this matter. In addition, other text-based features should be studied to complement the description of short signals, such as the ones in this work. Results could also be improved by optimizing the parameters of the text-based model, namely the best N-gram to use and which *stopwords* to remove from the classification process. In addition, the text-based approach should possibly give insights in the interpretability of the signals, that is, understanding why signals are different between each other. This could be possible by identifying the relevant keywords (patterns) and searching them over the signal with weight values for each pattern [50].

Acknowledgements. This project has received funding from the European Research Council (ERC) under the EU Horizon 2020 research and innovation programme [grant reference SCENT-ERC-2014-STG-639123, (2015-2022)] and by national funds from FCT - Fundação para a Ciência e a Tecnologia, I.P., in the scope of the project UIDP/04378/2020 and UIDB/04378/2020 of the Research Unit on Applied Molecular Biosciences - UCIBIO and the project LA/P/0140/2020 of the Associate Laboratory Institute for Health and Bioeconomy - i4HB, which is financed by national funds from financed by FCT/MEC (UID/Multi/04378/2019). This work was also partly supported by Fundação para a Ciência e Tecnologia, under PhD grant PD/BDE/142816/2018.

References

1. A study of an electronic nose for detection of lung cancer based on a virtual saw gas sensors array and imaging recognition method, author = Chen, Xing and Cao, Mingfu and Li, Yi and Hu, Weijun and Wang, Ping and Ying, Kejing and Pan, Hongming, year = 2005, journal = Measurement Science and Technology, volume = 16, number = 8, pages = 1535–1546, doi = https://doi.org/10.1088/0957-0233/16/8/001, issn = 0957-0233, url = https://iopscience.iop.org/article/10.1088/0957-0233/16/8/001, keywords = Breath detection, Electronic nose, Lung cancer, Non-invasive detection, Virtual sensors array

2. Alves., R., Rodrigues., J., Ramou., E., Palma., S., Roque., A., Gamboa., H.: Classification of volatile compounds with morphological analysis of e-nose response. In: Proceedings of the 15th International Joint Conference on Biomedical Engineering Systems and Technologies - BIOSIGNALS, pp. 31–39. INSTICC, SciTePress (2022). https://doi.org/10.5220/0010827200003123

3. Bos, L.D.J., Sterk, P.J., Schultz, M.J.: Volatile metabolites of pathogens: a systematic review. PLoS Pathog. 9(5), e1003311 (2013). https://doi.org/10.1371/journal.ppat.1003311, https://dx.plos.org/10.1371/journal.ppat.1003311

4. Bruins, M., Rahim, Z., Bos, A., van de Sande, W.W., Endtz, H.P., van Belkum, A.: Diagnosis of active tuberculosis by e-nose analysis of exhaled air. Tuberculosis 93(2), 232–238 (2013). https://doi.org/10.1016/j.tube.2012.10.002, https://linkinghub.elsevier.com/retrieve/pii/S1472979212001898

5. Capelli, L., et al.: Application and uses of electronic noses for clinical diagnosis on urine samples: a review. Sensors 16(10), 1708 (2016). https://doi.org/10.3390/s16101708, http://www.mdpi.com/1424-8220/16/10/1708

6. Chandler, R., Das, A., Gibson, T., Dutta, R.: Detection of oil pollution in seawater: biosecurity prevention using electronic nose technology. In: 2015 31st IEEE International Conference on Data Engineering Workshops. vol. 2015-June, pp. 98–100. IEEE (2015). https://doi.org/10.1109/ICDEW.2015.7129554, http://ieeexplore.ieee.org/document/7129554/

7. Chen, L.Y., et al.: Development of an electronic-nose system for fruit maturity and quality monitoring. In: 2018 IEEE International Conference on Applied System Invention (ICASI), pp. 1129–1130. IEEE (2018). https://doi.org/10.1109/ICASI.2018.8394481, https://ieeexplore.ieee.org/document/8394481/

8. Coronel Teixeira, R., et al.: The potential of a portable, point-of-care electronic nose to diagnose tuberculosis. J. Infect. 75(5), 441–447 (2017). https://doi.org/10.1016/j.jinf.2017.08.003, https://linkinghub.elsevier.com/retrieve/pii/S0163445317302608

9. D'Amico, A., et al.: An investigation on electronic nose diagnosis of lung cancer. Lung Cancer 68(2), 170–176 (2010). https://doi.org/10.1016/j.lungcan.2009.11.003, https://linkinghub.elsevier.com/retrieve/pii/S0169500209005807

10. Di Natale, C., Macagnano, A., Martinelli, E., Paolesse, R., D'Arcangelo, G., Roscioni, C., Finazzi-Agrò, A., D'Amico, A.: Lung cancer identification by the analysis of breath by means of an array of non-selective gas sensors. Biosens. Bioelectron. **18**(10), 1209–1218 (2003). https://doi.org/10.1016/S0956-5663(03)00086-1, https://linkinghub.elsevier.com/retrieve/pii/S0956566303000861

11. Dragonieri, S., Pennazza, G., Carratu, P., Resta, O.: Electronic nose technology in respiratory diseases. Lung **195**(2), 157–165 (2017). https://doi.org/10.1007/s00408-017-9987-3

12. Dragonieri, S., et al.: An electronic nose in the discrimination of patients with asthma and controls. J. Allergy Clin. Immunol. **120**(4), 856–862 (2007). https://doi.org/10.1016/j.jaci.2007.05.043, https://linkinghub.elsevier.com/retrieve/pii/S009167490701038X

13. Dutta, R., Hines, E.L., Gardner, J.W., Boilot, P.: Bacteria classification using Cyranose 320 electronic nose. BioMed. Eng. OnLine **1**(1), 4 (2002). https://doi.org/10.1186/1475-925X-1-4, https://biomedical-engineering-online.biomedcentral.com/articles/10.1186/1475-925X-1-4

14. Esteves, C., et al.: Effect of film thickness in gelatin hybrid gels for artificial olfaction. Mater. Today Bio 1(December 2018), 100002 (2019). https://doi.org/10.1016/j.mtbio.2019.100002, https://linkinghub.elsevier.com/retrieve/pii/S2590006418300401

15. Faouzi, J., Janati, H.: pyts: a python package for time series classification. J. Mach. Learn. Res. **21**(46), 1–6 (2020). http://jmlr.org/papers/v21/19-763.html

16. Fens, N., et al.: Exhaled breath profiling enables discrimination of chronic obstructive pulmonary disease and asthma. Am. J. Respir. Critic. Care Med. **180**(11), 1076–1082 (2009). https://doi.org/10.1164/rccm.200906-0939OC, http://www.atsjournals.org/doi/abs/10.1164/rccm.200906-0939OC

17. Frazão, J., Palma, S.I.C.J., Costa, H.M.A., Alves, C., Roque, A.C.A., Silveira, M.: Optical gas sensing with liquid crystal droplets and convolutional neural networks. Sensors **21**(8), 2854 (2021). https://doi.org/10.3390/s21082854, https://www.mdpi.com/1424-8220/21/8/2854/htm

18. HaCohen-Kerner, Y., Miller, D., Yigal, Y.: The influence of preprocessing on text classification using a bag-of-words representation. PLOS ONE **15**(5), 1–22 (2020). https://doi.org/10.1371/journal.pone.0232525, https://doi.org/10.1371/journal.pone.0232525

19. He, Q., et al.: Classification of electronic nose data in wound infection detection based on PSO-SVM combined with wavelet transform. Intell. Autom. Soft Comput. **18**(7), 967–979 (2012). https://doi.org/10.1080/10798587.2012.10643302, http://autosoftjournal.net/paperShow.php?paper=10643302

20. Hockstein, N.G., Thaler, E.R., Lin, Y., Lee, D.D., Hanson, C.W.: Correlation of pneumonia score with electronic nose signature: a prospective study. Ann. Otol. Rhinol. Laryngol. **114**(7), 504–508 (2005). https://doi.org/10.1177/000348940511400702, http://journals.sagepub.com/doi/10.1177/000348940511400702

21. Hockstein, N.G., Thaler, E.R., Torigian, D., Miller, W.T., Deffenderfer, O., Hanson, C.W.: Diagnosis of pneumonia with an electronic nose: correlation of vapor signature with chest computed tomography scan findings. Laryngoscope **114**(10), 1701–1705 (2004). https://doi.org/10.1097/00005537-200410000-00005, http://doi.wiley.com/10.1097/00005537-200410000-00005

22. Hu, W., et al.: Electronic noses: from advanced materials to sensors aided with data processing. Adv. Mater. Technol. **4**(2), 1–38 (2018). https://doi.org/10.1002/admt.201800488, https://onlinelibrary.wiley.com/doi/abs/10.1002/admt.201800488

23. Hussain, A., et al.: Tunable gas sensing gels by cooperative assembly. Adv. Funct. Mater. **27**(27), 1700803 (2017). https://doi.org/10.1002/adfm.201700803, http://doi.wiley.com/10.1002/adfm.201700803

24. Jian, Y., et al.: Artificially intelligent olfaction for fast and noninvasive diagnosis of bladder cancer from urine. ACS Sens. **7**(6), 1720–1731 (2022). https://doi.org/10.1021/acssensors. 2c00467, https://doi.org/10.1021/acssensors.2c00467, pMID: 35613367

25. Karakaya, D., Ulucan, O., Turkan, M.: Electronic nose and its applications: a survey. Int. J. Autom. Comput. **17**(2), 179–209 (2020). https://doi.org/10.1007/s11633-019-1212-9, http:// link.springer.com/10.1007/s11633-019-1212-9

26. Keogh, E., Lonardi, S., Ratanamahatana, C.A.: Towards parameter-free data mining. In: Proceedings of the Tenth ACM SIGKDD International Conference on Knowledge Discovery and Data Mining, pp. 206–215. KDD 2004, Association for Computing Machinery, New York, NY, USA (2004). https://doi.org/10.1145/1014052.1014077

27. van Keulen, K.E., Jansen, M.E., Schrauwen, R.W.M., Kolkman, J.J., Siersema, P.D.: Volatile organic compounds in breath can serve as a non-invasive diagnostic biomarker for the detection of advanced adenomas and colorectal cancer. Aliment. Pharmacol. Ther. **51**(3), 334–346 (2020). https://doi.org/10.1111/apt.15622, http://doi.wiley.com/10.1111/apt.15622

28. Kodogiannis, V., Lygouras, J., Tarczynski, A., Chowdrey, H.: Artificial odor discrimination system using electronic nose and neural networks for the identification of urinary tract infection. IEEE Trans. Inf. Technol. Biomed. **12**(6), 707–713 (2008). https://doi.org/10.1109/ TITB.2008.917928, http://ieeexplore.ieee.org/document/4526692/

29. Lee, Y.S., Joo, B.S., Choi, N.J., Lim, J.O., Huh, J.S., Lee, D.D.: Visible optical sensing of ammonia based on polyaniline film. Sens. Actuators B: Chem. **93**(1–3), 148–152 (2003). https://doi.org/10.1016/S0925-4005(03)00207-7, https://linkinghub.elsevier. com/retrieve/pii/S0925400503002077

30. Liang, Z., Tian, F., Zhang, C., Sun, H., Liu, X., Yang, S.X.: A correlated information removing based interference suppression technique in electronic nose for detection of bacteria. Analytica Chimica Acta **986**, 145–152 (2017). https://doi.org/10.1016/j.aca.2017.07.028, http://dx.doi.org/10.1016/j.aca.2017.07.028

31. Liddell, K.: Smell as a diagnostic marker. Postgrad. Med. J. **52**(605), 136–138 (1976). https://doi.org/10.1136/pgmj.52.605.136, https://pmj.bmj.com/lookup/doi/10.1136/pgmj.52. 605.136

32. Lin, J., Keogh, E., Wei, L., Lonardi, S.: Experiencing sax: a novel symbolic representation of time series. Data Min. Knowl. Discov. **15**, 107–144 (2007). https://doi.org/10.1007/s10618-007-0064-z

33. Lin, J., Khade, R., Li, Y.: Rotation-invariant similarity in time series using bag-of-patterns representation. J. Intell. Inf. Syst. **39**(2), 287–315 (2012). https://doi.org/10.1007/s10844-012-0196-5

34. Moens, M., et al.: Fast identification of ten clinically important micro-organisms using an electronic nose. Lett. Appl. Microbiol. **42**(2), 121–126 (2006). https://doi.org/10.1111/ j.1472-765X.2005.01822.x, http://doi.wiley.com/10.1111/j.1472-765X.2005.01822.x

35. Pádua, A.C., Palma, S., Gruber, J., Gamboa, H., Roque, A.C.: Design and evolution of an opto-electronic device for VOCs detection. In: BIODEVICES 2018–11th International Conference on Biomedical Electronics and Devices, Proceedings; Part of 11th International Joint Conference on Biomedical Engineering Systems and Technologies, BIOSTEC 2018 1(Biostec), pp. 48–55 (2018). https://doi.org/10.5220/0006558100480055

36. Pavlou, A.K., Magan, N., Jones, J.M., Brown, J., Klatser, P., Turner, A.P.: Detection of Mycobacterium tuberculosis (TB) in vitro and in situ using an electronic nose in combination with a neural network system. Biosens. Bioelectron. **20**(3), 538–544 (2004). https://doi.org/10.1016/j.bios.2004.03.002, https://linkinghub.elsevier.com/retrieve/ pii/S0956566304001204

37. Persaud, K., Dodd, G.: Analysis of discrimination mechanisms in the mammalian olfactory system using a model nose. Nature **299**(5881), 352–355 (1982). https://doi.org/10.1038/ 299352a0, http://www.nature.com/articles/299352a0

38. Pinto, J., et al.: Urinary volatilomics unveils a candidate biomarker panel for non-invasive detection of clear cell renal cell carcinoma. J. Proteome Res. **20**(6), 3068–3077 (2021). https://doi.org/10.1021/acs.jproteome.0c00936, https://pubs.acs.org/doi/10.1021/acs.jproteome.0c00936

39. Raspagliesi, F., Bogani, G., Benedetti, S., Grassi, S., Ferla, S., Buratti, S.: Detection of ovarian cancer through exhaled breath by electronic nose: a prospective study. Cancers **12**(9), 1–13 (2020). https://doi.org/10.3390/cancers12092408

40. Röck, F., Barsan, N., Weimar, U.: Electronic nose: current status and future trends. Chem. Rev. **108**(2), 705–725 (2008). https://doi.org/10.1021/cr068121q, https://pubs.acs.org/doi/10.1021/cr068121q

41. Rodrigues, J., Folgado, D., Belo, D., Gamboa, H.: SSTS: a syntactic tool for pattern search on time series. Inf. Process. Manage. **56**(1), 61–76 (2019). https://doi.org/10.1016/j.ipm.2018.09.001, https://www.sciencedirect.com/science/article/pii/S0306457318302577

42. Saidi, T., Zaim, O., Moufid, M., El Bari, N., Ionescu, R., Bouchikhi, B.: Exhaled breath analysis using electronic nose and gas chromatography–mass spectrometry for non-invasive diagnosis of chronic kidney disease, diabetes mellitus and healthy subjects. Sens. Actuat. B: Chem. **257**, 178–188 (2018). https://doi.org/10.1016/j.snb.2017.10.178, http://dx.doi.org/10.1016/j.snb.2017.10.178

43. Santonico, M., et al.: In situ detection of lung cancer volatile fingerprints using broncho-scopic air-sampling. Lung Cancer **77**(1), 46–50 (2012). https://doi.org/10.1016/j.lungcan.2011.12.010, https://linkinghub.elsevier.com/retrieve/pii/S016950021100674X

44. Santos, G., Alves, C., Pádua, A., Palma, S., Gamboa, H., Roque, A.: An optimized e-nose for efficient volatile sensing and discrimination. In: Proceedings of the 12th International Joint Conference on Biomedical Engineering Systems and Technologies, pp. 36–46. SCITEPRESS - Science and Technology Publications (2019). https://doi.org/10.5220/0007390700360046, http://www.scitepress.org/DigitalLibrary/Link.aspx?doi=10.5220/0007390700360046

45. Santos, J., et al.: Electronic nose for the identification of pig feeding and ripening time in Iberian hams. Meat Sci. **66**(3), 727–732 (2004). https://doi.org/10.1016/j.meatsci.2003.07.005, https://linkinghub.elsevier.com/retrieve/pii/S0309174003001955

46. Schäfer, P.: The BOSS is concerned with time series classification in the presence of noise. Data Min. Knowl. Disc. **29**(6), 1505–1530 (2014). https://doi.org/10.1007/s10618-014-0377-7

47. Schäfer, P., Leser, U.: Fast and accurate time series classification with weasel, pp. 637–646. Association for Computing Machinery, New York, NY, USA (2017). https://doi.org/10.1145/3132847.3132980

48. van der Schee, M.P., Fens, N., Buijze, H., Top, R., van der Poll, T., Sterk, P.J.: Diagnostic value of exhaled breath analysis in tuberculosis. In: D96. WHAT'S NEW IN TUBERCU-LOSIS DIAGNOSTICS. pp. A6510–A6510. American Thoracic Society (2012). https://doi.org/10.1164/ajrccm-conference.2012.185.1_MeetingAbstracts.A6510, http://www.atsjournals.org/doi/abs/10.1164/ajrccm-conference.2012.185.1_MeetingAbstracts.A6510

49. Schnabel, R., et al.: Analysis of volatile organic compounds in exhaled breath to diagnose ventilator-associated pneumonia. Sci. Rep. **5**(1), 17179 (2015). https://doi.org/10.1038/srep17179, http://www.nature.com/articles/srep17179

50. Senin, P., Malinchik, S.: Sax-vsm: interpretable time series classification using sax and vector space model (2013). https://doi.org/10.1109/ICDM.2013.52

51. de Vries, R., et al.: Integration of electronic nose technology with spirometry: validation of a new approach for exhaled breath analysis. J. Breath Res. **9**(4), 046001 (2015). https://doi.org/10.1088/1752-7155/9/4/046001, https://iopscience.iop.org/article/10.1088/1752-7155/9/4/046001

140   R. Alves et al.

52. Wilson, A.D., Baietto, M.: Advances in electronic-nose technologies developed for biomedical applications. Sensors **11**(1), 1105–1176 (2011). https://doi.org/10.3390/s110101105, http://www.mdpi.com/1424-8220/11/1/1105

53. Wong, D.M., et al.: Development of a breath detection method based e-nose system for lung cancer identification. In: 2018 IEEE International Conference on Applied System Invention (ICASI), pp. 1119–1120. IEEE (2018). https://doi.org/10.1109/ICASI.2018.8394477, https://ieeexplore.ieee.org/document/8394477/

54. Yang, H.Y., Wang, Y.C., Peng, H.Y., Huang, C.H.: Breath biopsy of breast cancer using sensor array signals and machine learning analysis. Sci. Rep. **11**(1), 103 (2021). https://doi.org/10.1038/s41598-020-80570-0, http://www.nature.com/articles/s41598-020-80570-0

55. Ye, L., Keogh, E.: Time series shapelets: a new primitive for data mining. In: Proceedings of the 15th ACM SIGKDD International Conference on Knowledge Discovery and Data Mining, pp. 947–956. KDD 2009, Association for Computing Machinery, New York, NY, USA (2009). https://doi.org/10.1145/1557019.1557122

High-Level Features for Human Activity Recognition and Modeling

Yale Hartmann$^{(\boxtimes)}$, Hui Liu , and Tanja Schultz

Cognitive Systems Lab, University of Bremen, Bremen, Germany
{yale.hartmann,hui.liu,tanja.schultz}@uni-bremen.de
http://csl.uni-bremen.de/

Abstract. High-Level Features (HLF) are a novel way of describing and processing human activities. Each feature captures an interpretable aspect of activities,
and a unique combination of HLFs defines an activity. In this article, we propose and evaluate a concise set of six HLFs on and across the CSL-SHARE and
UniMiB SHAR datasets, showing that HLFs can be successfully extracted with
machine learning methods and that in this HLF-space activities can be classified
across datasets as well as in imbalanced and few-shot learning settings. Furthermore, we illustrate how classification errors can be attributed to specific HLF
extractors. In person-independent 5-fold cross-validations, the proposed HLFs
are extracted from 68% up to 99% balanced accuracy, and activity classification
achieves 89.7% (CSL-SHARE) and 67.3% (UniMiB SHAR) accuracy. Imbalanced and few-shot learning results are promising, with the latter converging
quickly. In a person-dependent evaluation across both datasets, 78% accuracy is
achieved. These results demonstrate the possibilities and advantages of the proposed high-level, extensible, and interpretable feature space.

Keywords: Human activity recognition · High-level features · Interpretable
machine learning · Wearable sensors

1 Background and Related Works

Human activity recognition (HAR), an important research topic for today's modern life,
involves proven machine learning (ML) algorithms for related tasks, including biosignal (pre-)processing, feature extraction and selection, unsupervised data segmentation,
and activity modeling approaches, as the classic and the state-of-the-art HAR research
pipelines portray [7,28,45]. A suitable algorithm and a high recognition rate are prerequisites for HAR applications to work smoothly [25]. Forefront research works in
non-traditional areas, such as device-free HAR [11], the effect of validation methods
on HAR performance [6], advanced sensing techniques applicable to HAR [5], and
interactive and interpretable online HAR [18], have been emerging.

In most research settings, the domain related to machine learning has received more
attention from researchers, focusing on solving the following two problems:

- Which ML approaches are more applicable for the study's objectives, such as activity patterns, application scenarios, and datasets?

A. C. A. Roque et al. (Eds.): BIOSTEC 2022, CCIS 1814, pp. 141–163, 2023.
https://doi.org/10.1007/978-3-031-38854-5_8

– What topological and parametric adjustments should be made to the applied ML approaches to obtain better results (accuracy)?

The first query was fully attended to, and field-related addressed. HAR has been effectively studied on various well-established machine learning models such as Long Short-Term Memory (LSTM) [38,53], Basic and Deep Neural Networks [23,37,50], Convolutional Neural Networks [13,24,38,42,52,55], Recurrent Neural Networks [2,9,21,36,38,44], and Hidden Markov Models (HMM) [29,33,40], among others. More sophisticated modeling schemes based on mature ML models, such as Residual Neural Networks [19,22,32,47] and Hierarchical Hidden Markov Models [54], have also been applied to HAR. With the basic research of these ML models in the field of HAR, the second problem mentioned above has also received favorable attention and is usually solved based on model reformulation, parameter tuning, feature investigation, and iterative optimization [1,2,16,30,41,48].

Noticeably, the vast majority of HAR studies listed above tend to be closely related to, or even just about, ML models. In other words, researchers involved may not care about or cannot effectively investigate the kinematic and physiological implications of "activity" as a study object for human **activity** recognition. In these studies, "human activity" is more of a signal set than a sport or kinesiological phenomenon. Similar deficiencies have been better recognized and addressed in other fields of ML-based pattern recognition. For instance, the mechanics of human voice production has been extensively studied, leading to excellent automatic speech recognition models, such as the three-state HMM-based Bakis-model [3] constructing phonemes by imitating phonetics in segmenting the pronunciation. Each sub-phoneme, represented as one state (begin/middle/end), models a phoneme part, improving the model generalizability and extendability for efficient training and decoding while reflecting the phonetic and biological significance. Moving from audio to video, the physiological model of the human eye's stereo vision has been commonly applied to image/video recognition [10,43].

Looking back at HAR, there is a paucity of literature linking human kinesiology, somatology, physiology, or sportology to ML models. While these connections should be feasible and pivotal, how they are studied requires crossing interdisciplinary divides. A simple attempt in a statistical sense is to derive a reasonable duration based on big data for every single motion in daily life and common sports, providing reference in data segmentation, signal windowing, and modeling [31]. The recently proposed motion units [27] approach is another step forward in bridging the gap from movement science to machine learning, which partitions each human activity into a sequence of shared, meaningful, and activity distinguishing states, analog to phonemes in speech recognition, endowing HAR modeling with operability, interpretability, generalizability, and expandability.

As an exhaustive follow-up to our earlier conference publication [15], this article elaborates on our novel method for practical knowledge incorporation from other fields into HAR, facilitating non-ML experts for developing recognition systems. We propose a feasible approach to allow researchers to design high-level activity properties with their respective possible values, such as Backwards/Neutral/Forwards. Such a set of features, extracted with classifiers, can be optimized or transformed into feature functions in further stages, e.g., with the help of ML experts. A necessary condition for the proposed setup to work well is that each activity is divergent from all other activities on at least one property, which enables the classification to be performed effectively with an easily attributable featuring error discovery and a well interpretable feature space.

The following article includes a further in-depth elaboration of the High-level Features, Error Attribution, and reiterated High-level Features compared to [18]. Furthermore, all experiments have been re-run, and new few-shot experiments were added. All experiments are run on the CSL-SHARE [26], and UniMiB SHAR [35] datasets. These datasets deploy different sensor carriers (knee-bandage and smartphone), sensors and sensor positions (EMG, goniometer, accelerometer, and gyroscope around the knee and accelerometer in different trouser pockets), and mostly different activities with a few shared ones ("jump", "walk", "going up stairs", among others). These properties make the two datasets a perfect fit to demonstrate the utility of High-level Features for Human Activity Recognition.

2 High-Level Features

In this work, we propose a set of High-Level Features along with how to extract and utilize them in multiple tasks like classification, few-shot learning, and dataset combination.

2.1 Concept

High-Level Features describe properties of human activities independent of the sensor setup used to record them in a human interpretable way. For instance, one HLF entitled *Back/Front* might encode if a person is moving along the frontal direction, e.g., forward, no-movement, or backward. This feature value is assigned based on activity initially, and the association from sensor data to feature value is learned using classification algorithms (see Sect. 3). Therefore, the activity "Walk" will be assigned the *Back/Front* value of *Forward*, while "Walk Back" will be assigned *Backward*, and "Walk sideways" is *Neutral* in the frontal direction.

The feature development is based on the activity target and activity knowledge rather than the sensor data. Therefore, in some sensor setups, they might be impossible to extract. For instance, a sensor setup based on a single IMU can likely not extract the muscle force produced during jumps or bench presses, as the force is dependent not only on the acceleration with which it is moved but also the weight stemmed. Nevertheless, the muscles produce this force during both activities and should be modeled accordingly.

We propose developing these descriptive HLFs such that each activity has a unique combination of feature values. Uniqueness has multiple benefits: activity classification and zero-shot learning are straightforward. Furthermore, this leads to unambiguous activity definitions. Uniqueness means that the one-hot encoded feature value vectors can be looked up in a table for classification. At the same time, uniqueness implies that two activities with identical features must be identical, or another property must distinguish them. Vice versa, a unique combination of feature values implies a specific activity. Both are tremendously helpful for developing HLFs: the first allows thinking about differences between activity pairs, and the latter allows checking how well the features can scale. If most combinations are impossible, it might make sense to re-think the features.

We propose treating the feature extraction as a classification task, thereby learning the relationship between data and defined feature values in a data-driven fashion. One could either use a single classifier to predict all feature values utilizing the possible interdependence between features or treat them as independent by training a different classifier per HLF. Both can be achieved with any machine learning classifier, with different benefits. Here we focus on the latter due to its extensibility and flexibility of adding or removing features by excluding or training classifiers, as well as the ability to attribute errors made during classification to a specific feature extractor.

Feature extraction is sensor and dataset-dependent due to the classification procedure. However, classification in the extracted high-level feature space is sensor-independent due to its knowledge-driven and activity-based design. This independence has multiple advantages: (1) the feature design is not limited to a specific dataset, which results in scalable and meaningful features, (2) in this feature space, we can combine multiple datasets for comparison, classification, and modeling, and (3) the feature extraction itself can be adjusted to each datasets specifics, like sampling-rates, missing values, or sensors.

2.2   Proposed High-Level Features

We proposed the HLF concept along with eight specific features in our previous work [18]. Here, we further developed this into a more concise HLF-set utilizing the previously mentioned error propagation (see Sect. 5). We developed six High-Level Features: *Back/Front*, *Left/Right*, *Up/Down*, *Force*, *Knee*, and *Impact*.

Back/Front. describes if the person moved along the sagittal plane. For instance, because they walk forward or sit in a moving car. It can hold three different values: *Back*, *Neutral*, and *Forward*. Note that *Neutral* does not imply the person is sitting still. They could be moving to either side or up and down, just not forward or backward.

Left/Right. similarly describes movement along the frontal plane. However, it can take multiple values, describing the subtlety of the movement: *Left-extreme* (large left movement in short time), *Left*, *Left-slightly* (subtle left movement in long time), *Neutral*, *Right-slightly*, *Right*, *Right-extreme*, and *Any* (indicating there is movement, but not clearly defined). As discussed previously, these are required to distinguish left/right shuffles from left/right curves and slight curves.

Up/Down. describes movement along the transverse plane. It can take the values *Down*, *Neutral*, *Up*, and *Updown*. The latter is required to describe jumps, during which the body initially goes up and sinks back down again. Currently, the HLFs are extracted as one value for the whole segmented activity and, therefore, a trade-off in modeling is required for jumps. One solution would be to aim for *Up/Down* to model the starting movement of an activity, in which case jump would be assigned *Up*. The same argument goes for the ending of a movement. Neither truly captures the movement of the jump activity, which is why we opted to use the special case *UpDown* for now. The best solution would be to model HLFs in sequences which values may change over time. We discuss this further in Sect. 8.

Force. describes the force the upper (right) leg muscles need to generate during this activity. It can take the values *N.a./None* (no notable usage of the muscles), *Low*, *Medium*, and *High*. This HLF is primarily required to distinguish jumping with one and jumping with two legs but also supports distinguishing multiple other activities.

Knee. describes the movement or posture of the knees during the activity and is mainly required to distinguish the only two static activities in the two used datasets: stand and sit. It can take the values *Bent* or *Straight* (for postures) as well as *Move* and *Falter* (for movements). Additionally, it can take the values *Left knee first* and *Right knee first*, which brings the total different values for the *Knee* HLF up to six. The latter two are technically a special case of the *Move* value and are currently required due to activity distinctions in the CSL-SHARE dataset.

Impact. describes the amount or quality of impacts broadly. For falls, it takes the value *One*, as in one larger impact when hitting the ground. Special cases are if the person is hitting something during the fall but still hitting the ground (UniMiB SHAR: "HittingObstacle"), in which case it can take the value *Two*. Similarly, the person falling might soften the fall by extending their arms, for which the value *Softened* is chosen. During static activities, the feature may take the value *N.a./None*, and during gait-related activities *Several*. Therefore, resulting in five different values for *Impact*.

2.3   HLF Assignments

The full HLF assignment table across both datasets is depicted in Fig. 1. Each column displays an activity's unique feature value combination, while each row displays the feature values across all activities. For easier readability, the table is color coded. Note that the color is only consistent in each row. *Back* in *Back/Front* is coded dark blue for all *Backs* in this feature, while dark blue for *Up/Down* is used for all *Ups*.

Figure 1 shows that each activity in this feature space is uniquely coded and that multiple clusters of activities exist with similar feature values. For instance, the gait-related activities share most features except *Left/Right* and *Knee*.

Plotting the distance between activities in this new feature space reveals these clusters further. Figure 2 shows the distance between each pair of activities, with red regions indicating low distance and blue regions high distance. The distance is measured as the number of feature values in which a pair of activities differ, which correlates to the euclidean distance of the one-hot encoded feature values per activity.

The main clusters emerge for falls and gait-based activities. Furthermore, it can be observed that the V-Cut and Spin activities create their own clusters as well as share most of their features with each other. More interesting is that the falls are less dissimilar to the more static activities like sitting, standing, or sitting down than the gait and sports-related activities. Intuitively this makes sense, as falls are no active activities and thus

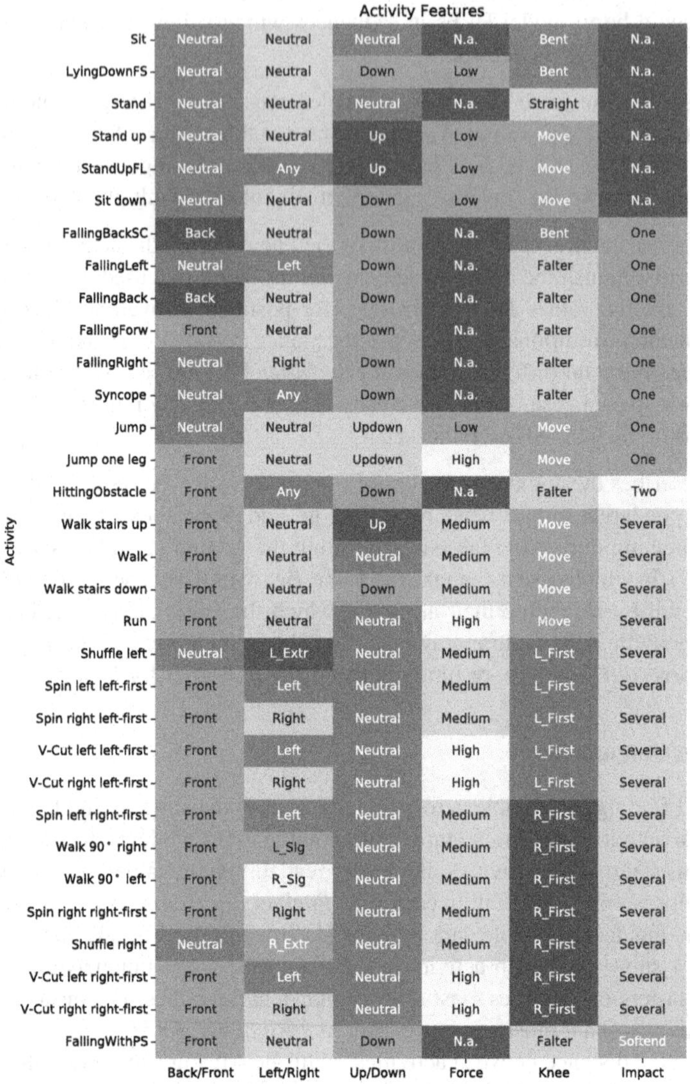

Activity	Back/Front	Left/Right	Up/Down	Force	Knee	Impact
Sit	Neutral	Neutral	Neutral	N.a.	Bent	N.a.
LyingDownFS	Neutral	Neutral	Down	Low	Bent	N.a.
Stand	Neutral	Neutral	Neutral	N.a.	Straight	N.a.
Stand up	Neutral	Neutral	Up	Low	Move	N.a.
StandUpFL	Neutral	Any	Up	Low	Move	N.a.
Sit down	Neutral	Neutral	Down	Low	Move	N.a.
FallingBackSC	Back	Neutral	Down	N.a.	Bent	One
FallingLeft	Neutral	Left	Down	N.a.	Falter	One
FallingBack	Back	Neutral	Down	N.a.	Falter	One
FallingForw	Front	Neutral	Down	N.a.	Falter	One
FallingRight	Neutral	Right	Down	N.a.	Falter	One
Syncope	Neutral	Any	Down	N.a.	Falter	One
Jump	Neutral	Neutral	Updown	Low	Move	One
Jump one leg	Front	Neutral	Updown	High	Move	One
HittingObstacle	Front	Any	Down	N.a.	Falter	Two
Walk stairs up	Front	Neutral	Up	Medium	Move	Several
Walk	Front	Neutral	Neutral	Medium	Move	Several
Walk stairs down	Front	Neutral	Down	Medium	Move	Several
Run	Front	Neutral	Neutral	High	Move	Several
Shuffle left	Neutral	L_Extr	Neutral	Medium	L_First	Several
Spin left left-first	Front	Left	Neutral	Medium	L_First	Several
Spin right left-first	Front	Right	Neutral	Medium	L_First	Several
V-Cut left left-first	Front	Left	Neutral	High	L_First	Several
V-Cut right left-first	Front	Right	Neutral	High	L_First	Several
Spin left right-first	Front	Left	Neutral	Medium	R_First	Several
Walk 90° right	Front	L_Slg	Neutral	Medium	R_First	Several
Walk 90° left	Front	R_Slg	Neutral	Medium	R_First	Several
Spin right right-first	Front	Right	Neutral	Medium	R_First	Several
Shuffle right	Neutral	R_Extr	Neutral	Medium	R_First	Several
V-Cut left right-first	Front	Left	Neutral	High	R_First	Several
V-Cut right right-first	Front	Right	Neutral	High	R_First	Several
FallingWithPS	Front	Neutral	Down	N.a.	Falter	Softend

Fig. 1. HLFs per activity. The color is coded per feature values per row, with no intentional meaning of color between rows.

do not require muscle force and are always *Neutral* in either *Back/Front* or *Left/Right*, while the gait-based activities will seldom be *Neutral* in the *Back/Front* HLF. One could roughly group activities based on these HLFs into three categories: fall, gait-based, and lounge. Note that these observations span two separate datasets because the HLFs design is based on the activities rather than the sensor data of these two datasets.

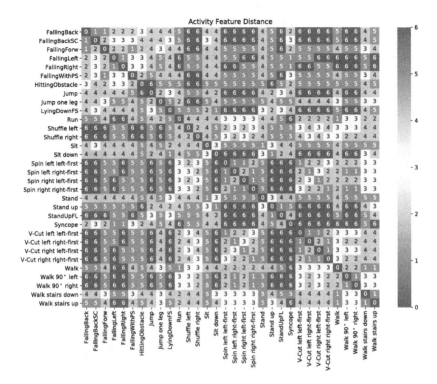

Fig. 2. Distance between activities within the HLF-space. Measured as the number of distinguishing feature values.

3   Feature Extraction

Correct extraction of the High-Level Features from given sensor data is crucial for any further task, including classification and analysis. We treat feature extraction as a classification task for each feature separately. Therefore, the machine learning task is to learn the relationship between the sensory data of an activity to its assigned categorical feature value for each HLF. As discussed in Sect. 2, one could also utilize a single larger extractor. However, we opted for the extensibility, explainability, and the possibility of attributing classification errors to specific feature extractors instead of the single large one when utilizing multiple independent feature extractors.

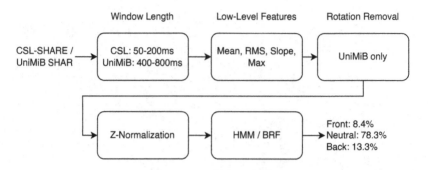

Window Length   Low-Level Features   Rotation Removal

Fig. 3. HLF Extractor pipeline with preprocessing and classification stages.

Figure 3 depicts the HLF extractors. The initial sequence is windowed, four features are extracted (Mean, RMS, Slope, Max), and the whole sequence is normalized. In the case of the UniMiB SHAR dataset, a simple rotation removal is employed to mitigate the different phone positions, as described in [17]. Lastly, two classifiers are tested: a Hidden Markov Model and a Balanced Random Forest (BRF) [8]. The former fully supports sequences, and the latter is trained on a fixed vector length of the first 50 low-level features. On the UniMiB SHAR dataset, this entails the full sequence (as all sequences are 3 s long), and on the CSL-SHARE, this translates to the first half second.

Our previous work deployed out-of-the-box Random Forests, BRFs, and HMMs with only slight parameter tuning for each HLF [15]. Very similar, we evaluated HMMs and BRFs here, tuning both slightly to treat them as mostly out-of-the-box. The BRF is chosen here as with the proposed HLF assignment each HLF has one or two dominant and multiple less-represented values due to the datasets' activities, and humans preferring to walk forward instead of backward, as seen in Fig. 4.

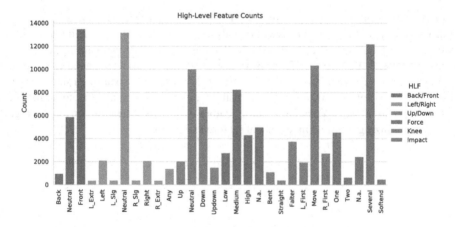

Fig. 4. Number of samples for each feature value across datasets. The color indicates the values' corresponding HLF.

The Balanced Random Forests are tuned as to the window length and overlap for each HLF. Tuning resulted in window lengths of 50ms (CSL-SHARE) and 800ms (UniMiB SHAR), with 80% overlap to perform best. The HMMs are tuned for window length and overlap, and two general-purpose topologies were tested. The first topology plainly uses three states for each HLF target value. The second topology has a target-specific second to fourth state and shares its initial and fifth state across all HLF values. This design aims to allow the HMM to pick the most representative 3-phase subsequence for each HLF by allowing the first and last state to take arbitrary portions off of the sequence, leaving the middle states to distinguish between targets. Parameter tuning revealed 100ms and 200ms, depending on HLF (CSL-SHARE), 400ms (UniMiB SHAR) window length and 80% overlap to work best. Both topologies performed well and were mostly on par on the CSL-SHARE dataset. The plain three states outperformed the shared topology on the UniMiB SHAR consistently. This performance contrasts [17] and will be investigated further in future work.

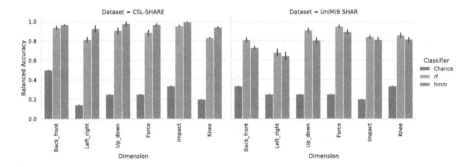

Fig. 5. Summarized HLF extraction performance from 5-fold person-independent evaluation, listing HMMs, BRFs, and chance level. Metric is the balanced accuracy.

For each of the six HLFs and each dataset, a 5-Fold person-independent cross-validation was conducted. The balanced accuracy is used as a metric, as each HLF typically contains one dominant and multiple underrepresented feature values, as seen in Fig. 4. All cross-validation results, including the chance level, are summarized in Fig. 5. Both classifiers significantly outperform the chance level. The HMM consistently is better than the BRF on the CSL-SHARE, while the opposite holds on the UniMiB SHAR dataset. Performance on the CSL-SHARE dataset ranges from 92% (*Left/Right*) to 99% (*Impact*) and ranges from 68% (*Left/Right*) to 94% (*Force*) balanced accuracy on the UniMiB SHAR dataset. In both cases, each single feature extraction performance is higher or close to state-of-the-art classification balanced accuracy. While very encouraging, note that error propagates, and the final classification performance is below state-of-the-art.

4   Activity Classification

Activity Classification in this HLF space is straightforward. There are two main options: utilizing the unique combination property to look up the activity based on the extracted

features or training another classifier in this new space. The former is especially interesting for zero-shot learning or error attribution (see Sect. 5), while the latter has the
potential to counter-balance difficulties in extracted HLFs.

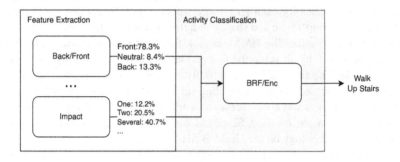

Fig. 6. Classifier stages with HLF extractors.

Figure 6 depicts the classification process. The HLFs are extracted as described in
Sect. 3 and are configured to return the probability for each possible HLF value, e.g.,
the *Back/Front* extractor will return how likely the Front/Neutral/Back values are given
a sensor data sequence. We found the extra information of the classifier confidences
benefited the final classification, but of course, a one-hot encoding from the extractors
would also be possible. All HLF probabilities are then stacked into a single feature
vector given to the classifier.

The encoding classifier calculates the euclidean distance between the given vector
and each activity, represented as stacked one-hot encoding of the assigned HLFs, and
picks the closest one. This approach allows zero-shot activity prediction. Given the
extracted features and definition of unseen activities, the classifier can predict them.
Furthermore, with the encoding classifier, classification errors can be attributed to the
different features. If walking was predicted to be walking a curve left, the reason for the
misclassification must be the *Left/Right* HLF.

The BRF classifier is simply trained to learn the relation between the stacked probabilities and the activity label. The BRF may learn to counter-balance the difficulties
from the extractors by associating and counteracting low confidences of HLF extractions.

Activity classification in this high-level feature space is evaluated in a 5-fold person-
independent evaluation using the accuracy and balanced accuracy as metrics. The HLF
Extractors are configured with the previously found hyperparameters (see Sect. 3) but
are retrained inside the 5-fold cross-validation. Retraining is important to ensure the
high-level extractors have not been trained on test samples, thus overestimating the
final classification performance. Both a BRF-based and an encoding-based classifier
are evaluated.

The final classification performance with the BRF-based classifier is 89.7% (CSL-
SHARE) and 67.3% accuracy (UniMiB SHAR). These accuracies trail the previously
reported 93.7% (CSL-SHARE) and 77.0% accuracy (UniMiB SHAR) in a leave-one-
person-out cross-validation [17]. While 5-fold person-independent cross-validation can

underestimate the performance due to a limitation in available training data compared to a leave-one-person-out validation, the results from Sect. 6 indicate that the errors are not made because of too little data. [17] employed (low-level) feature space transformations using a combination of HMMs and an LDA, which should be evaluated with the high-level feature extraction in future work.

The final classification performance with the Encoding-based classifier is 88.1% (CSL-SHARE) and 66.4% accuracy (UniMiB SHAR). These are slightly lower than with the BRF classifier. However, the following analysis mainly focuses on the encoding-based classifier as the interpretation and the relation between final classification and HLFs are solely based on to the HLF extraction.

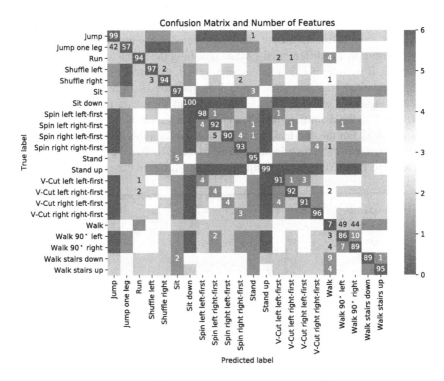

Fig. 7. Blended confusion and distance matrix for the Encoding-based classifier on the CSL-SHARE dataset. The color indicates distance, and values indicate the percentage of cases. (Color figure online)

Figure 7 shows the confusion matrix for the CSL-SHARE dataset blended with the distance matrix shown previously. The color indicates feature distance, and the number indicates the percentage of cases. The main error is that walking in a straight line is often predicted to be walking 90° left/right in three steps. The other cluster of errors happens within the spin activities as well as between the spins and their v-cut counterparts. Notably, almost all errors occur between low to medium-distance activities (colored red).

Figure 8 shows the blended matrix for the UniMiB SHAR dataset. Similar to CSL-SHARE, most errors occur between low-distance activities. There are three main clusters of errors: between types of falls, between walking and walking the stairs, and then between in the distinction between sitting and lying. The confusion within the falls on this dataset has been reported previously [17]. Interestingly at no time falling forward is correctly predicted; instead, falling left/right and syncope seem to sink most falls. The last cluster is especially interesting as sitting down is mainly misclassified as lying down from sitting, and standing up is mostly confused with standing up from lying, but standing up (from lying) is misclassified as lying down from sitting.

5 Error Attribution

Activity classification is never perfect, and one interesting question is why a misclassification was made. In the High-Level Feature space with unique feature combinations for activities, the classification error can be attributed to the underlying feature extraction by determining the different HLFs distinguishing the actual and predicted activity. For example, if walking is classified as walking left, this error can be attributed to the *Left/Right* and *Knee* HLF, as these are the distinguishing HLFs between the two activities. Encoding-based classifiers render this straightforward, as the distance from the extracted HLF to the definition of walk and between the extracted HLF to walking left is the same in all but the distinguishing HLFs. Therefore, this misclassification occurs due to the erroneous extraction in at least one of these HLFs. The following error attribution analysis is based on the encoding-based classification experiment from Sect. 4.

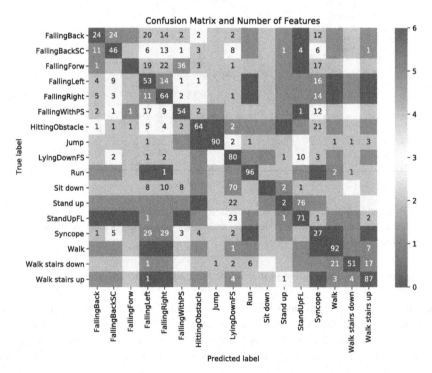

Fig. 8. Blended confusion and distance matrix for the Encoding-based classifier on the UniMiB SHAR dataset. The color indicates distance, and values indicate the percentage of cases.

Figure 9 shows the number of times a distinguishing feature was wrongly extracted during the experiment on CSL-SHARE. Distinguishing here means that this HLF value differs between the true and the predicted activity. Wrongly extracted features that are not part of the distinguishing set between the two confused activities are ignored as they did not influence the classification. The color and upper number indicate the number of times the HLF was wrongly extracted divided by the total number of these activities, while the number in brackets divides by the number of errors. That is to say, the former indicates the impact on the global accuracy while the latter indicates how many errors this HLF is partial in. Take jumping with one leg: 41% of its instances are classified as something else due to the *Back/Front* feature not being *Forward*. *Back/Front* is wrongly extracted in 95% of the cases where jumping with one leg was confused.

The two main errors on the CSL-SHARE dataset are the *Left/Right* and *Knee* HLF extractions causing walking to be misclassified in almost all instances, as well as *Back/Front* (in combination with *Force*), causing jumping with one leg to be confused with jumping with two legs.

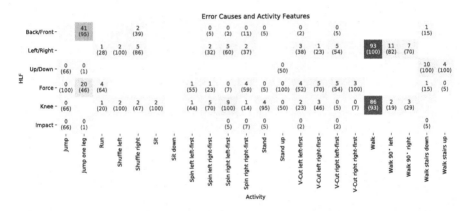

Fig. 9. Errors in activity distinguishing HLF extractors on the CSL-SHARE dataset. Color and upper value indicate the percentage of cases of all true activities. Value in brackets indicates the percentage of cases of all misclassified activities.

The walking activity is most often confused with walking in a slight curve (see Fig. 9). Figure 10 shows that in 93% of all actual walking activities, the *Left/Right* feature was incorrectly extracted and that in 100% of misclassified walks the *Left/Right* feature was incorrect. Indicating that these two features are tough to extract for this activity, which implies that either the HLF assignment needs to be reconsidered, further sensory data included, or further development of the extractor is necessary. This particular difficulty has occurred within other works [17] as well, but on a much smaller scale, meaning that clearer sensor data is likely helpful, but more importantly, the extraction and HLF assignment need to be further investigated. The confusion around jump with one leg mainly stems from the *Back/Front* feature, but *Force* also plays a role. Possibly because jumping with one leg is moving forward, but not the same way as walking is and thus is not far away from *Neutral* either, which includes jumping in place which as an activity is not far away from jumping with two legs.

Figure 10 shows the error causes on the UniMiB SHAR dataset. The leading error is that the extracted *Knee* feature in sit down does not match the defined one. Looking closer reveals multiple clusters: *Left/Right* is misclassified in most errors made on the falls. As these are mostly descriptive on the HLF assignment, this likely is a problem in the extraction being confused by the different device orientations present in the UniMiB SHAR dataset. Similarly, *Left/Right* and *Knee* are very present in the activities in and around standing and sitting. Lastly, *Up/Down* is causing problems in classifying walking down stairs, which makes sense as this is a walking-based activity and the only one in the *Down* group along with all falls with vastly different sensor data making it hard to find commonalities on how to extract these features.

6   Few-Shot Learning

Few-shot, zero-shot, and learning with imbalanced data are essential tasks in Human Activity Recognition, as many activities cannot be extensively recorded. A typical example is falling for which little or mostly simulated data exist. Nevertheless, falls are crucial to be recognized accurately. The proposed HLF extraction and classification have a significant advantage here, as data is shared across activities via the HLFs grouping.

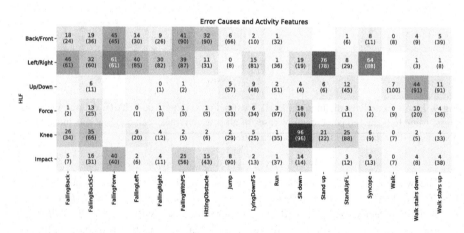

Fig. 10. Errors in activity distinguishing HLF extractors on the UniMiB SHAR dataset. Color and upper value indicate the percentage of cases of all true activities. Value in brackets indicates the percentage of cases of all misclassified activities.

6.1 Imbalanced Learning

Simulated imbalanced data experiments are adapted from our previous work and re-run in this new feature space and hyperparameters [15]. For each activity, the classifier is evaluated as in Sect. 4, except that from that activity, only a subset of randomly chosen samples is kept simulating a highly imbalanced dataset. Four metrics are recorded: the overall accuracy per fold and three low-resource activity-specific metrics. Namely, the f1 score of that activity only, the percentage of correctly extracted one-hot HLF vectors, and lastly the mean errors in HLF extraction.

The results for the imbalanced experiments are depicted in Fig. 11 and are consistently a few percentage points higher than previously reported [15]. Accordingly, while very promising further improvement in the HLF extraction across sensor data from different activities is required.

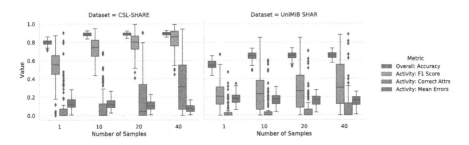

Fig. 11. Imbalanced performance on CSL-SHARE and UniMiB SHAR datasets. Averaged across 5-fold person-independent cross-validation and rotating low-resourced activity.

6.2 Few-Shot Learning

Few-Shot learning experiments investigate how little data is required to achieve good performance and if fewer than the recorded data might suffice. Similar to the imbalanced experiment, the proposed method has an advantage due to data sharing. The *Back/Front*s value *Neutral* is associated with multiple activities sensor data.

A 5-fold person-independent cross-validation is run. Similar to the imbalanced case, the training data is subsampled. Here $n \in \{1, 10, 20, 40, 80, 150, 300\}$ sequences are sampled from each activity. In the case of $n = 1$, the full feature extraction and final classification are trained on 22 (CSL-SHARE) and 17 (UniMiB SHAR) samples and evaluated on the full test split. For comparison: in the above classification experiments (see Sect. 4), 310 (CSL-SHARE) and 550 (UniMiB SHAR) training samples existed per activity per fold. Note that the UniMiB SHARE dataset is imbalanced, and some activities might already be fully present in earlier stages.

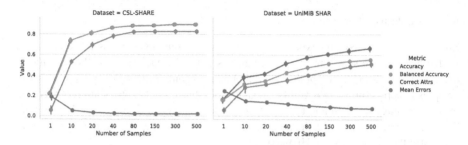

Fig. 12. Few-shot performance on CSL-SHARE and UniMiB SHAR datasets. Averaged across 5-fold person-independent cross-validation and for increasing numbers of sampled sequences.

Figure 12 shows the accuracy, balanced accuracy, the percentage of fully correct extracted HLF values, and the mean HLF extraction errors for each evaluated sampled subsets training-fold. The classifier on the CSL-SHARE dataset converges very quickly after around 40 samples per activity, while the classifier on the UniMiB SHAR dataset converges steadily after 40 samples per activity. Note that the percentage of fully correct extracted features in this experiment is calculated over all activities, while in the imbalanced experiments above, it is calculated over the activity in question alone.

The difference is stark: while in the imbalanced experiment, the median of fully extracted feature values was at a maximum of 35% (CSL-SHARE, 40 samples), in the few-shot experiment, it reached a mean of almost 80% after 40 samples while having a much lower standard deviation. Therefore, indicating a problem in feature extraction for these highly imbalanced cases. These results are encouraging for good classification performance on small datasets.

7   Dataset Combination

Sensor choices along with feature choices in HAR typically follow the specific activities that should be discriminated. Even comparing the same activity like "walking" across datasets is impossible as soon as different sensors or sensor positions were chosen. However, comparing activities across sensor setups is of high interest and supports understanding the activities as well as their modeling. The following experiment focuses on classification in this high-level feature space, comparison and design are discussed in Sect. 2, and further experiments are planned for future work.

The HLFs are by design sensor independent, allowing to combine multiple datasets in this space and, thus, enabling comparison and classification of the different activities. The transformation into the HLF space is achieved by having two dataset-dependent feature extractions with the same HLFs. The extracted and stacked vectors then have the same dimension across datasets, meaning that the activity classification step is trained on these vectors to predict the original dataset-specific activity labels. Not unlike an interpretable equivalent to swapping the first layers of a Neural Network depending on input while keeping the last layers fixed. The activity-level classification is, therefore, independent of the dataset, which means that now "V-Cuts" (CSL-SHARE) need to be distinguished from "Falls" (UniMiB SHAR). At the same time, both datasets have shared activities like "Walk" resulting in more samples compared to each individual dataset.

The following experiment combines the CSL-SHARE and UniMiB SHAR datasets in a classification experiment. It is not easy to ensure the occurrence of an activity that only exists in one dataset to be in both the training and test set but from different people in a person-independent evaluation across datasets. The main problem is an activity only occurring in the test set as is the case in zero-shot learning. Therefore, a 10-fold person-dependent stratified evaluation scheme is deployed.

The resulting 78% accuracy with both the Encoding and BRF-based HLF classifier is in the middle between the 88% on the CSL-SHARE and the 67% on the UniMiB SHAR dataset (see Sect. 4). This result is noteworthy with the scheme being person-dependent instead of person-independent.

The blended confusion matrix for the encoding-based classifier is shown in Fig. 13. The only difference for the activities occurring in only one dataset (like "FallingBack" or "Walk 90° left") is the person-dependent evaluation and, therefore, feature extraction. Accordingly, it is reasonable to attribute the better performance of falling forward/left/right, and walking 90° left/right to the evaluation scheme. Data of a person

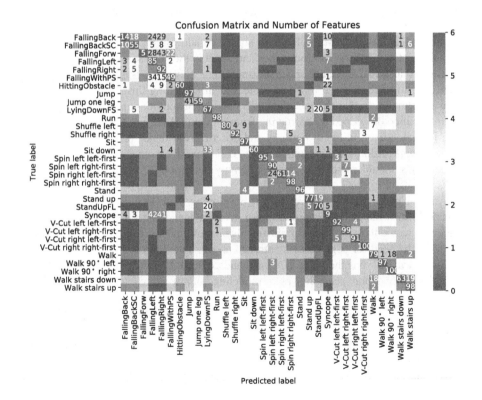

Fig. 13. Blended confusion and distance matrix for the Encoding-based classifier on the combined CSL-SHARE and UniMiB SHAR dataset. The color indicates distance, and values indicate the percentage of cases.

might be present in both train and test set, resulting in person-dependent subtleties to be picked up and included in the HLF extraction. However, it is also noteworthy that shuffle left/right, lying down from sitting, and syncope perform significantly worse. This might be due to hyperparameter settings being optimized for independence but requires further investigation. Nevertheless, some activities' misclassifications remain. Especially falling left/right and syncope remain sink states, and lying down from sitting is often confused with standing up from lying. Future work should involve both optimization and analysis of person-dependent HLF extraction and a person-independent dataset combination evaluation. For instance, by pairing participants across datasets to ensure activities in the test set are present in training prior.

This dataset combination demonstrates that combining datasets with this method is possible, which creates a foundation to find commonalities and suited features for activities across different settings.

8 Future Work

The results from the HLF extraction and the different classification experiments, on each dataset separately, imbalanced and few-shot, as well as on both datasets combined, are very encouraging and show the feasibility and possibilities with these HLFs and within this feature space. Multiple points should be addressed to improve these results, catch up to state-of-the-art performances and develop the HLF space further.

The proposed HLF feature space has more than eleven thousand unique combinations. Not all of those have to be possible, but investigating this further and naming more of them will further enhance the understanding of activities and HLFs. High-level features will be developed by borrowing from previous HAR work [27], sports knowledge [34], and even utilizing findings and criteria from dance [12] from decades of previous work. Additionally, extending the HLF to work on other datasets with different activities should ensure more robust activity definitions as well as more versatile HLFs.

Another major part for future work is developing these HLFs to return sequences of probabilities rather than compressing a given sequence into a single vector. HLF sequences would have multiple significant advantages, including online recognition and removing the need for edge cases mentioned above. Take jumping, which currently in the *Up/Down* HLF has the value *Updown*, and could then simply be first up and then down. Not only a more sensible way of modeling but also more expressive and precise over time. Similarly, the *Knee* HLF values used to indicate the starting foot would benefit from more precise time information, as this could be transformed to model which knee is in front as the more general case of the starting foot.

There are multiple challenges with extracting HLFs as sequences. The main challenges include learning the sensor data to HLF relationship, different sampling rates across datasets, and reconsidering the uniqueness property and categorical values requirement. Addressing the learning challenge, one approach could be to change the ground truth labeling from being a single value per sequence to a sequence itself. However, this labeling is a lot more time-consuming, and in cases of data recordings without videos might not even be possible. Another approach could be to develop a classifier that implicitly learns the sequence to value relationship. LSTM hidden states come to mind, but it might be hard to ensure interpretability, otherwise, the need for HLF definitions is void. The different sampling rates mainly play a role in comparison across datasets and could be addressed by re-sampling or interpolation. Classification with sequence models is not affected as much, as models like HMMs do model order over time and are not affected by different speeds of HLF changes. Furthermore, the slow nature of HLFs might counteract the sampling rates. The uniqueness property might be addressed by condensing the sequence HLFs by removing duplicates or directly calculating the Levenshtein distance, as long as the HLFs remain categorical. Extracting sequences of HLFs rather than vectors promises more expressive and precise activity definitions, and its implications and modeling requirements will be further investigated.

The HLFs might benefit from supporting ordered or even numerical HLFs in addition to categorical ones. Take the *Left/Right* HLF, which has an ordering and intensity (Extreme Left, Left, Slight Left), which a classifier might explicitly learn. Implicitly this is likely already learned via the returned probabilities. If the classifier cannot surely distinguish between *Extreme Left* and *Left*, both of these probabilities will be high, indicating the true value to be somewhere in between. Nevertheless, explicitly modeling this might further enhance the HLFs. In the same wake, it might make sense to reconsider the *N.a.* and *Any* values present in multiple HLFs.

Further investigating the learned HLF extractors and how they arrive at their predictions is another major point. One of the substantial advantages of the proposed HLFs and their extraction mechanism is the fast and knowledge-based target assignment. The main assumption is that extractors can utilize the extra information by extracting the shared commonality across different activity labels. Some classifiers might be better at this than others, and there is no restriction enforcing this currently. The classifiers might subspace the sensor data by classifying the activity and grouping, say walk and walk left. This does not change the usefulness of combing the datasets via the HLF space, as knowledge engineering still provides multiple benefits. However, the benefit will be greatly improved, especially in the few-shot and imbalanced classification experiments, the more the classifiers can extract the specific attribute.

These and other topics, including estimating a performance ceiling with neural networks and extending to further datasets and modalities, are future work for these high-level features.

9   Conclusion

High-Level Features (HLFs) are a novel way of describing human activities via unique combinations of high-level human interpretable features. The nature of HLFs being defined based on activities rather than sensor data makes the extracted features comparable and combinable across datasets with different sensor setups.

In this article, we further elaborated and extended our initial HLFs and proposed six HLFs, *Back/Front*, *Left/Right*, *Up/Down*, *Force*, *Knee*, and *Impact*. We then demonstrated how to extract these with BRFs and HMMs and showed that classification in this feature space works well in standard settings, as well as imbalanced, few-shot settings and across datasets. The feature extraction worked very well with accuracies of at least

92% (CSL-SHARE) and 68% accuracy (UniMiB SHAR) and up to 99% (CSL-SHARE) and 94% accuracy (UniMiB SHAR) in a 5-fold person-independent cross-validation. The classification experiments showed that classification in the HLF-space works very well, with 89.7% (CSL-SHARE) and 67.3% (UniMiB SHAR) accuracy. Although currently behind state-of-the-art (93.7% CSL-SHARE, 77.0% UniMiB SHAR), the results are promising and stand out due to the possibility of understanding why an error was made and to attribute it to a combination of HLF extractors. The imbalanced and few-shot learning experiments showed how sharing data between activities with multiple HLF extractors supports learning with little or imbalanced data. In the case of imbalanced data, improvements can likely be made by further investigating the feature extractors and how they partition the low-level feature space in these cases. At the same time, few-shot learning converged very quickly on the CSL-SHARE dataset and more slowly on the UniMiB SHAR dataset, only requiring 10% (CSL-SHARE) of available data to perform on par with the full data for training. Both experiments indicate that further evaluation of preprocessing techniques and classifiers to only pay attention to the correct portions of the sensor data for this particular HLF should further enhance HLF extraction. The experiment on dataset combination as well as the analysis of activity distances in the HLF-space demonstrated the usefulness for cross-sensor-setup comparison, classification, and HLF design.

The next steps are clear: extend to more datasets and reiterate the activities' definition by adjusting and reconsidering the HLF value assignments. Furthermore, neural networks and further low-level feature processing will need to be evaluated, and the actual learnings of the HLF extractors will be investigated to improve the scalability of these HLFs further. At the same time, we want to extend the HLFs to sequence modeling to enable more precise activity descriptions. All of this is to improve performance and expressive power while not losing the option for non-ML experts to understand the extracted high-level features.

Acknowledgements. Many thanks to Steffen Lahrberg for his contributions, ideas, and handcrafted feature functions in the initial paper on High-Level Features [15]. Furthermore, a large thank you to all toolboxes: SciPy [49], NumPy [14], scikit-learn [39], Matplotlib [20], Seaborn [51], TSFEL [4], and our in-house decoder BioKIT [46].

References

1. Amma, C., Gehrig, D., Schultz, T.: Airwriting recognition using wearable motion sensors. In: First Augmented Human International Conference, p. 10. ACM (2010)
2. Arifoglu, D., Bouchachia, A.: Activity recognition and abnormal behaviour detection with recurrent neural networks. Procedia Comput. Sci. **110**, 86–93 (2017)
3. Bakis, R.: Continuous speech recognition via centisecond acoustic states. J. Acoust. Soc. Am. **59**(S1), S97–S97 (1976)
4. Barandas, M., et al.: TSFEL: time series feature extraction library. SoftwareX **11**, 100456 (2020)
5. Bian, S., Liu, M., Zhou, B., Lukowicz, P.: The state-of-the-art sensing techniques in human activity recognition: a survey. Sensors **22**(12), 4596 (2022)
6. Bragança, H., Colonna, J.G., Oliveira, H.A.B.F., Souto, E.: How validation methodology influences human activity recognition mobile systems. Sensors **22**(6), 2360 (2022)

7. Bulling, A., Blanke, U., Schiele, B.: A tutorial on human activity recognition using body-worn inertial sensors. ACM Comput. Surv. (CSUR) **46**(3), 1–33 (2014)
8. Chen, C., Liaw, A., Breiman, L.: Using random forest to learn imbalanced data. Technical report (2004)
9. Deng, Z., Vahdat, A., Hu, H., Mori, G.: Structure inference machines: Recurrent neural networks for analyzing relations in group activity recognition. In: Proceedings of the IEEE Conference on Computer Vision and Pattern Recognition, pp. 4772–4781 (2016)
10. Dickinson, S.J., Leonardis, A., Schiele, B., Tarr, M.J.: Object Categorization: Computer and Human Vision Perspectives. Cambridge University Press, Cambridge (2009)
11. Ding, X., Hu, C., Xie, W., Zhong, Y., Yang, J., Jiang, T.: Device-free multi-location human activity recognition using deep complex network. Sensors **22**(16), 6178 (2022)
12. Guest, A.H.: Labanotation: Or, Kinetography Laban : the System of Analyzing and Recording Movement, no. 27. Taylor & Francis (1977). http://books.google.com/books?id=Tq1YRDuJnvYC&pgis=1
13. Ha, S., Yun, J.M., Choi, S.: Multi-modal convolutional neural networks for activity recognition. In: SMC 2015 - IEEE International Conference on Systems, Man, and Cybernetics, pp. 3017–3022. IEEE (2015)
14. Harris, C.R., et al.: Array programming with NumPy. Nature **585**(7825), 357–362 (2020)
15. Hartmann, Y., Liu, H., Lahrberg, S., Schultz, T.: Interpretable high-level features for human activity recognition. In: Proceedings of the 15th International Joint Conference on Biomedical Engineering Systems and Technologies, pp. 40–49. SCITEPRESS - Science and Technology Publications (2022)
16. Hartmann, Y., Liu, H., Schultz, T.: Feature space reduction for multimodal human activity recognition. In: Proceedings of the 13th International Joint Conference on Biomedical Engineering Systems and Technologies - Volume 4: BIOSIGNALS, pp. 135–140. INSTICC, SciTePress (2020)
17. Hartmann, Y., Liu, H., Schultz, T.: Feature space reduction for human activity recognition based on multi-channel biosignals. In: Proceedings of the 14th International Joint Conference on Biomedical Engineering Systems and Technologies, pp. 215–222. INSTICC, SciTePress (2021)
18. Hartmann, Y., Liu, H., Schultz, T.: Interactive and interpretable online human activity recognition. In: 2022 IEEE International Conference on Pervasive Computing and Communications Workshops and Other Affiliated Events (PerCom Workshops), pp. 109–111. IEEE, Pisa (2022)
19. He, K., Zhang, X., Ren, S., Sun, J.: Deep residual learning for image recognition. In: CVPR 2016 - IEEE Conference on Computer Vision and Pattern Recognition, pp. 770–778 (2016)
20. Hunter, J.D.: Matplotlib: a 2D graphics environment. Comput. Sci. Eng. **9**(3), 90–95 (2007). http://ieeexplore.ieee.org/document/4160265/
21. Inoue, M., Inoue, S., Nishida, T.: Deep recurrent neural network for mobile human activity recognition with high throughput. Artif. Life Robot. **23**(2), 173–185 (2018)
22. Keshavarzian, A., Sharifian, S., Seyedin, S.: Modified deep residual network architecture deployed on serverless framework of IoT platform based on human activity recognition application. Futur. Gener. Comput. Syst. **101**, 14–28 (2019)
23. Kwon, Y., Kang, K., Bae, C.: Analysis and evaluation of smartphone-based human activity recognition using a neural network approach. In: IJCNN 2015 - International Joint Conference on Neural Networks, pp. 1–5. IEEE (2015)
24. Lee, S.M., Yoon, S.M., Cho, H.: Human activity recognition from accelerometer data using convolutional neural network. In: BIGCOMP 2017 - IEEE International Conference on Big Data and Smart Computing, pp. 131–134. IEEE (2017)
25. Liu, H.: Biosignal processing and activity modeling for multimodal human activity recognition. Ph.D. thesis, University of Bremen (2021)

26. Liu, H., Hartmann, Y., Schultz, T.: CSL-SHARE: a multimodal wearable sensor-based human activity dataset. Front. Comput. Sci. (2021)
27. Liu, H., Hartmann, Y., Schultz, T.: Motion units: generalized sequence modeling of human activities for sensor-based activity recognition. In: EUSIPCO 2021–29th European Signal Processing Conference. IEEE (2021)
28. Liu, H., Hartmann, Y., Schultz, T.: A practical wearable sensor-based human activity recognition research pipeline. In: Proceedings of the 15th International Joint Conference on Biomedical Engineering Systems and Technologies - Volume 5: HEALTHINF, pp. 847–856 (2022)
29. Liu, H., Schultz, T.: ASK: a framework for data acquisition and activity recognition. In: Proceedings of the 11th International Joint Conference on Biomedical Engineering Systems and Technologies - Volume 3: BIOSIGNALS, pp. 262–268. INSTICC, SciTePress (2018)
30. Liu, H., Schultz, T.: A wearable real-time human activity recognition system using biosensors integrated into a knee bandage. In: Proceedings of the 12th International Joint Conference on Biomedical Engineering Systems and Technologies - Volume 1: BIODEVICES, pp. 47–55. INSTICC, SciTePress (2019)
31. Liu, H., Schultz, T.: How long are various types of daily activities? Statistical analysis of a multimodal wearable sensor-based human activity dataset. In: Proceedings of the 15th International Joint Conference on Biomedical Engineering Systems and Technologies - Volume 5: HEALTHINF, pp. 680–688 (2022)
32. Long, J., Sun, W., Yang, Z., Raymond, O.I.: Asymmetric residual neural network for accurate human activity recognition. Information 10(6), 203 (2019)
33. Lukowicz, P., et al.: Recognizing workshop activity using body worn microphones and accelerometers. In: Ferscha, A., Mattern, F. (eds.) Pervasive 2004. LNCS, vol. 3001, pp. 18–32. Springer, Heidelberg (2004). https://doi.org/10.1007/978-3-540-24646-6_2
34. Meinel, K., Schnabel, G.: Bewegungslehre - Sportmotorik: Abriß einer Theorie der sportlichen Motorik unter pädagogischem Aspekt. Meyer & Meyer Verlag, Aachen, 12, ergänzte auflage edn. (1987). https://suche.suub.uni-bremen.de/peid=B80288025
35. Micucci, D., Mobilio, M., Napoletano, P.: UniMiB SHAR: a dataset for human activity recognition using acceleration data from smartphones. Appl. Sci. 7(10), 1101 (2017)
36. Murad, A., Pyun, J.Y.: Deep recurrent neural networks for human activity recognition. Sensors 17(11), 2556 (2017)
37. Oniga, S., Sütő, J.: Human activity recognition using neural networks. In: Proceedings of the 15th International Carpathian Control Conference, pp. 403–406. IEEE (2014)
38. Ordóñez, F.J., Roggen, D.: Deep convolutional and LSTM recurrent neural networks for multimodal wearable activity recognition. Sensors 16(1), 115 (2016)
39. Pedregosa, F., et al.: Scikit-learn: machine Learning in Python. J. Mach. Learn. Res. 12(85), 2825–2830 (2011). http://jmlr.org/papers/v12/pedregosa11a.html
40. Ronao, C.A., Cho, S.B.: Human activity recognition using smartphone sensors with two-stage continuous hidden Markov models. In: ICNC 2014–10th International Conference on Natural Computation, pp. 681–686. IEEE (2014)
41. Ronao, C.A., Cho, S.B.: Human activity recognition with smartphone sensors using deep learning neural networks. Expert Syst. Appl. 59, 235–244 (2016)
42. Ronaoo, C.A., Cho, S.B.: Evaluation of deep convolutional neural network architectures for human activity recognition with smartphone sensors. J. Korean Inf. Sci. Soc. 858–860 (2015)
43. Scheirer, W.J., Anthony, S.E., Nakayama, K., Cox, D.D.: Perceptual annotation: measuring human vision to improve computer vision. IEEE Trans. Pattern Anal. Mach. Intell. 36(8), 1679–1686 (2014)
44. Singh, D., Merdivan, E., Psychoula, I., Kropf, J., Hanke, S., Geist, M., Holzinger, A.: Human activity recognition using recurrent neural networks. In: Holzinger, A., Kieseberg, P., Tjoa, A.M., Weippl, E. (eds.) CD-MAKE 2017. LNCS, vol. 10410, pp. 267–274. Springer, Cham (2017). https://doi.org/10.1007/978-3-319-66808-6_18

45. Straczkiewicz, M., James, P., Onnela, J.P.: A systematic review of smartphone-based human activity recognition methods for health research. NPJ Digit. Med. **4**(1), 148 (2021)

46. Telaar, D., et al.: BioKIT - Real-time decoder for biosignal processing. In: Proceedings of the Annual Conference of the International Speech Communication Association, INTER-SPEECH, pp. 2650–2654 (2014)

47. Tuncer, T., Ertam, F., Dogan, S., Aydemir, E., Pławiak, P.: Ensemble residual network-based gender and activity recognition method with signals. J. Supercomput. **76**(3), 2119–2138 (2020). https://doi.org/10.1007/s11227-020-03205-1

48. Uddin, M.Z., Thang, N.D., Kim, J.T., Kim, T.S.: Human activity recognition using body joint-angle features and hidden Markov model. ETRI J. **33**(4), 569–579 (2011)

49. Virtanen, P., et al.: SciPy 1.0: fundamental algorithms for scientific computing in Python. Nat. Methods **17**(3), 261–272 (2020)

50. Wang, J., Chen, Y., Hao, S., Peng, X., Hu, L.: Deep learning for sensor-based activity recognition: a survey. Pattern Recogn. Lett. **119**, 3–11 (2019)

51. Waskom, M.L.: seaborn: statistical data visualization. J. Open Sour. Softw. **6**(60), 3021 (2021)

52. Yang, J., Nguyen, M.N., San, P.P., Li, X., Krishnaswamy, S.: Deep convolutional neural networks on multichannel time series for human activity recognition. In: IJCAI, vol. 15, pp. 3995–4001. Buenos Aires, Argentina (2015)

53. Yang, S.H., Baek, D.G., Thapa, K.: Semi-supervised adversarial learning using LSTM for human activity recognition. Sensors **22**(13), 4755 (2022)

54. Youngblood, G.M., Cook, D.J.: Data mining for hierarchical model creation. IEEE Trans. Syst. Man Cybern. Part C (Appl. and Rev.) **37**(4), 561–572 (2007)

55. Zeng, M., et al.: Convolutional neural networks for human activity recognition using mobile sensors. In: MOBICASE 2014–6th International Conference on Mobile Computing, Applications and Services, pp. 197–205. IEEE (2014)

Data Augmentation Based on Virtual Wrist Devices for Fall Detection

Inês Carvalho[1], Eduarda Vaz[1], Heitor Cardoso[1,2], and Plinio Moreno[1,2(✉)] [iD]

[1] Instituto Superior Técnico, Universidade de Lisboa, 1049-001 Lisboa, Portugal
[2] Institute for Systems and Robotics, 1049-001 Lisboa, Portugal
`plinio@isr.tecnico.ulisboa.pt`

Abstract. Fall detection based on machine learning algorithms require data samples that have larger risks to gather than other similar topics such as the recognition of Activities of Daily Life (ADL). In this work we aim to detect falls using wrist devices, which have sensors such as accelerometers, gyroscopes and/or magnetometers. In this context, we aim to reduce risks and add a larger number of data samples to an existing fall detection dataset, by using simulated wrist band devices. We resort to two simulation approaches for data augmentation: (i) Virtual characters based on Motion Capture technology aimed at computer games, and (ii) fall simulation by the application of forces on an animated character. We present an evaluation of the data augmentation, which selects the real-life samples as the testing set. On the selected machine learning algorithms, k Nearest Neighbors and Decision Tree got classification improvements by using the augmented data, which shows the promising results of created samples for fall detection.

Keywords: Fall detection · Data augmentation · Wrist band devices

1 Introduction

The increase of average life expectancy, social and cultural changes have led to an increased number of autonomous elderly population that live alone, bringing social and healthcare challenges because of the difficulty of monitoring and following fall occurrences and their impact on healthcare systems and independent living [10]. Recent developments on sensing devices have brought small wearable gadgets that include sensors for fast and accurate fall detection. Wristbands and watches have accelerometers, gyroscopes and orientation sensors that provide features for robust fall detection based on Machine Learning. However, robust detection of falls based on Machine learning algorithms requires large amounts of data that covers all the possible daily activities as well as different types of realistic falls. To increase the generalization capabilities and robustness, the generation of new data samples (i.e. data augmentation) is a viable approach to improve the classification models.

Data augmentation is a common tool in machine learning, which allow classifiers to deal with bias on the dataset [12,20], reduce the difference between the distributions of the training data and the application domain data, and generalize better to small transformations on the input values [13]. In the case of vision-based fall detection, data augmentation has been applied to generate fall data with occluded regions [25]. In the case

A. C. A. Roque et al. (Eds.): BIOSTEC 2022, CCIS 1814, pp. 164–178, 2023.
https://doi.org/10.1007/978-3-031-38854-5_9

of time-series fall detection using 1-D convolutional networks, data augmentation has been used to increase robustness to shifts in the time axis and rotations in the 3D space [13]. In the context of this work, data augmentation is defined as the addition of samples based on virtual wrist devices from two sources: (i) Actors (i.e. game characters) that execute motions in a motion capture (i.e. MoCap) environment [23] and (ii) the physics-based simulation of a human body falling [6]. By adding virtual samples, we expect to: (i) Improve the overall classification performance and (ii) improve the classification on the initial (real-world) data samples. Thus, the baseline of this work corresponds to the classifiers trained with the real-world wristband data from by [17, 18], which we want to improve by adding new samples to the models. The models trained with mixed data samples from real-world and virtual wristbands are evaluated on: (i) The mixed dataset and (ii) the real-world samples.

2 Related Work

Falls are characterized by larger accelerations of the center-of-mass of a person, which motivated the most compelling fall dataset available, SisFall [22]. SisFall introduces a dataset of falls and ADLs acquired with a device attached to the waist of participants, which incorporate acceleration and gyroscope data. The dataset contains 19 types of ADLs (performed by young and elderly participants) and 15 types of falls (performed mostly by young participants). A straightforward threshold-based classifier was applied on this work, achieving up to 96% accuracy in detecting falls. However, validation testing with the elderly significantly reduced the fall detection performance of the features tested, as algorithms trained on data from young people tended to bias the thresholds upwards in amplitude. This type of result makes evident the need to include data from older people in the training phase. Several works have applied more complex machine learning algorithms on this dataset [4, 14, 21] such as Convolutional Neural Networks and Recurrent Neural Networks. Although several works have shown promising results using the SisFall dataset, its applicability to the majority of the population requires that people agree to wear the sensor on the waist. Smartwatches and wristbands are a better option, because wearing a device on the wrist is easier to agree on, and does not have the stigma of wearing a heath monitoring device [24].

Considering the future availability of multiple type of sensors in smart homes and buildings, [15] presents a dataset that considers RGB cameras, infrared sensors, and accelerometers and gyroscopes at several locations of the body of the person. The scenario is similar to the one of the SisFall dataset [22], but adds on the multiple sensors in the environment. [15] shows that the additional information of the multi-modal sensors provides better fall detection results than using single-mode sensors. In a follow-up [11] propose to detect the falls on the dataset by [15] using Neural Network architectures, which improve further the performance of fall detection. Although we aim to detect falls as well, the dataset of [15] and the fall detection of [11], their application is limited to the smart-home environment, where the computational complexity needs to be moved to a centralized server. As stated in the introduction, our application scenario considers that the only available device is a wristband device for fall detection.

Other recent approaches have placed a set of motion tracking devices, where each tracking device is composed of a 3 axis accelerometer, 3 axis gyroscope and 3 axis magnetometer. Each device is placed on a different body part (chest, waist, wrist and ankle), and the group of devices are connected via bluetooth to a smart phone. The 17 participants recruited, performed 8 ADLs and 3 types of falls [5]. The main goal of the dataset was to evaluate which body parts provide the appropriate information for fall detection. They conclude that the chest and waist locations provide the most informative motion features for fall detection [19], which corroborates the sensor placing design of SisFall dataset.

The work exposed in [17, 18] is the most recent on fall detection using only wrist devices, which is not a common configuration in the literature. For this protocol, twenty-two young adults were involved, repeating each activity three times. A total of twelve different activities were studied, where half of them are related to fall simulation and half simulate activities of daily life. After evaluating five different machine learning methods, the best result was presented by the k-NN method, resulting in 99% accuracy. In light of this result, it is shown that machine learning approaches with the proper motion decomposition are potentially capable of achieving optimal results for a fall detection system based on a wrist-worn device. The dataset and approach presented in [17, 18] is the basic building block of our approach, so we propose to augment this dataset with virtual wrist devices. The second building block of this work is the dataset presented in [23], which creates a virtual wrist device by computing accelerations at the wrist of actors. The motion of the real-life actors correspond to avatars for game characters. The virtual wrist device dataset is utilized as a challenging testing dataset. In this work we evaluate the virtual dataset in a data augmentation approach, verifying the classification improvement on the initial real-life dataset in [17, 18]. In [6] is presented another approach that aims to generate data samples of falls by using physics simulation. We consider this approach as the third building block, verifying the classification improvement on the initial real-life dataset in in [17, 18].

3   Approach

Fall detection is addressed as a binary classification problem, where fall samples are considered as the positive class. In this work, a data sample corresponds to a recorded sequence of sensor values while an user is doing an activity. The raw sensor values are 3-dimensional acceleration and 3-dimensional orientation measured on the wrist, which are utilized for feature computation.

The features for every time instant include accelerations, velocities and displacements, computed at the sensor's reference frame and at the inertial reference frame (based on the 3D orientation). The magnitude of accelerations, velocities and displacements are averaged over fixed intervals of time. In addition, vertical components of acceleration, velocity and displacement are estimated using the orientation. Finally, for each recording (i.e. data sample), mean and maximum values of the (vertical) accelerations, velocities and displacements are arranged in various configurations as input features. Those input features are fed into the following classifiers: K-nearest neighbors (KNN) [9], Linear Discriminant Analysis (LDA) [8], Decision Trees (DT) [3], Logistic Regression (LR) [2] and Support-Vector Machine (SVM) [7]. We evaluate the accuracy of the classifiers by computing the average and standard deviation of the k-fold cross-validation method. To evaluate the data augmentation approach based on virtual environments, we consider three data sources for the training set: (i) The real-life wrist sensor from [17,18], (ii) the virtual device from actors in [23] and (iii) the physics based fall simulation in [6]. We train models with augmented versions of the initial dataset. Then we evaluate the impact of data augmentation by computing classification accuracy on the real-life wrist sensor data that belongs to the testset.

3.1 Feature Computation

Raw acceleration values (X, Y and Z) are filtered using a median filter to reduce the noise. Then, we follow the same approach as in [17,18] that at each sample, computes the average value of each acceleration component over one second. The basis of all the features is then the magnitude of the filtered and averaged acceleration (i.e. Total Acceleration, TA). Finally, for each sequence the mean and maximum TA values are the basic features for each sequence to be classified.

Based on the TA values of a sequence, velocity and displacement features are computed through integration (i.e. Total Velocity, TV; and Total Displacement, TD). Similar to TA-based features, mean and maximum values are obtained for each sequence.

The 3D orientation provides the sensor orientation with respect to the earth, where usually the Z component (i.e. vertical component) corresponds to the majority of the acceleration during fall occurrences. In addition to TA, TV and TD, we obtain the vertical component of these features, adding the Vertical Acceleration (VA), Vertical Velocity (VV) and Vertical Displacement (VD) to the set of available features. The final set of features includes: TA, TV, TD, VA, VV and VD.

3.2 Classifiers

Since the feature space is low dimensional and the total number of samples of the augmented dataset is 1052, we resort to conventional machine learning algorithms that have good learning rates and work robustly on these conditions [1], such as K-nearest neighbors, Decision Trees and Logistic Regression. We also consider Linear Discriminant Analysis and Support-Vector Machine that uses the Radial Basis Function kernel.

4   Datasets

In this work we consider three sources of data: (i) The wrist-based device dataset by [17,18], (ii) the virtual dataset from characters in Unity presented in [23], and (iii) the simulated syncope and forward fall in [6]. With these three data sources we evaluate the impact of data augmentation on the wrist-based (real-life) dataset. Ideally, all models that use augmented datasets should improve the classification performance on the wrist-based (real-life) device. We consider three incremental data augmentation scenarios to evaluate the impact of our approach, where the testset across scenarios is the same: data from the real-life wrist-based device. The training set of the three scenarios are as follows: (i) Data from the real-life wrist device data, (ii) data from the real-life and unity characters, and (iii) training with samples from all datasets. We compute the classification performance on the same samples for all scenarios. We explain each source of data in the following subsections.

4.1   Wrist Device (WD) - Arduino-Based

The dataset by [18] designs a wristband based on an GY-80 device[1] connected to an Arduino UNO, which is connected by cable to a desktop computer (see Fig. 1). The data recorded during the execution of the activities includes 3D accelerations, 3D rotational velocities and 3D magnetic field information. The dataset protocol summarized in Table 1, considers Activities of Daily Life (ADL) in the non-fall class, and four types of fall.

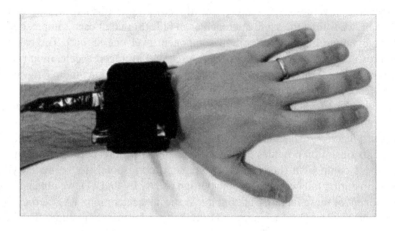

Fig. 1. Handcrafted wrist device designed in [18]. Extracted from the M.Sc. Thesis in [18].

The dataset contains various types of falls and a reduced set of non-fall activities (ADLs), which are oriented towards the elderly use-case scenario. Falls such as trip-based falls and syncope[2] falls are not considered in this dataset. In addition, other non-fall activities such workout exercises, gestures and idle are not included in this dataset.

4.2   Virtual Device from Characters in Unity (VDC)

The work presented in [23] implements an Unity environment that includes several characters from Mixamo, to generate sensor data for fall detection. For each character, a predefined motion as listed in Table 2 is executed. While the motion is executed in the Unity environment, the linear and angular motion statistics are computed for emulating the accelerometer and gyroscope. The data generated includes: (i) 3D accelerometer, (ii) 3D gyroscope and (iii) 3D orientation.

During the execution of the animation, Unity provides the pose (i.e. position x and orientation matrix A) of the wrist with respect to the world frame. Then, backward

---

[1] Referred to as Inertial Measurement Unit (IMU).
[2] Fainting due to cardiovascular abnormalities.

Table 1. Summary of activities and number of samples per class of the WD dataset [18]. Twenty two subjects participated in the recordings and each subject performed every activity three times, which yields 792 samples.

Class	Activity
Fall 18 samples/person	Forward fall
	Backward fall
	Sideways to device's side
	Sideways to no-device side
	Fall after waist clockwise rotation
	Fall after waist counterclockwise rotation
Non-fall 18 samples/person	Walking
	Clapping
	Open and close door
	Moving object
	Tying a shoe
	Sitting on chair

Table 2. Summary of activities and number of samples per class of the VDC dataset. LH denotes the character wears the device on the Left Hand and RH on the Right Hand. Total number of samples is 162.

Class	Activity	Hand
Fall 32 samples	Trip fall	11 LH, 11 RH
	Syncope fall	5 LH, 5 RH
Non-fall 130 samples	Workout exercises	13 LH, 13 RH
	Daily Living exercises	6 LH, 6 RH
	Gestures	11 LH, 11 RH
	Walking	15 LH, 15 RH
	Idle	20 LH, 20 RH

differences are computed to obtain the linear velocity ($\mathbf{v}$), linear acceleration ($\mathbf{a}$) and angular velocity (ω):

$$\mathbf{v}(t) = \frac{\Delta \mathbf{x}(t)}{\Delta t} \tag{1}$$

$$\mathbf{a}(t) = \frac{\Delta \mathbf{v}(t)}{\Delta t} \tag{2}$$

$$\omega(t) = \frac{\Delta \mathbf{A}}{\Delta t} \mathbf{A}. \tag{3}$$

The finite differences in Eqs. (1-3) provide the sensor values for each animated character.

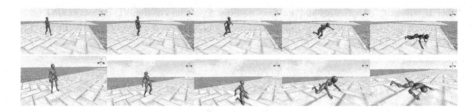

Fig. 2. Visualization of the sequence of frames of VDC fall types in [23]. The top row shows the character during a trip fall and the bottom row shows the character during the syncope fall.

Regarding the falling class, in [23] are considered two new types of falls: Trip and syncope. Pictures from the animated characters for these type of falls are shown in Fig. 2. Regarding the non-falling class, the ADLs considered are as follows:

- Workout Exercises: Air squats, burpee, running, jumping jacks, Frisbee throw, dribble
- Gestures: pointing, praying, waving, writing, handshake
- Idle: Bored balancing while stand, idle stand, idle sit, idle talking on the phone, idle laying
- Walking: Walking with a walker, walking forward, walking backward, walking and turn 180, walking injured
- Daily Living Exercises: Crouch to stand, stairs ascending and descending, standing up

Table 2 summarizes the Unity dataset classes and its corresponding activities per class. The dataset is parsed into a JSON [16] file that contains the simulated sensor values and their corresponding activity type and class label for all the 162 samples.

4.3 Virtual Device from Simulations in Unity (VDS)

The dataset in [23] has more non-falling samples that fall samples, which creates a bias on the machine learning models. To balance the dataset and include another approach to generate fall samples, we include data generated from the physics simulation approach presented in [6].

The work in [6] focuses on forward and syncope falls on a humanoid that has the limb sizes and motion limitations of an average elderly person. The fall simulation starts with an prerecorded motion of the limbs (i.e. animation) that is not affected by the physics engine up until the fall event occurs (See example in Fig. 3). In the case of a forward fall, right after there is any collision with the humanoid, the animation is deactivated and the physics engine is activated. Then, a force is applied on the trunk element and after few milliseconds upward forces are applied on the arms. In the case of a syncope fall, the humanoid is executing one of several ADLs, and at some point the animation is deactivated and the physics engine is activated. Then, a small forward force is applied to the humanoid. In order to have variations on the behavior and the sensor measurements, random variations of the force magnitude and orientation (i.e. noise) are added to the applied forces. Similarly to [23], the simulated sensor values

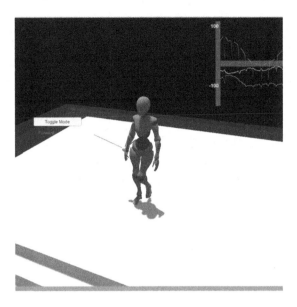

Fig. 3. Visualization of the simulation environment presented in [6]. In the screenshot, the humanoid is executing the walking animation, and when the stairs cause the fall, the physics engine will start to act.

of acceleration are estimated by finite differences. We modified the output of the simulator to store the orientation values, which allow to compute vertical components of acceleration, velocity and displacement.

5   Experiments

In the experiments presented in [23] and [6], the goal is to use the generated data samples as the testing set. This approach aims to verify the generalization properties of the models trained with real-life samples and the plausibility of using the generated samples as data with distribution shift[3]. In both works they obtain accuracy values similar between the created samples and the real-life ones, showing that the generated data can be used as another testing set. In this work we aim to evaluate the generated data as part of a data augmentation approach, where we want to develop models that improve the classification accuracy on the initial real-life samples. To evaluate this approach, we compute the classification scores on the testset of the WD dataset [17]. As training samples, we have three incremental setups: (i) Using only the WD data samples [17], (ii) using WD and VDC data samples [23] and (iii) using WD, VDC and VDS [6].

The evaluation measures include accuracy, sensitivity (i.e. true positive rate) and specificity (i.e. true negative rate). In the case of fall detection the ideal target is not missing the occurrence of a fall event (i.e. highest sensitivity). If we have competing algorithms with similar accuracy, we prefer the approach with higher sensitivity. The

---

[3] Samples that are not close to the training samples in the feature space.

feature sets and their corresponding classifiers used in [17], are summarized in Table 3. The selected features correspond to the best accuracy result. We also consider the complete set of features, to have a better view of the classification trends with the augmented datasets.

Table 3. Feature sets and classifiers from [17].

Feature set	Classifier
VA, VV, VD	k-NN
TA, VA, TV	LDA
VA, TV	LR
VA, TV	DT
VA, TV	SVM
TA, TV, TD, VA, VV, VD	All features

We follow the k-fold cross-validation method to evaluate the deviations from the average values of accuracy, sensitivity and specificity as shown in Table 4.

5.1   Baseline Model and Results from [23]

Table shows the classification results presented in [23]. The best model is the DT classifier with Vertical Acceleration and Total Velocity as features, considering its high mean accuracy and sensitivity values while having a low deviation from the corresponding means. Following DT, we have SVM and LDA with similar accuracy values, but SVM has a higher sensitivity.

Table 4. Evaluation of different machine learning methods for [17] dataset. Sensitivity (Sens.), Specificity (Spec.) and Accuracy (Acc.) results. These results were previously presented in [23].

Algorithm	Sens. (%)	Spec. (%)	Acc. (%)
k-NN	$92,66 \pm 4,03$	$84,32 \pm 7,06$	$88,02 \pm 4,60$
LDA	$91,68 \pm 4,33$	$\mathbf{93,94 \pm 3,42}$	$92,05 \pm 3,41$
LR	$89,04 \pm 4,17$	$93,48 \pm 3,11$	$90,65 \pm 2,62$
DT	$92,93 \pm 3,35$	$93,16 \pm 3,65$	$\mathbf{93,06 \pm 2,13}$
SVM	$\mathbf{93,91 \pm 4,28}$	$90,39 \pm 4,56$	$92,05 \pm 2,93$

To verify the variance of the classification result with respect to the selection of the k-fold sets, we run the same experiment shown in Table 4, but changing the sets for the k-fold cross-validation. We expect to have a similar accuracy values and ordering of the classification algorithms. In Table 5 we observe a small decrease (between 1% and 2%)

Table 5. Evaluation of different machine learning methods for [17] dataset. Sensitivity (Sens.), Specificity (Spec.) and Accuracy (Acc.) results.

Algorithm	Sens. (%)	Spec. (%)	Acc. (%)
k-NN	88,12 ± 5,77	83,49 ± 4,92	85,97 ± 3,96
LDA	82,20 ± 6,01	**94,58 ± 4,12**	88,38 ± 3,54
LR	87,47 ± 5,15	93,05 ± 4,63	90,39 ± 2,91
DT	91,25 ± 3,01	91,23 ± 3,41	**91,41 ± 1,94**
SVM	**92,29 ± 3,40**	89,24 ± 4,96	90,90 ± 2,72

in all the performance metrics, and the best accuracy is obtained with the DT algorithm. Best specificity is obtained with LDA and best sensitivity with SVM. Thus, the results are consistent but with a decreased performance.

In addition, the best classifier (using the WD data) of each cross-validation test shown in Tables 4-5 was selected to run on the testing set on the VDC dataset. To obtain more comprehensive results, we run all the models for all the cross-validation sets, which are shown in Table 6 along with the results presented previously in [23]. We note that the best performance is obtained with the k-NN algorithm (using VA, VV and VD features), having the best sensitivity, specificity and accuracy. The main difference with the best selected classifier k-NN is the specificity, which was not good on the previous results but in the k-fold test shows better average values.

Table 6. Results after applying the machine learning models obtained by training with the WD [17] dataset and testing on the VDC dataset. Sensitivity (Sens.), Specificity (Spec.) and Accuracy (Acc.) results. On each cell the left hand side result corresponds to the best model from the cross-validation that was previously presented in [23]. On the right hand side the average of running the test for all the models from the cross-validation sets.

Algorithm	Sens. (%)	Spec. (%)	Acc. (%)
k-NN	**100 (95,41 ± 10,28)**	64,62 (**75,46 ± 10,86**)	71,61 (**82,87 ± 8,45**)
LDA	40,63 (80,01 ± 1,50)	63,08 (40,03 ± 20,31)	58,64 (34,66 ± 13,83)
LR	90,63 (85,01 ± 15,50)	35,39 (25,01 ± 10,50)	46,30 (33,44 ± 13,03)
DT	53,13 (89,71 ± 25,46)	**77,69** (41,94 ± 23,83)	**72,84** (42,34 ± 29,85)
SVM	68,75 (42,34 ± 25,97)	66,15 (52,68 ± 23,87)	66,66 (39,75 ± 17,50)

5.2 Data Augmentation Tests - Testing Set from WD Data

In this set of experiments, we follow the k-fold cross-validation approach and show the classification results just on the VD testing set (i.e. part of the VD data that belongs to the testing set on that k-fold partition). We conducted tests using five different classifiers (K-NN, LDA, LR, DT and SVM), and using two types of features: (i) The selected features for each classifier as shown in Table 3 and (ii) all the features as shown on the last row of Table 3. We want to evaluate if the same classification trends apply for these two types of features.

Table 7 shows the results of the k-NN algorithm. Note that by adding the VDC dataset (WD + VDC), average sensitivity improves while the standard deviation decreases. In addition, accuracy improves or maintain similar values to WD while the standard deviation decreases. Thus, adding the VCD data to WD data brings improvements on classifying the real-life data of WD, which shows that we can add the data of the virtual device to improve the classification on the real-life data. By adding the VDS dataset, we observe a different result for each type of features: (i) On selected features, accuracy reduces slightly (i.e. almost constant), sensitivity reduces and specificity has a slight increase, and (ii) on all features, sensitivity increases, specificity reduces and accuracy reduces. In general, we see that adding the virtual data brings less variance to the classifier while keeping the classification accuracy at similar values.

Table 7. Classification results of the **K-nearest neighbors** (k-NN) algorithm obtained by using three different training sets (WD [17], VDC [23] and VDS [6]) and one test set (WD [17]). Sensitivity (Sens.), Specificity (Spec.) and Accuracy (Acc.) results.

Features	Training Dataset	Sens. (%)	Spec. (%)	Acc. (%)
VA,VV,VD	WD + VDC + VDS	88,65 ± 5,09	84,60 ± 3,00	86,74 ± 2,49
	WD + VDC	89,33 ± 4,75	84,35 ± 2,13	86,81 ± 2,39
	WD	88,13 ± 5,77	83,49 ± 4,92	85,97 ± 3,96
All	WD + VDC + VDS	93,23 ± 2,16	86,27 ± 3,69	89,84 ± 2,02
	WD + VDC	93,02 ± 3,18	87,38 ± 5,91	90,25 ± 3,36
	WD	92,55 ± 3,20	87,71 ± 7,73	90,28 ± 4,34

Table 8 shows the results of the Decision Tree (DT) algorithm. The DT classifier attains a very good performance with accuracy, sensibility and specificity around the 90%. We observe a similar trend to the k-NN classifier, where the WD+VDC models bring improvements with respect to WD. In difference to k-NN classifier, the standard deviation increases. By adding the VDS dataset, the classification variance is slightly reduced as well as the accuracy. In general, we see that adding the virtual data brings less variance to the classifier while keeping the classification accuracy at similar values, which is the same trend as the k-NN classifier.

Table 9 shows the results of the SVM classifier. In general, the addition of virtual data samples causes a performance drop around 3%, and an increase of the classification variance. In this case, the kernel parameters were not changed across experiments, which shows that extensive search of the RBF kernel parameters is needed to improve the performance using the augmented datasets.

Table 10 shows the results of the LDA algorithm. The addition of VDC data reduces by a large margin the classification metrics (5%-6%) on the WD dataset. The VDC data reduces the specificity by a large margin, which means that linear separation of

Table 8. Classification results of the **Decision Tree** (DT) algorithm obtained by using three different training sets (WD [17], VDC [23] and VDS [6]) and one test set (WD [17]). Sensitivity (Sens.), Specificity (Spec.) and Accuracy (Acc.) results.

Features	Training Dataset	Sens. (%)	Spec. (%)	Acc. (%)
VA,TV	WD + VDC + VDS	89,41 ± 4,75	90,24 ± 3,58	89,75 ± 2,83
	WD + VDC	91,29 ± 4,15	92,46 ± 3,12	91,95 ± 3,11
	WD	91,26 ± 3,01	91,23 ± 3,41	91,42 ± 1,94
All	WD + VDC + VDS	89,62 ± 4,46	91,24 ± 2,90	90,21 ± 1,99
	WD + VDC	89,94 ± 3,27	91,65 ± 2,02	90,78 ± 2,02
	WD	90,46 ± 6,02	90,54 ± 3,79	90,65 ± 3,22

Table 9. Classification results of the **Support Vector Machine** (SVM) algorithm obtained by using three different training sets (WD [17], VDC [23] and VDS [6]) and one test set (WD [17]). Sensitivity (Sens.), Specificity (Spec.) and Accuracy (Acc.) results.

Features	Training Dataset	Sens. (%)	Spec. (%)	Acc. (%)
VA,TV	WD + VDC + VDS	89,11 ± 3,32	86,21 ± 4,87	87,61 ± 2,60
	WD + VDC	90,80 ± 5,08	84,54 ± 5,19	87,69 ± 3,62
	WD	92,29 ± 3,40	89,24 ± 4,97	90,90 ± 2,72
All	WD + VDC + VDS	88,25 ± 5,79	87,18 ± 4,26	87,77 ± 3,45
	WD + VDC	90,32 ± 4,57	83,97 ± 4,32	87,19 ± 2,79
	WD	93,40 ± 3,84	89,24 ± 4,71	91,40 ± 3,21

Table 10. Classification results of the **Linear Discriminant Analysis** (LDA) algorithm obtained by using three different training sets (WD [17], VDC [23] and VDS [6]) and one test set (WD [17]). Sensitivity (Sens.), Specificity (Spec.) and Accuracy (Acc.) results.

Features	Training Dataset	Sens. (%)	Spec. (%)	Acc. (%)
TA, VA,TV	WD + VDC + VDS	85,18 ± 5,99	81,84 ± 4,29	83,60 ± 2,68
	WD + VDC	79,90 ± 5,25	82,79 ± 4,54	81,29 ± 2,40
	WD	82,20 ± 6,01	94,58 ± 4,12	88,38 ± 3,54
All	WD + VDC + VDS	82,70 ± 6,77	85,12 ± 3,78	84,04 ± 4,05
	WD + VDC	80,32 ± 5,62	84,46 ± 4,42	82,39 ± 2,99
	WD	81,17 ± 4,27	94,07 ± 4,42	87,62 ± 3,50

the augmented dataset is more difficult. Nevertheless, the addition of VDS samples increases the performance by 2%.

Table 11 shows the results of the LR algorithm. In this case is clear the performance decrease after adding the virtual wrist devices from VDC and VDS (around 12% for selected features and around 8% for all features). It is also clear that adding the VDS dataset brings improvements, which are larger on the selected features case and very

Table 11. Classification results of the **Logistic Regression** (LR) algorithm obtained by using three different training sets (WD [17], VDC [23] and VDS [6]) and one test set (WD [17]). Sensitivity (Sens.), Specificity (Spec.) and Accuracy (Acc.) results.

Features	Training Dataset	Sens. (%)	Spec. (%)	Acc. (%)
VA,TV	WD + VDC + VDS	83,34 ± 6,69	80,64 ± 5,87	82,01 ± 4,50
	WD + VDC	75,75 ± 4,19	81,92 ± 6,75	78,88 ± 3,60
	WD	87,48 ± 5,15	93,05 ± 4,64	90,40 ± 2,91
All	WD + VDC + VDS	79,97 ± 5,50	84,88 ± 3,79	82,61 ± 2,80
	WD + VDC	79,64 ± 5,68	84,94 ± 4,52	82,28 ± 3,40
	WD	87,38 ± 3,43	93,01 ± 4,76	90,27 ± 2,55

small on the all-features case. In general, the data augmentation procedure does not improve the results of the LR algorithm, assuming the same set of parameters.

6 Conclusions

Considering the risks involved in recording datasets for fall detection, we propose an approach to evaluate data augmentation for fall detection, based on data generated from virtual wrist devices. Previous works have addressed the creation of data from virtual environments and simulations, but their application is limited to use the generated samples as a testing set. In this work we go further, by including the generated samples on the training set, which is a type of data augmentation. We evaluate the data augmentation by computing the classification scores on the initial real-life data samples. Our goal is to verify the impact of the new created samples on the classification scores of the real-life data samples. On the one hand, we observe that for k-NN and DT classifiers, the addition of the created samples have a positive effect on the classification scores, either by improving the average scores and/or reducing the variances. This is a very good result, because this created data samples can be added to existing classifiers without any extra effort. On the other hand, we observe that for SVM, LR and LDA, the addition of the created samples reduces the average scores most of the times. On the case of these three classifiers, an extra step of parameter tunning would be needed in order to improve the classification scores with the added samples. Future work should consider joining multiple real-life existing datasets (e.g. [5, 15, 17]) with the virtual ones (e.g. [6, 23]).

Acknowledgements. This publication has been partially funded by the project LARSyS - FCT Project UIDB/50009/2020 and the project and by the project IntelligentCare - Intelligent Multimorbidity Management System (Reference LISBOA-01-0247-FEDER-045948), which is cofinanced by the ERDF - European Regional Development Fund through the Lisbon Portugal Regional Operational Program - LISBOA 2020 and by the Portuguese Foundation for Science and Technology - FCT under CMU Portugal

References

1. Adadi, A.: A survey on data-efficient algorithms in big data era. J. Big Data **8**(1), 1–54 (2021)
2. Berkson, J.: Application of the logistic function to bio-assay. J. Am. Stat. Assoc. **39**(227), 357–365 (1944)
3. Breiman, L., Friedman, J.H., Olshen, R.A., Stone, C.J.: Classification and regression trees. Routledge (2017)
4. Casilari, E., Lora-Rivera, R., García-Lagos, F.: A study on the application of convolutional neural networks to fall detection evaluated with multiple public datasets. Sensors **20**(5), 1466 (2020)
5. Casilari, E., Santoyo-Ramón, J.A., Cano-García, J.M.: Umafall: a multisensor dataset for the research on automatic fall detection. Procedia Comput. Sci. **110**, 32–39 (2017). 14th International Conference on Mobile Systems and Pervasive Computing (MobiSPC 2017) / 12th International Conference on Future Networks and Communications (FNC 2017)/Affiliated Workshops
6. Collado-Villaverde, A., Cobos, M., Muñoz, P., Barrero, D.F.: A simulator to support machine learning-based wearable fall detection systems. Electronics **9**(11), 1831 (2020)
7. Cortes, C., Vapnik, V.: Support-vector networks. Mach. Learn. **20**(3), 273–297 (1995)
8. Fisher, R.A.: The use of multiple measurements in taxonomic problems. Ann. Eugen. **7**(2), 179–188 (1936)
9. Fix, E., Hodges, J.J.: Discriminatory analysis. nonparametric discrimination: consistency properties. Technical report, University of California, Berkeley (1951)
10. Fuster, V.: Changing demographics: a new approach to global health care due to the aging population (2017)
11. Galvão, Y.M., Ferreira, J., Albuquerque, V.A., Barros, P., Fernandes, B.J.: A multimodal approach using deep learning for fall detection. Expert Syst. Appl. **168**, 114226 (2021)
12. Jaipuria, N., et al.: Deflating dataset bias using synthetic data augmentation. In: Proceedings of the IEEE/CVF Conference on Computer Vision and Pattern Recognition (CVPR) Workshops (2020)
13. Kraft, D., Srinivasan, K., Bieber, G.: Deep learning based fall detection algorithms for embedded systems, smartwatches, and IoT devices using accelerometers. Technologies **8**(4), 72 (2020)
14. Luna-Perejón, F., Domínguez-Morales, M.J., Civit-Balcells, A.: Wearable fall detector using recurrent neural networks. Sensors **19**(22), 4885 (2019)
15. Martínez-Villaseñor, L., Ponce, H., Brieva, J., Moya-Albor, E., Núñez-Martínez, J., Peñafort-Asturiano, C.: Up-fall detection dataset: a multimodal approach. Sensors **19**(9), 1988 (2019)
16. Pezoa, F., Reutter, J.L., Suarez, F., Ugarte, M., Vrgoč, D.: Foundations of JSON schema. In: Proceedings of the 25th International Conference on World Wide Web, pp. 263–273. International World Wide Web Conferences Steering Committee (2016)
17. de Quadros, T., Lazzaretti, A.E., Schneider, F.K.: A movement decomposition and machine learning-based fall detection system using wrist wearable device. IEEE Sens. J. **18**(12), 5082–5089 (2018)
18. Quadros, T., et al.: Development and evaluation of an elderly fall detection system based on a wearable device located at wrist. Master's thesis, Universidade Tecnológica Federal do Paraná (2017)
19. Santoyo-Ramón, J.A., Casilari, E., Cano-García, J.M.: Analysis of a smartphone-based architecture with multiple mobility sensors for fall detection with supervised learning. Sensors **18**(4), 1155 (2018)
20. Shorten, C., Khoshgoftaar, T.M.: A survey on image data augmentation for deep learning. J. Big Data **6**(1), 1–48 (2019)

21. Sucerquia, A., López, J.D., Vargas-Bonilla, J.F.: Real-life/real-time elderly fall detection with a triaxial accelerometer. Sensors **18**(4), 1101 (2018)
22. Sucerquia, A., López, J.D., Vargas-Bonilla, J.F.: SisFall: a fall and movement dataset. Sensors **17**(1), 198 (2017)
23. Vaz., E., Cardoso., H., Moreno., P.: Evaluation of fall detection approaches based on virtual devices: leveraging on motion capture data in unity environments. In: Proceedings of the 15th International Joint Conference on Biomedical Engineering Systems and Technologies - BIOSIGNALS, pp. 50–56. INSTICC, SciTePress (2022)
24. Wang, H., Tao, D., Yu, N., Qu, X.: Understanding consumer acceptance of healthcare wearable devices: an integrated model of UTAUT and TTF. Int. J. Med. Inform. **139**, 104156 (2020)
25. Zhao, Y., Gao, Y., Zhai, J., Li, D.: A data augmentation strategy for skeleton-based fall detection. In: 2021 China Automation Congress (CAC), pp. 7188–7193 (2021)

Propagation of Response Signals Registered in *EEG* Under Photostimulation

S. Bozhokin ⓘ, I. Suslova$^{(\boxtimes)}$ ⓘ, and D. Tarakanov

Peter the Great Polytechnic University, Polytechnicheskaya Str,29, Saint-Petersburg, Russia
ibsus@mail.ru

Abstract. The electroencephalogram of the brain (*EEG*) is considered as a set of electrical activity bursts generated by neuronal ensembles. Each *EEG* burst is modeled as a superposition of elementary non-stationary signals (*ENS*). The advantage of this model is in the possibility to obtain analytical results by using the continuous wavelet transform (*CWT*). A model of a biological medium is proposed taking into account the dispersion phenomenon. The dispersion leads to the fact that a wave disturbance of an arbitrary shape (*EEG* burst) undergoes changes as it propagates through the certain medium. Using the Debye model of the dielectric permittivity of a biological medium, an expression for changing the shape of a burst propagating in the brain is found. For a group of subjects exposed to photostimulation with different frequencies, we calculated the frequency composition, times of occurrence and velocities of *EEG* bursts moving along the cerebral cortex. To process *EEG*, the continuous wavelet transform and techniques for analyzing spectral integrals are used.

Keywords: *EEG* bursts · Continuous wavelet transform · Brain · photostimulation

1 Introduction

The traditional and most common non-invasive method for studying the electrical activity of the brain is the recording of an electroencephalogram (*EEG*) signal [1–5] from many channels of a cerebral cortex in various spectral ranges. It is known that the *EEG* recording is the essentially non-stationary signal [1–6]. Even at rest, in the absence of any external stimuli, we observe numerous temporary bursts that form certain patterns of oscillatory activity.

The structure of the *EEG* represents different forms of oscillatory patterns associated with the electrical activity of neuronal ensembles and reflecting the functional states of the brain [7–9]. The work [10] shows that the amplitude, temporal, and spatial characteristics of segments of neural activity indicate the rate of formation, lifetime, and decay rate of neural ensembles. According to [10], the duration of quasi-stationary segments of alpha activity is approximately 300–350 ms, depending on the channel. This value is approximately three times more than the characteristic period of alpha oscillations of 100 ms (10 Hz). This estimate indicates a strong non-stationarity of *EEG* signal. Such

A. C. A. Roque et al. (Eds.): BIOSTEC 2022, CCIS 1814, pp. 179–198, 2023.
https://doi.org/10.1007/978-3-031-38854-5_10

a non-stationary *EEG* signal recorded from each brain channel can be represented as a system of bursts, each of which is characterized by its time of appearance, duration, and the behavior of the local frequency in a certain spectral range [11, 12]. Even at rest, the *EEG* shows numerous temporal bursts. These spontaneous changes in the electrical activity of neural ensembles can be associated with the processes of their synchronization and desynchronization, which, in turn, can be caused by the peculiarities of the mental state of each subject [13].

Multichannel *EEG* recordings show travelling of electrical activity maxima along different trajectories. This movement can be interpreted as a wave propagation in a certain direction along the cerebral cortex [14–20]. In {20] the wave trajectories in the range of α-rhythm originating mainly in the frontal or occipital region are calculated. The trajectories of these waves always cross the central areas of the brain. The characteristic velocity of such waves is 2.1 ± 0.29 m/s.

Traveling waves can perform many functions, reflecting the internal state of the brain or responses to external stimuli [20–23]. In [18] the study of memory mechanisms identified traveling waves at different frequencies for different electrode configurations in a wide frequency range (from 2 to 15 Hz). It has been shown that traveling waves propagate mainly from the posterior to anterior regions of the brain [18, 24].

Cognitive processes are accompanied by the transformation of neural ensembles into smaller and more stable micro-ensembles of local synchronization [10, 25]. It is believed that high-frequency oscillations in the range of β - rhythm, which are a reflection of cognitive processes, are determined by the synchronous activity of relatively small neural ensembles [10, 25]. In the low-frequency range, large neural ensembles are involved in the oscillatory process [13, 26]. A short-term increase in the correlation of signals from different channels indicates the synchronization of activity in the corresponding areas of the cerebral cortex. Such an increase indicates the establishment of functional connections in the brain necessary for solving certain problems [27].

One of the most difficult tasks in *EEG* processing is to determine the spatial and temporal localization of sources of neuron activity from signals recorded on the outer surface of the skull. Such a problem belongs to inverse problems of mathematical physics [1, 28, 29]. Even in the case of the most simplified model of sources in the form of electric dipoles located in a homogeneous sphere, the problem does not have a unique solution. The problems of restoring activity sources from experimental data and ways to solve them are considered in the works [30, 31].

When solving any problems of wave propagation caused by the electrical activity of the brain, the problem of modeling the medium of propagation arises. This requires additional anatomical information that can be obtained using *MRI* or *CT* [32]. The wave pattern is distorted when waves pass through the bones of the skull, skin, and other conductive media [28, 33, 34]. The real topology of the cortex is individual and has a complex structure with a large number of convolutions and furrows. In addition, it is necessary to take into account the anisotropy of brain conductivity [35, 36]. Thus, modeling the medium of wave propagation is a separate problem to properly mapping the trajectories of disturbances in the cerebral cortex.

The properties of the wave propagation medium can lead to the appearance of a time delay as a reaction of the medium to a wave disturbance (temporal dispersion), or cause the influence of neighboring points on the process in a given point in the space (spatial dispersion) [37–39].

Travelling waves (*TW*) velocities in various spectral ranges are calculated in [40], and it is shown that, on average, alpha waves are faster than theta waves: 6.5 ± 0.9 m/s for alpha waves and 4.0 ± 0.9 m/s for theta waves, with the ratio between them 1.6 ± 0.5. That is, waves of higher frequency propagate faster than waves of lower frequency, which is generally consistent with the study [41]. According to the theory of diffuse signal transmission through the nervous tissue [35, 42], the pathway consists of many fibers with different conduction velocities. *TW* are associated with switching activity of various brain centers [41]. With each such switch, a burst of neuronal activity, being compact at the beginning, stretches in time and decreases in amplitude due to the dispersion of the medium. The phase velocities of each configuration of waves in the cerebral cortex significantly depend on the dispersion of the medium, which can lead to variations in the time of arrival of certain types of disturbances at fixed points of the cortex associated with the location of the recording electrodes. In theoretical terms, if we consider a wave pattern as some bursts of activity moving along the cerebral cortex, characterized by certain dissipative properties, then the effect of temporal dispersion on the velocity and shape of wave patterns will be determined by the properties of the mathematical model of each burst [11] and the type of dispersion relation.

The temporal characteristics of the response to a rhythmic visual stimulus can characterize the features of *TW* propagation in a dispersive medium. Mathematical analysis of *EEG* recordings during photostimulation in [43, 44] gives the times of assimilation and forgetting of rhythms, as well as the times characterizing the delay of the *EEG* signal relative to the flashes of photostimulation signal.

The functional connections in the brain are dynamically formed and rebuilt in different parts of the brain during the performance of cognitive tasks, under the influence of external stimuli, and even at rest [45–48]. Registration of data on the electrical activity of the brain in the form of non-stationary *EEG* signals or time series makes it possible to study functional relationships using various methods [21]. The most well-known methods to study the relationship between the activity of different parts of the brain in different spectral ranges are: spectral methods (the fast Fourier transform; wavelet transform [11, 12, 18, 40, 43]; method of informational entropy (mutual information) [49]-[51]; neural network methods [52–55]. It should be noted that the wavelet transform has undoubted advantages over the method of the windowed (fast) Fourier transform due to the absence of the need to select the window width. As a rule, the selection of the window width requires preliminary information about the properties of the signal, which is a separate task.

The present work involves the study of the velocity and direction of electrical activity waves in the cerebral cortex during photostimulation. The method to study the changes in the form and rhythmic structure of brain activity patterns is based on multilevel modeling: representing the *EEG* signal as a system of Gaussian-type signals and considering the brain as a biological dissipative medium with time dispersion. The bursts of activity recorded in *EEG* channels are modeled by the superposition of elementary non-stationary signals (*ENS*) [11]. In [12] the model of *EEG* bursts as a nonlinear approximation of Gaussian peaks moving at certain velocities in certain directions was used to map brain activity waves travelling in the cerebral cortex. In the work [12], the spontaneous *EEG* of a healthy subject at rest was processed. No specific properties of the brain as a medium of wave propagation were assumed in [12]. The present article introduces brain model as a special wave propagation medium by setting its dispersion properties. The main difference between this work and [12] is that we use photostimulation to analyze the propagation of *TW* along the cerebral cortex. Mathematical techniques of the continuous wavelet transform (*CWT*) with the Morlet mother wavelet function applied in this article allow us to study correctly the rhythm assimilation processes and calculate the velocities of *EEG* bursts propagation. The use of the proposed models together with the wavelet transform makes it possible to obtain analytical results and compare them with numerical results.

2 Dispersion Phenomenon in the Propagation of Disturbances in Biological Media

Wave dispersion is a phenomenon associated with the difference in phase velocity V_p and group velocity V_g of signals depending on their wavelength λ or wave vector k ($\lambda = 2\pi/k$). The dispersion of waves leads to the fact that a wave disturbance of an arbitrary shape undergoes changes as it propagates. To describe the dispersion, the so-called dispersion equation is introduced, which is the dependence of the wave frequency $\omega\left(\vec{k}\right)$ on the wave vector $\vec{k}$. In an isotropic medium, in which there is no dependence on the direction of wave propagation, the dispersion equation is simplified, and the angular frequency $\omega(k)$ of the wave depends only on the modulus of the wave vector. Knowing the dispersion relation $\omega(k)$, one can find the dependence of phase velocity $V_p = \omega/k$ and group velocity $V_g = \frac{d\omega}{dk}$ on frequency or wavelength. Wave dispersion is related either to the presence of a time delay in the reaction of the medium to a wave disturbance (temporal dispersion), or to an influence of neighboring points on a fixed point in space (spatial dispersion) [37, 56–58].

The purpose of this section is to study analytically the change in shape of an elementary non-stationary signal (*ENS*) $Z_L(t)$ [11]

$$Z_L(t) = \frac{b_L}{2\sqrt{\pi}\,\tau_L} exp\left[-\frac{(t-t_L)^2}{4\tau_L^2}\right] cos\left[2\pi f_L(t-t_L) + \alpha_L\right], \tag{1}$$

propagating in a dissipative biological medium (*DBM*) with temporal dispersion. This signal (1) in the absence of dispersion has the form of a harmonic oscillation with the Gaussian envelope. The superposition of such *ENS* (1) can serve as a mathematical model of brain activity bursts [11]. Elementary non-stationary signal (*ENS*) is characterized by five quantity parameters: amplitude b_L, harmonic oscillation frequency f_L, phase α_L, time localization of the center $t = t_L$, and time duration τ_L. The Fourier image $\overline{Z}_L(\omega)$ of (1) takes the form

$$\overline{Z}_L(\Omega) = \frac{1}{2}b_L exp\left(-\frac{i\Omega t_L}{\tau_L}\right)\left\{exp\left[-(\Omega-\Omega_L)^2 + i\alpha_L\right] + exp\left[-(\Omega+\Omega_L)^2 - i\alpha_L\right]\right\}, \tag{2}$$

where $\Omega = \omega\tau_L$, $\Omega_L = \omega_L\tau_L$, $\omega = 2\pi f$, $\omega_L = 2\pi f_L$.

Let us assume that a dissipative biological substance (medium) (*DBM*) with temporal dispersion and complex-valued wave vector $\hat{k}(\omega)$, occupies one-dimensional space with a positive value of one-dimensional coordinate $x \geq 0$. The signal $Z_L(x, t)$ propagating in such a medium depends on the coordinate x and time t:

$$Z_L(x, t) = \int_{-\infty}^{\infty} \overline{Z}_L(\omega) exp\left[i\left(\omega t - \hat{k}(\omega)x\right)\right]\frac{d\omega}{2\pi}. \qquad (3)$$

In a particular case $x = 0$, there is one-to-one correspondence between the original signal function and its Fourier component: $Z_L(t) \Leftrightarrow \overline{Z}_L(\omega)$. If *ENS* propagates in a vacuum, the quantity $\hat{k}$ becomes a real valued $\hat{k} \to k = \omega/c$, where c is the velocity of light and $Z_L(x, t) = Z_L(t - x/c)$. This means that in a vacuum, *ENS* does not change its shape or frequency, and propagates in the positive direction of x-axis with the velocity equal to c. The formula (3) is valid for a low amplitude signal assuming that spectral components with different frequencies ω propagate independently of each other.

The dispersion law for *DBM*, which determines the dependence of the complex-valued wave vector $\hat{k}(\omega)$ on frequency ω, has the form $\hat{k}^2 = \frac{\omega^2\hat{\varepsilon}(\omega)}{c^2}$. To describe analytically the complex permittivity of the medium $\hat{\varepsilon}(\omega)$ as a function of the angular frequency ω, we use the Debye formula [58]–[60]:

$$\hat{\varepsilon}(\omega) = \varepsilon_\infty + \frac{\varepsilon_A - \varepsilon_\infty}{1 + i\omega\tau_A} + \frac{\varepsilon_B - \varepsilon_\infty}{1 + i\omega\tau_B}. \qquad (4)$$

Time dispersion $\hat{\varepsilon}(\omega)$ (4) shows the delay of polarization processes in response to an electromagnetic disturbance. The quantities τ_A and τ_B are the time intervals characterizing the relaxation of *DBM* to the equilibrium state. Dependences $\hat{\varepsilon}(\omega)$ of many dielectric media can be approximated by selecting the constant real values ε_∞, ε_A, ε_B, τ_A, τ_B. For definiteness, we will assume that $\tau_B > \tau_A$. The value ε_∞ is determined from the limit expression $\varepsilon_\infty = lim\varepsilon(\omega)|_{\omega\tau_B \gg 1}$. Using (4), one can obtain an expression for both the real $\varepsilon(\omega)_{Re}$ and imaginary $\varepsilon(\omega)_{Im}$ parts of the complex permittivity $\hat{\varepsilon}(\omega) = \varepsilon_{Re}(\omega) - i\varepsilon_{Im}(\omega)$. For the real and imaginary parts of the permittivity, the conditions $\varepsilon_{Re}(\omega) = \varepsilon_{Re}(-\omega)$ and $\varepsilon_{Im}(\omega) = -\varepsilon_{Im}(-\omega)$ are satisfied. For further study of *ENS* change while propagating in *DBM*, we will assume that the dependence $\hat{\varepsilon}(\omega)$ is known.

The works [60, 61] present graphs of both real $\varepsilon_{Re}(\omega)$ and imaginary parts $\varepsilon_{Im}(\omega)$ for such biological media as: muscle tissue, fat, skin, blood, brain. Figure 1 presents the plots of $\varepsilon_{Re}(\omega)$ and $\varepsilon_{Im}(\omega)$ for *DBM* with $\varepsilon_A = 1 \cdot 10^2$, $\varepsilon_B = 9 \cdot 10^2$, $\varepsilon_\infty = 1$, $\tau_A = 10^{-11}s$, $\tau_B = 5 \cdot 10^{-8}s$. Such numerical parameters correspond to the graph $\hat{\varepsilon}(\omega)$ given in [60] for the brain as *DBM*.

To calculate the integral (3), instead of the complex wave vector $\hat{k}(\omega)$, we introduce the complex refractive index $\hat{n}(\omega) = n_{Re}(\omega) - in_{Im}(\omega)$ using the relation $\hat{k}(\omega) = \omega\hat{n}(\omega)/c$. The real part $n_{Re}(\omega)$ will characterize the change in the velocity of signal propagation $V(\omega) = c/n_{Re}(\omega)$. The imaginary part $n_{Im}(\omega)$ will characterize the damping of the Fourier component with x.

$$Z_L(x, t) = \int_{-\infty}^{\infty} \overline{Z}_L(\omega) exp\left[i\omega\left(t - \frac{xn_{Re}(\omega)}{c}\right) - \frac{\omega n_{Im}(\omega)x}{c}\right]\frac{d\omega}{2\pi} \qquad (5)$$

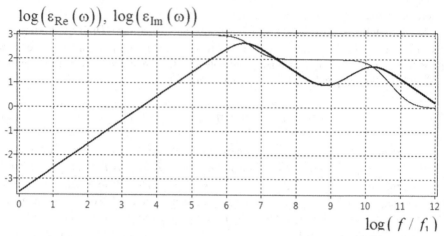

$\log\left(\varepsilon_{Re}(\omega)\right), \log\left(\varepsilon_{Im}(\omega)\right)$

$\log\left(f/f_1\right)$

Fig. 1. $\mathrm{Log}(\varepsilon_{Re}(\omega))$(thin line) and $\log(\varepsilon_{Im}(\omega))$(bold line) depending on $\log\left(\frac{f}{f_1}\right)$ at $f_1 = 1$ Hz.

The dispersion law giving the relation between $\hat{\varepsilon}(\omega)$ and $\hat{n}(\omega)$ has the form $\hat{\varepsilon}(\omega) = \hat{n}^2(\omega)$. By equating the real and imaginary parts of the dispersion law, one can obtain the formulas for $n_{Re}(\omega)$ and $n_{Im}(\omega)$ through the known values $\varepsilon_{Re}(\omega)$ and $\varepsilon_{Im}(\omega)$:

$$n_{Re}(\omega) = \sqrt{\frac{\sqrt{\varepsilon_{Re}^2(\omega) + \varepsilon_{Im}^2(\omega)} + \varepsilon_{Re}(\omega)}{2}}, \tag{6}$$

$$n_{Im}(\omega) = \sqrt{\frac{\sqrt{\varepsilon_{Re}^2(\omega) + \varepsilon_{Im}^2(\omega)} - \varepsilon_{Re}(\omega)}{2}}. \tag{7}$$

In Fig. 2 we show the dependencies $n_{Re}(\omega)$ and $n_{Im}(\omega)$ on f. The calculations are based on $\hat{\varepsilon}(\omega)$ with specified parameters (4).

The analysis of $n_{Re}(\omega)$ at frequencies $\omega < 10^7$ *rad/s* ($f < 1.6 \cdot 10^6$ *Hz*) shows that the signal propagation velocity $V(\omega) = c/n_{Re}(\omega)$ practically coincides with the constant value $V_L = c/n_{Re}(0)$. Figure 1 shows that at frequencies $\omega < 10^7$ *rad/s*, the inequality $\frac{\varepsilon_{Re}(\omega)}{\varepsilon_{Im}(\omega)} << 1$ holds true. Therefore, the propagation of an electromagnetic wave in *DBM* occurs with small damping. We introduce time parameters τ_* and τ_V, to determine the wave vector k_D and dispersion velocity $V(\omega)$ for $\omega\tau_V << 1$:

$$\tau_* = \frac{\tau_B(\varepsilon_B - \varepsilon_\infty) + \tau_A(\varepsilon_A - \varepsilon_\infty)}{2\sqrt{\varepsilon_A + \varepsilon_B - \varepsilon_\infty}}, k_D = \frac{\omega_L^2 \tau_*}{c}, \tag{8}$$

$$\tau_V = \sqrt{\frac{[\tau_A^2(\varepsilon_A - \varepsilon_\infty) + \tau_B^2(\varepsilon_B - \varepsilon_\infty)]}{2(\varepsilon_A + \varepsilon_B - \varepsilon_\infty)}}; V(\omega) = V_L\left(1 + \omega^2\tau_V^2\right). \tag{9}$$

The imaginary part $n_{Im}(\omega)$ of the refractive index is characterized by a linear dependence on frequencyω:$n_{Im}(\omega) \approx \varepsilon_{Im}(\omega)/(2\sqrt{\varepsilon_{Re}(\omega)}) \approx \omega\tau_*$. The term associated with

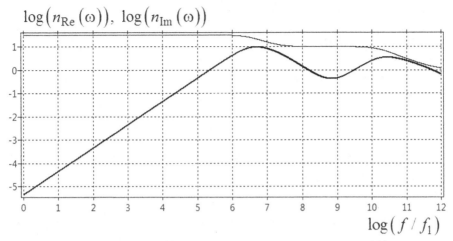

$$\log\left(n_{Re}(\omega)\right), \ \log\left(n_{Im}(\omega)\right)$$

$$\log\left(f/f_1\right)$$

Fig. 2. $Log(n_{Re}(\omega))$ (thin line) and $log(n_{Im}(\omega))$(bold line) depending on $log\left(\frac{f}{f_1}\right)$ at $f_1 = 1Hz$.

signal attenuation $Z_L(x, t)$ in the expression (6) can be represented as $\omega x n_{Im}(\omega)/c = \omega^2 k_D x/\omega_L^2$. The analysis of signal Fourier component $\overline{Z}_L(\omega)$ (3) shows that frequencies $\omega \approx \omega_L$ give the main contribution to the integral (6) since $\Omega_L \tau_L = 2\pi f_L \tau_L >> 1$. This is due to the fact that *ENS* oscillation period $T_L = 1/f_L$ is much less than the charac-teristic decay time τ_L of the Gaussian envelope of the signal:$T_L << \tau_L$. The ratio of the imaginary part of the wave vector $k_{Im} = \omega^2 k_D/\omega_L^2$ to its real part $k_{Re} = \omega/V_L$ at frequencies $\omega \approx \omega_L$ equals to$k_{Im}/k_{Re} \approx k_D V_L/\omega_L$.

Let us estimate all quantities at the frequency of the *ENS* signal $\omega_L \approx 10^7 rad/s$ for *DBM* of the brain: $V_L = 0.95 \cdot 10^7 m/s$, $\tau_* \approx 7.1 \cdot 10^{-7} s$, $\tau_V = 3.35 \cdot 10^{-8} s$, $k_D \approx 2.4 \cdot 10^{-1}(\frac{1}{m})$, $k_{Im}/k_{Re} \approx 0.23$. For frequencies $\omega_L \leq 10^7 rad/s$, we can neglect the dependence of velocity $V(\omega)$ (9) on frequency ω. At the angular frequency $\omega_L \approx 10^2 rad/s$, which corresponds to the frequency $f_L \approx 15.9H z$ of *EEG* β − rhythm, the value k_D decreases by 10 orders of magnitude, and k_{Im}/k_{Re} becomes equal to $0.23 \cdot 10^{-5}$.

Under our assumptions regarding the behavior of $n_{Im}(\omega)$ and $n_{Re}(\omega)$, we can calculate analytically the form of the signal $Z_L(x, t)$ propagating in *DBM* of the brain:

$$Z_L(x, t) = \frac{b_L}{2\sqrt{\pi}\tau_L\Gamma_L(x)}exp\left[-\frac{k_D x}{\Gamma_L^2(x)} - \frac{\left(t - t_L - \frac{x}{V_L}\right)^2}{4\tau_L^2\Gamma_L^2(x)}\right]cos\left[\frac{2\pi f_L}{\Gamma_L^2(x)}\left(t - t_L - \frac{x}{V_L}\right) + \alpha_L\right],$$

(10)

$$\Gamma_L(x) = \sqrt{1 + \frac{k_D x}{\omega_L^2 \tau_L^2}}.$$

(11)

Important to note the features of signal propagation in a medium with this model of temporal dispersion. The signal amplitude $b_L(x)$ compared with the amplitude $b_L(0)$ decreases according to the law $b_L(x)/b_L = exp\left[-\frac{k_D x}{\Gamma_L^2(x)}\right]/\Gamma_L(x)$. At the time moment$t$, the signal localization center is at the point $t = t_L + \frac{x}{V_L}$. While signal propagating through DBM, the signal width $\tau_L(x)$ at a point x compared to the initial width $\tau_L(0)$ increases as $\tau_L(x) = \tau_L(0)\Gamma_L(x)$. The signal frequency $f_L(x)$ decreases as compared to the frequency at zero-point $f_L(0)$ according to the relation $f_L(x)/f_L = 1/\Gamma_L^2(x)$.

For ENS signal of frequency $\omega_L \approx 10^7 rad/s$ ($\omega_L\tau_L$=10) at the distance from the initial point $x = 1/k_D \approx 4.17m$, the signal amplitude will decrease approximately by a factor of $e = 2.72$. The multiplier $b_L(x)$ will decrease by 0.5%. The width of the signal envelope $\tau_L(x)$ will increase by 1%, and its frequency $f_L(x)$ will decrease by 1%.

As an example, we consider DBM with dispersion properties of the brain and study the propagation of the superposition $Z(x, t) = Z_L(x, t) + Z_M(x, t)$ of two ENS signals with a given parameters $\vec{L} = (b_L; f_L; t_L + x/V_L; \tau_L; \alpha_L)$ and $\vec{M} = (b_M; f_M; t_M - x/V_M; \tau_M; \alpha_M)$ (10). The first signal $Z_L(x, t)$ has time-center at t_L and propagates in the positive direction of x-axis with the velocity $V_L = V_0$. The second signal $Z_M(x, t)$ has localization at t_M and propagates in the opposite direction with the velocity $V_M = V_0$. For simplicity, let us assume that there is no fading in $DBM \rightarrow k_D = 0$ (8). The signals have the same unit amplitudes $b_L/(2\sqrt{\pi}\tau_L) = b_M/(2\sqrt{\pi}\tau_M)$=1. Time parameters τ_L and τ_M satisfy the relations $|t - t_L - x/V_0| << \tau_L$, $|t - t_M - x/V_0| << \tau_M$. The fulfillment of these inequalities means that the amplitudes of both ENS are equal for all considered values of coordinates x and times t. The frequencies of two signals f_L and f_M differ slightly: $f_L = f_0(1 + \varepsilon)$, $f_M = f_0(1 - \varepsilon)$, where the quantity f_0 has the dimension of frequency, and the dimensionless parameter ε is small $\varepsilon << 1$. Under such assumptions, the total signal $Z(x, t)$ can be considered as some beat signal, being a superposition of two oscillations with close frequencies

$$Z(x, t) = \tilde{Z}(x, t)cos\left(2\pi f_0 t - \frac{2\pi \varepsilon x}{\lambda_0} + \psi\right), \qquad (12)$$

$$\psi = \frac{\alpha_L + \alpha_M}{2} - \pi(f_L t_L + f_M t_M), \qquad (13)$$

$$\tilde{Z}(x, t) = 2cos\left(2\pi \varepsilon f_0 t - \frac{2\pi x}{\lambda_0} + \varphi\right), \qquad (14)$$

$$\varphi = \frac{\alpha_L - \alpha_M}{2} - \pi(f_L t_L - f_M t_M). \qquad (15)$$

The superposition signal $Z(x, t)$ (12) is represented as some oscillation form. The phase ψ (13) of such an oscillation changes only at large distances x satisfying the relation $\varepsilon x \geq \lambda_0$, where $\varepsilon << 1$; $\lambda_0 = V_0/f_0$ is the oscillation wavelength in DBM. The value $\tilde{Z}(x, t)$ (14) is the amplitude of oscillation slowly varying in space and time. The maximum of $\tilde{Z}(x, t)$ moves in DBM at a low velocity $V_{max} = \varepsilon V_0 \ll V_0$. The parameters φ (13) and ψ (15) are constant phases, which do not depend on the coordinate x and time t. Figure 3 shows the graph of the total signal at the parameters: $x = 0$, f_0=2Hz, ε=0.012, $f_L = f_0(1 + \varepsilon)$, $f_M = f_0(1 - \varepsilon)$, $t_L = 8/f_L$, $t_M = 16/f_M$, α_L=0, α_M=π, V_0=1 m/s, $\tau_L = \tau_M$=1000s. For the given parameters, we have the relation $\tilde{Z}(x = 0, t = 0) = 0$.

The maximum value $\tilde{Z}_{max}(x, t_{max}) = 2$, plotted for $x = 0$ is reached at time $t_{max}(0) = 1/4\varepsilon f_0 = 10.417$ s. Note that in a medium without dispersion under the condition $k_D = 0$

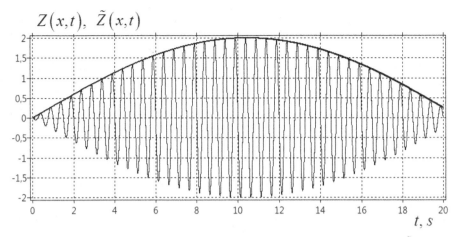

Fig. 3. Thin line shows $Z(0, t)$; bold line indicates the slowly changing amplitude $\tilde{Z}(0, t)$.

(8), the graph $\tilde{Z}(x, t)$ for $x > 0$ shifts to the right and does not change its shape. Maximum value $\tilde{Z}_{max}$ for a fixed value $x > 0$ takes place at a later time $t_x > t_{max}$. The values x and t_x relate to each other as $x = \varepsilon V_0(t_x - t_{max}(0))$. Thus, in DBM, the maximum amplitude $\tilde{Z}(x, t)$, as a result of the beats of two oscillations with close frequencies, propagates with the velocity $V_{max} = \varepsilon V_0$ much lower than the wave propagation velocity in the medium without dispersion.

Let us apply our results to explain the existence of traveling waves observed in EEG experiments. One of the possible mechanisms for the emergence of such waves is the appearance of stable wave packets. We can interpret slowly propagating wave packets as beats of two oscillations with the opposite directions of velocities and similar amplitudes and frequencies. It is known that the cerebral cortex is a heterogeneous medium in which both excited and unexcited neural ensembles coexist. In addition, the cerebral cortex has a complex relief with a lot of heterogeneities and convolutions. Many processes in the cerebral cortex are characterized by randomness. Such chaotic properties of the brain include: different directions of wave propagation, different amplitudes, frequencies, phases, times of occurrence, delay and decay times of oscillations. All this leads to the appearance act of stable wave packets with a certain fixed frequency. The moving maxima of the envelopes corresponding to such wave packets will form various traveling waves. The propagation trajectories of such envelopes can take a variety of forms.

3 *EEG* Bursts Propagating Under Photostimulation

Photostimulation (PHS) is a series of light pulses of a given frequency v_P and duration $T_P >> 1/v_p$, generated by a photoflash, which is used to study the process of mastering by the brain the external rhythm [43, 44, 61]–[64]. During PHS, neural ensembles of the brain reproduce the rhythm of external stimuli. Rhythmic light flashes cause a response in the visual cortex of the brain, both in the form of individual occipital spikes, and in the form of *EEG* changes with a frequency equal to or a multiple of the frequency of *PHS* (the phenomenon of rhythm assimilation) The state of specific brain pathways from the retina through the thalamic nuclei to the cortex, and the excitability of cortical neurons determine the process of assimilation. The response signals registered in *EEG* during photostimulation propagate along the cerebral cortex and reach the highest amplitudes in the occipital regions of the brain (channels $J = (O_1; O_z; O_2)$).

To study the non-stationary *EEG* signals during *PHS*, we use continuous wavelet transform (*CWT* - continuous wavelet transform) [65]–[77]. *CWT* image $V(v, t)$ has the form

$$V(v, t) = v \int_{-\infty}^{\infty} z(t\prime)\psi^*(v(t\prime - t))dt\prime. \tag{16}$$

CWT displays the original one-dimensional signal $z(t)$ on the plane of two arguments: time t and frequency v, characterizing the change in spectral properties of the signal over time. The value $v>0$ determines the scale of compression or expansion of the mother wavelet function $\psi(x)$. Argument t in (16) determines the wavelet localization in time. In the present work, we use the Morlet mother wavelet function [75, 76] given by the formula

$$\psi(x) = D_m exp\left(-\frac{x^2}{2m^2}\right)\left[exp(2\pi ix) - exp\left(-\Omega_m^2\right)\right], \tag{17}$$

$$D_m = \frac{(2\pi)^{1/4}}{\sqrt{\Omega_m\left(1 - 2exp\left(-\frac{3\Omega_m^2}{2}\right) + exp\left(-2\Omega_m^2\right)\right)}}. \tag{18}$$

The mother wavelet $\psi(x)$ must be well localized near the point $x=0$, have a zero mean value calculated over the entire interval of the variable $-\infty<x<\infty$, and have a unit norm. In (17)–(18), * - means complex conjugate; the value m plays the role of a control parameter, and $\Omega_m = m\pi\sqrt{2}$. At $m = 1$, the form of the wavelet transform given by (16) (proposed in [44]) correctly describes both the frequency position of the peaks $v_1 = f_L$, $v_2 = f_K$, and the amplitude relation between two harmonic signals $Z(t) = cos(2\pi f_K t) + cos(2\pi f_L t)$, having the same amplitude. The analytical *CWT* expression [75] for the elementary non-stationary signal *ENS* (1) shows that the value $|V(v, t)|$ correctly describes the amplitude behavior of *ENS* at $v = f_L$ at $m = 1$. Further, in processing the experimental *EEG* records during *PHS*, we will use the Morlet mother wavelet function (17) with $m = 1$.

We can derive for *CWT* the relation similar to the Parsevale equation of the Fourier analysis:

$$\int_{-\infty}^{\infty} z^2(t)dt = \frac{2}{C_\psi} \int_{-\infty}^{\infty} dt \int_0^{\infty} dv \frac{|V(v, t)|^2}{v}. \tag{19}$$

The Eq. (19) shows that the value

$$\varepsilon(v, t) = \frac{2}{C_\psi} \frac{|V(v, t)|^2}{v}, \tag{20}$$

characterizes the instantaneous distribution of a signal energy over frequencies v calculated at the moment of time t. The function $\varepsilon(v, t)$ (the local energy spectrum density of the signal) (20) characterizes the spectral properties of the signal at a given frequency v and time t. The constant $C_\Psi \approx 1$ is expressed in terms of the integral of the Fourier component of the mother wavelet [76].

To study the dynamics of occurrence and change of frequencies in non-stationary *EEG* signals, we introduce a spectral integral

$$E_\mu(t) = \frac{1}{\Delta v} \int\limits_{v_\mu - \Delta v/2}^{v_\mu + \Delta v/2} \varepsilon(v, t) dv. \qquad (21)$$

The value of $E_\mu(t)$ is the average value of the local density of the signal energy spectrum, integrated over the given spectral interval $\mu = \left[v_\mu - \Delta/2; v_\mu + \Delta/2\right]$, where v_μ is the center of the interval; Δ is the width of the interval.

The experimental data for the present study were obtained during photostimulation by a computer encephalograph at the NIIEM RAMS (Institute of Experimental Medicine) [44]. A prerequisite for the selection of subjects was the absence of a history of craniocerebral trauma and neuro-infections. Particular attention was paid to the *EEG* processing of the records from occipital channels (left O_1, central O_z, and right O_2). The recording electrodes were located according to the "10–20%" scheme.

For each subject ($N = 15$ people), the entire *EEG* recording session consisted of blocks differing from each other by a step change in v_p in the range $v_p = [8, 10, 14Hz]$. Such frequencies v_p lie within the $\alpha-$ range. Each block of the *EEG* data, having a total duration T and fixed *PHS* frequency equal to v_p, can be divided into three stages: the rest stage A in the interval $0 < t < t_A$, t_A is a moment of *PHS* switch-on; stage B in the interval $t_A < t < t_B$, t_B is a moment of *PHS* turn-off, and relaxation stage C in the interval $t_B < t < T$, T is a total observation interval. Each stage (A, B, C) lasted approximately 4-5s.

Let us study the effect of a photoflash operating at a frequency v_p on *TW* (traveling waves) propagation along the cerebral cortex. We calculate the spectral integrals $E_{PHS}(t)$ by integrating the local energy spectrum density of the *EEG* signal in a narrow frequency range $\mu = [v_p - \Delta, v_p + \Delta]$ near the *PHS* frequency v_p, where value $\Delta = 0.24Hz$. Such a narrow spectral interval μ makes it possible to analyze the propagation velocities of *TW* related to a certain *PHS* frequency $v_p = [8, 10, 14Hz]$.

Consider the *EEG* signal $z_J(t)$ from the channel $J = O_1$ registered from the subject N_1 (Fig. 4) during *PHS* with frequency $v_p = 8Hz$. *PHS* switch-on time $t_{on} = 1.75s$ and switch-off time $t_{of} = 5.75s$ are marked with vertical lines.

In Fig. 4 we can see three bursts of *EEG* activity at the frequencies $v \approx 8Hz$ with the maxima at the times $t_1 \approx 2.4s$, $t_2 \approx 3.9s$ and $t_3 \approx 6.3s$ marked by arrows. Note that the first burst, which occurs at $t_1 \approx 2.4s$, lags behind the start of the photoflare $t_{on}=1.75s$. The last burst, which has the maximum at $t_3 \approx 6.3s$, is observed already after the light flash is switched off at $t_{off} = 5.75s$. Quantitative parameters characterizing the lag of the *EEG* signals from the light flashes are given in [43].

The arrows in Fig. 5 mark the stage B ($t_{on}=1.75s$, $t_{off} = 5.75s$) during the *PHS* with frequency $v_P = 8Hz$. Three peaks of $|V_J(v, t)|$ in Fig. 5 at times $t_1 \approx 2.22s$, $t_2 \approx 4.0s$,

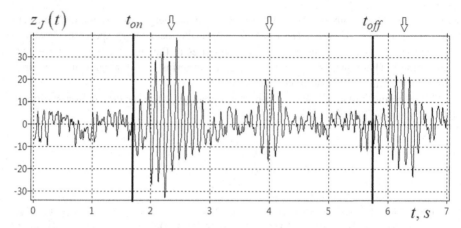

Fig. 4. *EEG* record $z_J(t)$ from the channel $J = O_1$ for N_1- subject depending on the time $t(s)$.

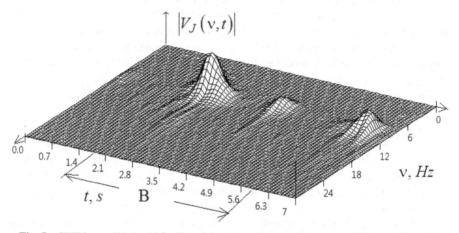

Fig. 5. *CWT* image $|V_J(\nu, t)|$ for N_1-subject depending on frequency $\nu(Hz)$, and time $t(s)$.

and $t_3 \approx 6.3s$ correspond to three *EEG* bursts in the record (Fig. 5). Wavelet analysis shows the appearance of other frequencies in the range $\nu \approx [6-18Hz]$. Figure 6 presents three spectral integrals $E_{PHS}(t)$ calculated for N_1-subject in a narrow frequency range $\mu = [\nu_p - \Delta, \nu_p + \Delta]$, where $\Delta = 0.25Hz$. We obtain the same data for N_1-subject making calculations for another two channels $J = O_z$ and $J = O_2$. Spectral integrals $E_{PHS}(t)$ for three occipital channels $J = \{O_1; O_2; O_z\}$ are shown in Fig. 6.

It is important to note that the maxima of all activity bursts shown in Fig. 6 are located at different time points. This is evidence for the bursts in a narrow frequency range $\mu = [\nu_p - \Delta, \nu_p + \Delta]$ moving along the surface of the brain at certain velocities V_{PHS}. An enlarged burst fragment centered at $t_1 \approx 2.22\ s$ is shown in Fig. 7.

The maximum values of $E_{PHS}(t)$ in each channel J are marked with bold dots: $t_1(O_2) = 2.108s$, $t_1(O_z) = 2.206s$, $t_1(O_1) = 2.226s$. The burst velocity V_{PHS} for a given frequency of photostimulation ν_P can be estimated by dividing the distance

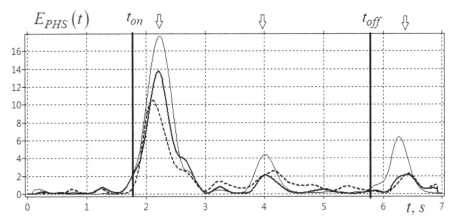

Fig. 6. Time dependence of spectral integrals $E_{PHS}(t)$ for N_1-subject at $\nu_P = 8Hz$. (Thin line corresponds to $J = O_1$; bold line → $J = O_z$; dotted line → $J = O_2$).

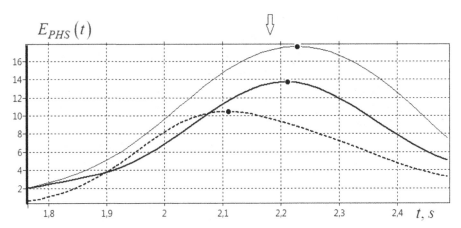

Fig. 7. Enlarged burst fragment centered at $t_1 \approx 2.22s$ for N_1-subject at $\nu_P = 8Hz$. (Thin line corresponds to $J = O_1$; bold line → $J = O_z$;dotted line→ $J = O_2$).

between channels $L \approx 5 \cdot 10^{-2}m$ on the difference in times of reaching the maximums. For the burst centered at $t_1 \approx 2.22s$, the *PHS* propagation velocities between the channels are: $V_{PHS}(O_2 \to O_z) \approx 0.498m/s$, $V_{PHS}(O_z \to O_1) \approx 0.493m/s$. The *EEG* bursts for N_1-subject centered at $t_2 \approx 4.0s$ and $t_3 \approx 6.3s$ are processed similarly. Averaging the propagation velocities for N_1-subject over three bursts, we obtain the mean value $\overline{V}_{PHS}(N_1) \approx 0.914\,m/s$

Consider the *EEG* signal $z_J(t)$ from the channel $J = O_1$ registered for the subject N_2 (Fig. 8) during *PHS* with the same frequency $\nu_p = 8Hz$. *PHS* switch-on time $t_{on} = 1.24s$ and switch-off time $t_{of} = 4.69s$ are marked with vertical lines.

The record of N_1-subject (Fig. 8), compared with N_2-subject (Fig. 4), shows a continuous burst of *EEG* activity in the time interval $[t_{on}; t_{off}]$. *CWT* image $|V_J(\nu, t)|$ for N_2-subject is shown in Fig. 9 ($\nu_p = 8Hz, J = O_1$).

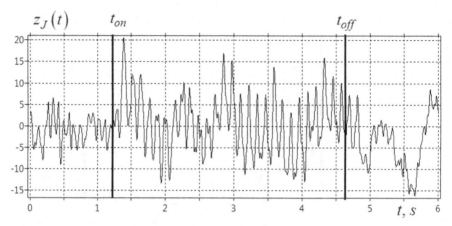

Fig. 8. *EEG* record $z_J(t)$ from the channel $J = O_1$ for N_2-subject depending on the time $t(s)$.

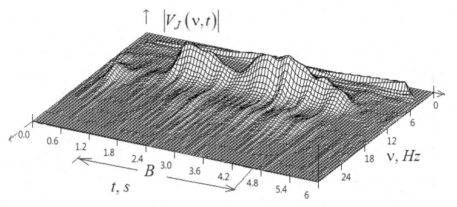

Fig. 9. *CWT* image $|V_J(\nu, t)|$ *depending on frequency* $\nu (Hz)$, *and time* $t(s)$ for N_2-subject.

Figure 9 for N_2-subject differs from Fig. 5 for N_1-subject by the presence of the activity burst at twice the photostimulation frequency $\nu \approx 2\nu_p = 16Hz$.

Note that for N_2-subject, we observe a continuous, trapezoidal level of external frequency ($\nu_P = 8Hz$) perception, against which we can detect separate small bursts (Fig. 10) of *EEG* activity. This mechanism of external frequency perception is different from that of N_2-subject, whose brain perceives an external perturbation with a frequency of ν_P=8 Hz and responds to it with a system of separate *EEG* bursts discrete in time (Fig. 6). The method for calculating velocities of *PHS* induced bursts for both tested subjects is the same.

Let us turn to the statistical processing of the observation results for $N = 15$ subjects exposed to photostimulation with discrete frequencies $\nu_p = [8, 10, 14Hz]$. The periods of photostimulation ($T_P \approx 4s$) alternate with periods of relaxation $T_R \approx 10s$. It should be noted that approximately 25% of the subjects showed a trapezoidal mechanism of mastering the external rhythm. The remaining 75% of the subjects responded to an external

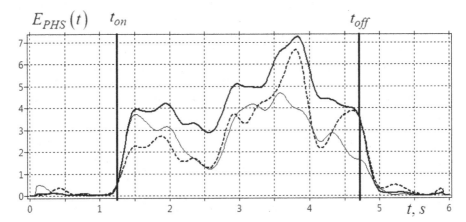

Fig. 10. Time dependence of spectral integrals $E_{PHS}(t)$ for N_2-subject at $v_P = 8Hz$. (Thin line corresponds to $J = O_1$; bold line $\rightarrow J = O_z$; dotted line$\rightarrow J = O_2$).

disturbance in the form of separate bursts of activity at the frequency of photostimulation v_P. At $v_P = 8Hz$, the mean velocity $< V_{PHS} >$ of PHS induced bursts averaged over all subjects and all photoflashes takes the value: $< V_{PHS} >= 0.96 \pm 0.41 m/s$; at $v_P = 10Hz$: $< V_{PHS} \geq 0.78 \pm 0.34 m/s$, and at $v_P = 14\ Hz$: $< V_{PHS} >= 1.25 \pm 0.59$ m/s.

4 Discussion and Conclusion

The article is devoted to the development of a mathematical model for the propagation of *EEG* activity bursts in the cerebral cortex during photostimulation. We consider electromagnetic disturbance propagating in a dissipative biological medium with temporal dispersion. Such wave forms can be modeled as a superposition of elementary non-stationary signals characterized by their own parameters: amplitude, frequency, localization center, amplitude envelope width and phase. If we take into account the dispersion of a biological medium, all these parameters start to change their values while signal propagating through this medium.

The biological medium is characterized by its dielectric constant $\varepsilon(\omega)$ depending on the angular frequency ω. To estimate the complex permittivity, we use the Debye model, which well describes the properties of such biological media as the brain, muscle tissue, blood, fat, etc. We determined the changes in all *ENS* parameters for the media with temporal dispersion. Some kind of beat representing the stable motion of two *ENS* with nearly the same frequencies is considered. The fact is that beats move with the velocity much less than the velocity of electromagnetic wave in the given medium. We showered that the beats, characterized by a certain frequency, occur in response to photostimulation. This process is facilitated by various, chaotic directions of wave propagation, their arbitrary amplitudes, frequencies, phases, times of occurrence, delay and damping times of oscillations.

The advantage of using photostimulation to study the propagation of *EEG* bursts along the cerebral cortex is that flashes of light of a certain frequency v_P force the brain to reproduce the oscillations with the frequencies close to ν_P. At the same time, the oscillatory forms with frequencies different from ν_P are suppressed. The narrow spectral interval makes it possible to analyze the propagation velocities of *EEG* disturbances in a small frequency range close to *PHS* frequency. The external frequency range ν_p can easily cover all $[\delta, \theta, \alpha, \beta, \gamma]$-ranges of *EEG* rhythm. Thus, we have the opportunities to analyze the trajectories and propagation velocities of disturbances at any fixed external frequency.

Continuous Wavelet Transform (*CWT*) using the Morlet mother wavelet function, is applied to process the non-stationary *EEG signal* during photostimulation with a frequency of ν_p. The *CWT* numerical calculation program for arbitrary signals is compared with *CWT* analytical expressions for ideal harmonic signals of the same amplitude and different frequencies, as well as with the analytical expression for the *ENS* signal. Spectral integrals $E_{PHS}(t)$ are used to analyze the propagation velocities of bursts travelling along the surface of the brain. The value of $E_{PHS}(t)$ is the local density of the signal spectrum integrated over a narrow frequency interval near the specified external frequency ν_p. Spectral integrals allowed us to calculate the delays in the arrival of the maxima of stimulus-induced wave forms into various *EEG* channels. For $N = 15$ subjects, we calculated the average velocities $< V_{PHS} >$ of the disturbances travelling along the cerebral cortex for different *PHS* frequencies $\nu_p = 8, 10, 14 Hz$. The characteristic average velocity is about 1 m/s.

The methods to study dynamic properties of travelling *EEG* bursts proposed in this article can be applied to the processing of experimental data related to the diagnosis of various diseases, as well as to the study the *EEG* rearrangements occurring during various functional tests.

Acknowledgment. The work was supported by the State Assignment for Fundamental Research (subject code FSEG -2020–0024).

References

1. Gnezditskii, V.V.: A Reverse EEG Problem and Clinical Electroencephalography. MEDpress-inform, Moscow (2004)
2. Nunez, P.L., Srinivasan, R.: Electric Fields of the Brain: The Neurophysics of EEG. 2nd edn. Oxford University Press (2006)
3. Ivanitsky, A.M., Ivanitsky, G.A., Nikolaev, A.R., Sysoeva, O.V.: Encyclopedia of Neuroscience. Electroencephalography. Springer, Cham (2009)
4. Tong,S., Thakor, N.: Quantitative EEG analysis methods and clinical applications. Artech House, Boston, London (2009)
5. Mecarelli, O. (ed.): Clinical Electroencephalography. Springer, Cham (2019). https://doi.org/10.1007/978-3-030-04573-9
6. Kaplan, A.Y., Fingelkurts, An.A., Fingelkurts, Al.A., Borisov, S.V., Darkhovsky, B.S.: Non-stationary nature of the brain activity as revealed by EEG/MEG: methodological, practical and conceptual challenges. Signal Proces. **85**, 2190–2212 (2005)
7. Borisyuk, R., Kazanovich, Y.: Oscillations and waves in the models of interactive neural populations. Biosystems **86**, 53–62 (2006)

8. Quiles, M.G., Wang, D., Zhaoc, L, Romeroc, R.A.F., Huang, D.S.: Selecting salient objects in real scenes: an oscillatory correlation model. Neural Netw. **24**, 54–64 (2011)
9. Chizlov, A.V., Graham, L.J.: Efficient evaluation of neuron populations receiving colored-noise current based on a refractory density method. Phys. Rev. E **77**, 011910 (2008)
10. Kaplan, A., Borisov, S.V.: Dynamic properties of segmental chaBoracteristics of EEG alpha activity in rest conditions and during cognitive tasks. Zhurnal Vysshei Nervnoi Deiatelnosti **53**(1), 22–32 (2003)
11. Bozhokin, S.V., Suslova, I.B.: Wavelet-based analysis of spectral rearrangements of EEG patterns and of non-stationary correlations. Phys. A **421**(1), 151–160 (2015)
12. Bozhokin, S.V., Suslova, I.B.: Wavelet-based method of mapping brain activity waves travelling in the cerebral cortex. In: Proceedings of the 15th International Joint Conference on Biomedical Systems and Technologies. BIOSIGNALS, vol.4, pp.63–73 (2022).https://doi.org/10.5220/0010888000003123
13. Hramov, A.E., Koronovskii, A.A., Makarov, V.A., Pavlov, A.N., Sitnikova, E.: Wavelets in Neuroscience. Springer Series in Synergetics. Springer-Verlag, Berlin (2015)
14. Hughes, J.R.: The phenomenon of travelling waves: a review. Clin. Electroencephalogr. **26**, 1–6 (1995)
15. Hindriks, R., van Putten, M.J., Deco, G.: Intra-cortical propagation of EEG alpha oscillations. Neuroimage **103**, 444–453 (2014)
16. Sato, T.K., Nauhaus, I., Carandini, M.: Traveling waves in visual cortex. Neuron **75**, 218–229 (2012)
17. Massimini, M., Huber, R., Ferrarelli, F., Hill, S., Tononi, G.: The sleep slow oscillation as a traveling wave. Neuroscience **24**(31), 6862–6870 (2004)
18. Bahramisharif, A., et al.: Propagating neocortical gamma bursts are coordinated by traveling alpha waves. J. Neurosci. **33**(48), 18849–18854 (2013)
19. Zhang, H., Watrous, A.J., Patel, A., Jacobs, J.: Theta and alpha oscillations are traveling waves in the human neocortex. Neuron **98**(6), 1269–1281 (2018). https://doi.org/10.1016/j.neuron.2018.05.019
20. Manjarrez, E., Vázquez, M., Flores, A.: Computing the center of mass for traveling alpha waves in the human brain. Brain Res. **1145**, 239–247 (2007)
21. Bhattacharya, S., Brincat, S.L., Lundqvist, M., Miller, E.K.: Traveling waves in the prefrontal cortex during working memory. PLoS Comput. Biol. **18**(1), e1009827 (2022). https://doi.org/10.1371/journal.pcbi.1009827
22. Muller, L., Chavane, F., Reynolds, J., Sejnowski, T.J.: Cortical travelling waves: mechanisms and computational principles. Nat. Rev. Neurosci. **19**(5), 255–268 (2018). https://doi.org/10.1038/nrn.2018.20
23. Buzsáki, G., Moser, E.I.: Memory, navigation and theta rhythm in the hippocampal-entorhinal system. Nat. Neurosci. **16**, 130–138 (2013)
24. Fries, P.: Rhythms for cognition: communication through coherence. Neuron **88**(1), 220–235 (2015). https://doi.org/10.1016/j.neuron.2015.09.034
25. Voytek, B., Canolty, R., Shestyuk, A., Crone, N., Parvizi, J., Knight, R.: Shifts in gamma phase–amplitude coupling frequency from theta to alpha over posterior cortex during visual tasks. Front. Hum. Neurosci. **4**, 191 (2010)
26. Buschman, T.J., Denovellis, E.L., Diogo, C., Bullcock, D., Miller, E.K.: Synchronous oscillatory neural ensembles for rules in the prefrontal cortex. Neuron **76**(1), 838–846 (2012)
27. Mysin, I.E., Kitchigina, V.F., Kazanovich, Y.: Modeling synchronous theta activity in the medial septum: key role of local communications between different cell populations. J. Comput. Neurosci. **39**(1), 1–16 (2015). https://doi.org/10.1007/s10827-015-0564-6
28. Nikolaev, A.R., Ivanitskii, G.A., Ivanitskii, A.M.: Studies of cortical interactions over short periods of time during the search for verbal associations. Physiol. Neurosci. Behav. Physiol. **31**(2), 119–132 (2004)

29. Schoffelen, J.-M., Gross, J.: Hum. Brain Mapp. **30**(6), 1857–1865 (2009). https://doi.org/10.1002/hbm.20745
30. Hassan, M., Wendling, F.: Electroencephalography source connectivity: aiming for high resolution of brain networks in time and space. IEEE Signal Process. Mag **35**(6), 81–96 (2018). https://doi.org/10.1109/MSP.2017.2777518
31. Baillet, S., Mosher, J.C., Leahy, R.M.: Electromagnetic brain mapping. IEEE Signal Process. Mag. **18**(6) 14–30 (2001)
32. Grech, R., et al.: Review on solving the inverse problem in EEG source analysis. J. Neuroeng. Rehabilit. **5**(1), 5–25 (2008). https://doi.org/10.1186/1743-0003-5-25
33. Shattuck, D.W., et al.: Magnetic resonance image tissue classification using a partial volume model. Neuroimage **13**(5), 856–876 (2001). https://doi.org/10.1006/nimg.2000.0730
34. Bastos, A.M., Schoffelen, J.-M.: A tutorial review of functional connectivity analysis methods and their interpretational pitfalls. Front. Syst. Neurosci. **9**, 1–23 (2016). https://doi.org/10.3389/fnsys.2015.00175
35. Hamedi, M., Salleh, S.H., Noor, A.M.: Electroencephalographic motor imagery brain connectivity analysis for BCI: a review. Neural. Comput. **28**(6), 999–1041 (2016). https://doi.org/10.1162/NECO_a_00838
36. da Silva, F.L.: Neural mechanisms underlying brain waves: from neural membranes to networks. Electroenceph. Clin. Neurophysiol **79**, 81–93 (1991)
37. Verkhlyutov, V.M., Balaev, V.V., Ushakov, V.L., Velichkovsky, B.M.: A novel methodology for simulation of EEG traveling waves on the folding surface of the human cerebral cortex. In: Kryzhanovsky, B., Dunin-Barkowski, W., Redko, V., Tiumentsev, Y. (eds.) NEUROINFORMATICS 2018. SCI, vol. 799, pp. 51–63. Springer, Cham (2019). https://doi.org/10.1007/978-3-030-01328-8_4
38. Toptygin, I.N.: Electromagnetic Phenomena in Matter - Statistical and Quantum Approaches. Wiley-VCH (2015)
39. Kalshchikov, A.A., Shtykov, V.V., Shalimova, E.V.: Direct method for estimating the distance traveled by a signal along the path with frequency dispersion. J. Radio Electron. **9**, 1–9 (2020). https://doi.org/10.30898/1684-1719.2020.9.1
40. Gavrilov, A., Kursitys A.: Distribution of Gaussian wave package with high frequency LFM filling in dissipative medium. Electron. J. Tech. Acoust. **4**, 1–14 (2012). https://www.ejta.org/en/2012
41. Patten, T.M., Rennie, C.J., Robinson, P.A., Gong, P.: Human cortical traveling waves: dynamical properties and correlations with responses. PLoS ONE **7**(6), e38392 (2012)
42. Robinson, P.A., Chen, P., Yang, L.: Physiologically based calculation of steady-state evoked potentials and cortical wave velocities. Biol. Cybern. **98**, 1–10 (2008)
43. Pfurtscheller, G., Lopes da Silva, F.H.: Event-related EEG/MEG synchronization and desynchronization: basic principles. Clin. Neurophysiol. **110**, 1842–1857 (1999)
44. Bozhokin, S.V.: Wavelet analysis of learning and forgetting of photostimulation rhythms for a nonstationary electroencephalogram. Tech. Phys. **55**(9), 1248–1256 (2010)
45. Bozhokin, S.V., Suvorov, N.B.: Wavelet analysis of transients of an electroencephalogram at photostimulation. Biomed. Radioelektron **3**, 21–25 (2008)
46. Bassett, D.S., et al.: Dynamic reconfiguration of human brain networks during learning. Proc. Natl. Acad. Sci. USA **108**(18), 7641–7646 (2011). https://doi.org/10.1073/pnas.1018985108
47. Braun, U., et al.: Dynamic reconfiguration of frontal brain networks during executive cognition in humans. Proc. Natl. Acad. Sci. USA **112**(37), 11678–11682 (2015). https://doi.org/10.1073/pnas.1422487112
48. Finc, K., et al.: Dynamic reconfiguration of functional brain networks during working memory training. Nat. Commun. **11**(1), 2435 (2020). https://doi.org/10.1038/s41467-020-15631-z
49. Maksimenko, V.A., et al.: Neural interactions in a spatially-distributed cortical network during perceptual decision making. Front. Behav. Neurosci. **13**, 220 (2019)

50. Cover, T.M., Thomas, J.A.: Elements of Information Theory. John Wiley and Sons, New York (2012)
51. Ioannides, A., et al.: Coupling of regional activation in a human brain during an object and face affect recognition task. Hum. Brain Mapp. **11**(2), 77–92 (2000)
52. Liu, L., Ioannides, A.A.: Spatiotemporal profiles of visual processing with and without primary visual cortex. Neuroimage **31**, 1726–1740 (2006). https://doi.org/10.1016/j.neuroimage. 2012.07.058
53. Ermentrout, B.: Neural networks as spatio-temporal pattern-forming systems. Rep Prog Phys **61**(4), 353–430 (1998)
54. Terman, D.H., Ermentrout, G.B., Yew, A.C.: Propagating activity patterns in thalamic neuronal networks. SIAM J. Appl. Math. **61**, 1578–1604 (2001)
55. Zheng, J., Lee, S., Zhou, Z.J.: A transient network of intrinsically bursting starburst cells underlies the generation of retinal waves. Nat. Neurosci. **9**, 363–371 (2006)
56. Villacorta-Atienza, J.A., Makarov, V.A.: Wave-processing of long-scale information by neuronal chains. PLoS ONE **8**(2), e57440 (2013). https://doi.org/10.1371/journal.pone.005 7440
57. Gavrilov, A., Kursitys, A.: Distribution of Gaussian wave package with high frequency LFM filling in dissipative medium. Electron. J. Tech. Acoust. **4**, 1–14 (2012). https://www.ejta.org/en/2012
58. Kittel, C.: Introduction to Solid State Physics, 8th edn. John Wiley, Hoboken (2021)
59. Lin, J.C.: Electromagnetic fields in biological systems. CRC Press, Taylor & Francis Group, London NY (2012)
60. Vendik, I.B., Vendik, O.G., Kozlov, D.S., Munina, I.G., Pleskachev, V.V.: Wireless monitoring of the biological object state at microwave frequencies: a review. Tech. Phys. **61**(1), 1–22 (2016)
61. Svyatogor, I.A., Dick, O.E., Nozdrachev, A.D., Guseva, N.L.: Analysis of changes in EEG patterns in response to rhythmic photic stimulation under various disruptions of the functional state of the central nervous system. Hum. Physiol. **41**(3), 261–268 (2015). https://doi.org/10. 1134/S0362119715030172
62. Trenité, D.K.N., Binnie, C.D., Harding, G.F.A., Wilkins, A.: Photic stimulation: standardization of screening methods. Epilepsia **40**, 75–79 (1999)
63. Boutros, N.N., Galderisi, S., Pogarell, O., Riggio, S.: Standard Electroencephalography in Clinical Psychiatry: A Practical Handbook. John Wiley & Sons, Hoboken (2011)
64. Trenité, D.K.N., et al.: Methodology of photic stimulation revisited: updated European algorithm for visual stimulation in the EEG laboratory. Epilepsia **53**(1), 16–24 (2012)
65. Mallat, S.: A Wavelet Tour of Signal Processing, 3rd edn. Academic Press, New York (2008)
66. Chui, C.K.: An Introduction to Wavelets. Academic Press, New York (1992)
67. Daubechies, I.: Ten Lectures on Wavelet. Society for industrial and applied mathematics. Society for Industrial and Applied Mathematics, Philadelphia (1992)
68. Chui, C.K., Jiang, O.: Applied Mathematics. Data Compression, Spectral Methods, Fourier Analysis, Wavelets and Applications. Mathematics Textbooks for Science and Engineering, v.2, Atlantis Press (2013)
69. Frick, P.G., Sokoloff, D.D., Stepanov, R.A.: Wavelets for the space-time structure analysis of physical fields. UFN **192**(1), 69–99 (2022)
70. Rhif, M., Abbes, A.B., Farah, I.R., Sang, Y.: Wavelet transform application for/in non-stationary time-series analysis: a review. Appl. Sci. **9**(7), 1345 (2019). https://doi.org/10. 3390/app9071345
71. Kaur, J., Kaur, A.: A review on analysis of EEG signals. In: Proceedings of International Conference on Advances in Computer Engineering and Applications, pp. 957–960. IEEE (2015)

72. Faust, O., Acharya, U.R., Adeli, H., Adeli, A.: Wavelet-based EEG processing for computer-aided seizure detection and epilepsy diagnosis. Seizure **26**, 56–64 (2015)

73. Addison, P. S.: The illustrated wavelet transform handbook: introductory theory and applications in science, engineering, medicine and finance. CRC press (2017)

74. Dick, O.E., Nozdrachev, A.D.: Application of methods of wavelet and recurrent analysis to studies of bioelectrical activity of the brain in moderate cognitive impairment. Hum. Physiol. **48**(2), 182–193 (2022)

75. Bozhokin, S.V.: Continuous wavelet transform and exactly solvable model of nonstationary signals. Tech. Phys. **57**(7), 900–906 (2012). https://doi.org/10.1134/S1063784212070067

76. Bozhokin, S.V., Zharko, S.V., Larionov, N.V., Litvinov, A.N., Sokolov, I.M.: Wavelet correlation of nonstationary signals. Tech. Phys. **62**(6), 837–845 (2017). https://doi.org/10.1134/S1063784217060068

77. Bozhokin, S.V., Sokolov, I.M.: Comparison of the wavelet and gabor transforms in the spectral analysis of nonstationary signals. Tech. Phys. **63**(12), 1711–1717 (2018). https://doi.org/10.1134/S1063784218120241

Mobile Tele-Dermatology Use Among University Students: A Pilot Study at Saint Joseph University (USJ)

Nabil Georges Badr$^{(\boxtimes)}$ ⓘ, Nanor Aroutine ⓘ, and Joumana Yeretzian ⓘ

Higher Institute of Public Health, Saint Joseph University, Beirut, Lebanon
nabil@itvaluepartner.com, nanor.aroutine@net.usj.edu.lb,
joumana.estephan@usj.edu.lb

Abstract. Due to its quick diagnosis and treatment plan, Tele-dermatology (TDM) had already gained the trust of patients and doctors by the turn of the twenty-first century. We therefore extend our pilot study into a descriptive inquiry to gain a good insight into the propensity of University Students in Lebanon to use Mobile Tele Dermatology (TDM). This paper is a continuation of the statistical analysis performed to determine the factors influencing the use of TDM by university students. We evaluate the connection between medical factors and TDM adoption, the influence of subjective norms and perceived risks, also in the contexts of social determinants, such as age and marital status. Result demonstrability showed as a strong predictor of adoption in both the statistical analysis and the descriptive inquiry in this paper. Both academics and practitioners should benefit from the extra observations and results of this pilot survey. A qualitative study is advised to build on this pilot and learn more about the factors influencing usage intention. This study can be expanded to a broader population with a range of ages and professions, offering a helpful comparison of the markets that can be served and the target audience that could offer information for both manufacturers and practitioners.

Keywords: Tele-dermatology · Technology Acceptance Model (TAM) · Mobile medical application · Skin cancer · Consumer Acceptance

1 Introduction

Access to care has improved as a result of decentralized, mobile, and personalized care [1]. Medical mobile applications are redefining the future of medical consultation; a trend that began at the turn of the century and was heavily emphasized during the COVID-19 pandemic [2]. Telehealth use spans the entire continuum of care, from acute to post-acute, urgent to routine management of healthy lifestyles. Even prior to the pandemic, physicians and patients began utilizing telehealth to treat a variety of conditions such as cancer [3], behavioral health [4], surgical recovery [5], substance abuse [6], home dialysis [7], and others.

A. C. A. Roque et al. (Eds.): BIOSTEC 2022, CCIS 1814, pp. 199–214, 2023.
https://doi.org/10.1007/978-3-031-38854-5_11

At the turn of the 21st century, Tele-dermatology (TDM) had already received acceptance among both patients and physicians due to the prompt diagnosis and management regimen that resulted from its use. The demand for telehealth is growing, particularly for diseases with an increasing incidence rate, such as cancer in general and skin cancer in particular, which claimed the life of 1 in 12 patient in 2021 [8]. Advancements in technology were exploited in an attempt to improve early detection of the disease and reduce its mortality rate through skin cancer screening and early identification of suspicious skin lesions that can potentially lead to skin cancer [9].

Mobile Tele-dermatology (TDM) is a medical application that can be used anywhere and anytime to help diagnose skin lesions [10, 11]. TDM was initially especially useful in rural areas [12], where dermatology services were typically handled by non-specialized healthcare personnel. The technology consists of having a remote attending practitioner evaluate images of a suspect skin area for diagnosis and treatment [13].

During the Covid-19 pandemic, patients were encouraged to resort to telehealth from the comfort of their homes [14], to avoid unnecessary clinical visits and minimize exposure to the virus and life threatening situations [15]. The use of medical applications increased by 50% compared to 2019 [16] and TDM became the alternative to in-person visits. TDM was considered effective in decreasing the risk of Covid-19 transmission by minimizing clinical visits and avoiding overcrowdings of the hospitals both in private and public facilities [17].

Worldwide, the younger generation has been fertile grounds for piloting mobile health technologies adoption, as they may be more open to try out mobile technology and related innovations [18, 19]. Among the patient population, undergraduate students (18+ of age) have taken up mobile application use [20, 21]. The literature sees TDM adoption through the lens of a practitioner [22] and most commonly from the provider's perspective [23], in the public sector [24], in the context of improving access to care [25] and guidance for implementation and use [26]. While TDM, a mobile application can bring care to a user's fingertips, not much attention has been given to review impetus of adoption and factors promoting TDM adoption in the young user group. We are therefore curious to explore.

2 Approach

In a related pilot study, we used the technology acceptance model to evaluate the factors influencing the acceptance of Tele-Dermatology (TDM) to diagnose skin lesions among the Lebanese students [27]. Our findings showed that, in general, 64% of students are ready to use Tele-Dermatology in their everyday life. In this paper, we extend the reporting of our findings to investigate this phenomenon through a descriptive elaboration, so that we could explore the dynamics of adoption beyond statistical evidence. Therefore, in this second paper, we summarize our findings from Aroutine et al., 2022 and examine those factors, found to predict the intention to use of TDM, and develop a descriptive review so that we gain a good insight into the propensity of University Students in Lebanon to use Mobile Tele Dermatology (TDM).

2.1 Summary of Our Statistical Pilot Study

The pilot study concluded on May 2021 at the University of Saint Joseph in Beirut Lebanon where 89 students from different faculties took part in a self-administered survey [27]. The survey questionnaire consisted of 2 parts and 27 questions (Appendix). The first part captured the demographic information (sex, age, field of education, marital status and employment) medical history of the participants. The second part of the questionnaire explored the TDM context using a 5-point Likert scale. The pilot study was completed and the answers were exported on an excel sheet. After data preparation, we used SMART PLS 3 for the statistical evaluation. Figure 1 shows our valid model - with outer loading factors – excerpt from our paper [27].

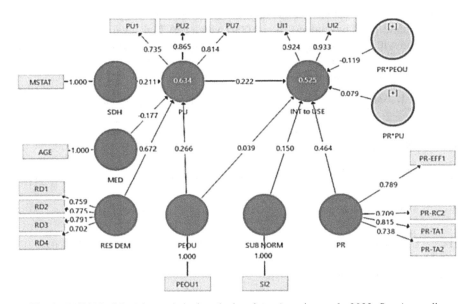

Fig. 1. Valid Model of the statistical analysis – from Aroutine et al., 2022; See Appendix.

To build the model of technology acceptance, we grounded our study on the extended TAM model to cover multiple contexts (TAM2, etc.), indicating the usage and acceptance behavior towards technology [28]. We developed our model to test the stated hypotheses and learn about TDM usage and factors of acceptance. Factors influencing the intention to use are therefore: Social determinants, medical factors, result demonstrability, perceived risk, subjective norms, perceived usefulness and perceived ease of use. For reference, we include an excerpt of our published paper, Aroutine et al., [27], listing the variables and the related Hypothesis.

For reporting and analysis purposes, we transformed the data captured on a Likert scale to binary variables, where neutral answers signified disagreement. That is, we regrouped the results as either Agree (4-Agree, 5-Strongly Agree), or Disagree (1-Strongly disagree, 2-Disagree, 3-Unsure). We differentiated between two outcomes: (1) "I will use Mobile TDM when it's offered to me," – which implies readiness now (Q.

23); and (2) "I will use Mobile TDM in my routine self-skin examination in the future" – which implies readiness in the future (Q. 24). The loading of INT USE (UI1 & UI2) respectively then assesses these outcomes, to their strengths and relevance in indicating the "intention to use".

2.2 Conclusions from Our Statistical Analysis

Summarizing the findings from our pilot study [27], our statistical analysis showed that marital status (Hypothesis H1); Results demonstrability (Hypothesis H3) and Perceived ease of use (Hypothesis H10) are antecedents to perceived usefulness and perceived risk, indicated by resistance to use, efficiency and technology anxiety predict our students' Intention to Use TDM (Hypothesis H4). Remarkably, the study results suggested that respondents linked "results demonstrability" (RES DEM) with perceived usefulness (PU) of mobile TDM by students (p = 0.000) with a very high level of confidence (t = 11.124) and with a very strong predictor of 67.2% (path coefficient = 0.672) – Table 1 is a reminder of the supported hypothesis from the study [27].

Table 1. Antecedents to TDM adoption in our pilot study - from Aroutine et al. [27].

Confirmed Hypothesis	Factors	Antecedents to	Statistical Significance (P Value)	Confidence level (t)	Predictability (Path Coefficient)
H1	Social determinants (SDH) such as marital status	Perceived Usefulness (PU)	p = 0.028	t = 2.209	21.1% (0.211)
H3	Results demonstrability (RES DEM)	Perceived Usefulness (PU)	p = 0.000	t = 11.124	67.2% (0.672)
H4	Perceived risk (PR)	Intention to Use (INT USE)	p = 0.000	t = 3.518	46.4% (0.464)
H10	Perceived ease of use (PEOU)	Perceived Usefulness (PU)	p = 0.002	t = 3.192	26.6% (0.266)

To note, according to the model R-values, the information presented in this study adequately describes the result. Our statistical study reflects 63.4 percent of the variability in the outcome for perceived usefulness and 52.5 percent of the variability in the outcome for intention to use [27]. These findings were supported by similar studies, where the proposed model explained 57.1 percent of the variation in young users' behavioral intention to use diabetes management apps and 56 percent of the variation in young users' behavioral intention to use a health information portal [29, 30]. The technology adoption theory accounts for a range in information technology use intentions of 17–53% based on findings from prior studies [31].

2.3 Sample Overview

The demographic characteristics of our sample are shown in Table 2. The participants were mostly single (n = 80, 90%) and female (n = 74, 83%) with an average age of 25. Around half of the participants were from the Faculty of Medicine (n = 42, 47%) and worked full time or part time, (n = 52, 58%). Four (4) participants had a history of skin cancer while 3 had a previously excised skin cancer [27].

Table 2. Sample description - from Aroutine et al. [27].

	Sample Distribution N= 89	
1- Gender	Male	17%
	Female	83%
2- Age	20 years or Less	25%
	Between 21 and 25	48%
	Between 26 and 30	13%
	Between 31 and 35	6%
	Between 36 and 40	2%
	Between 41 and 45	2%
	Between 46 and 50	3%
	Above 50	0%
3- Education	Business Management	6%
	Engineering and Sciences	16%
	Humanities	20%
	Medical & Health	47%
	Political Science - Law	4%
	Other	7%
4- Work	Part time	20%
	Full time	38%
	Other	42%
5- Status	Single	90%
	Married	10%

3 Descriptive Analysis Results

We identified social determinants as indicators of educational level, work and marital status[1]. The descriptive analysis found some relevance of education specialty, and marital status, etc. (Sect. 2, Table 2). In the statistical analysis [27], social determinants and results demonstrability such as marital status we connected to perceived usefulness and perceived risk to intention to use. Even though, the hypothesis related to subjective norms and medical factors were not confirmed, we still find it interesting for our descriptive inquiry to observe those independently. With that in mind, we proceed in this section to isolate each factor and continue with the descriptive analysis.

---

[1] https://www.who.int/health-topics/social-determinants-ofhealth#tab=tab_1.

3.1 Social Determinants - Age and Gender

Indications from the descriptive analysis (Tables 3 and 4) show that 77% of younger students (<= 20 years old) are ready to use TDM now. Both genders are more or less equally ready to embrace TDM now, but female students showed a higher intention to use TDM in the future (8% more than males). As mentioned and shown in previous studies in the literature, younger generations are more susceptible of using mobile technologies since they are more prone to use the internet [32] and innovate in their everyday life. Younger participants have shown readiness in embracing new eHealth technologies [33]. In our statistical analysis however, age and gender have not been shown as significant predictors of the antecedent relationship between social determinants (SDH) and perceived usefulness (PU) – They were reduced form the model [27] as their path coefficient was less than 0.707 [34], as we validated the final model in Fig. 1. Still, marital status was a stronger predictor of the relationship between social determinants (SDH) and perceived usefulness (PU).

3.2 Social Determinants - Age and Marital Status

Our statistical study showed that age is a significant predictor of perceived usefulness (PU). Reflecting the same, our descriptive observations (Table 3) point out that younger (21 - 25 years old), married male students, are ready to use TDM now (100%) while only a third of their married female classmates of the same age, are ready to use TDM now (33%) with two- thirds (67%) stating their intent to use it in the future.

Table 3. Descriptive Analysis – Demographics, Education Specialty and Time @ work.

Sample Profile (N=89)		Ready to Use Now (Q.23)	Future Intention (Q.24)
Gender	Male	60%	47%
	Female	65%	59%
Age	<=20 years of Age	77%	64%
	21 - 25	60%	56%
	26 - 30	67%	58%
	31 - 35	60%	60%
	36 - 40	0%	0%
	41 - 45	50%	50%
	46 - 50	67%	67%
Education	Business Management	60%	60%
	Engineering and Sciences	71%	50%
	Humanities	67%	67%
	Medical & Health	64%	62%
	Political Science - Law	50%	25%
	Other	50%	33%
Work Schedule	Part time	72%	56%
	Full time	68%	62%
	Other	57%	54%
Marital Status	Single	65%	56%
	Married	56%	67%

Among their older colleagues, all (100%) single male students, 26–30 years old and all (100%) married female students (31–35 years old) use it now and will continue to use it in the future (Table 4). Prior studies in the field of technology acceptance have shown that couples who were married used internet more frequently than the single ones, which is why they are more inclined to use mobile technologies and online health monitoring apps. In addition to that, eHealth literacy was found to be associated with computer characteristics knowledge, therefore the involvement in new conceptualized health technologies would be more accepted by people who use technologies and internet more frequently [46].

Table 4. Descriptive Analysis – Age, Gender and Marital Status.

Ready to Use Now (Q.23) / Future Intention (Q.24)	N= 89	Female				Male			
		Married		Single		Married		Single	
20 Years or younger	25%	100%	100%	84%	68%				
21 - 25	48%	33%	67%	62%	55%	100%		71%	57%
26 - 30	13%			60%	50%			100%	100%
31 - 35	6%	100%	100%	50%	50%				
36 - 40	2%								
41 - 45	2%							50%	
46 - 50	3%			100%	100%				50%

3.3 Education Specialty

The technology acceptance model developed by Davis et al. [32] supports education specialty that may indicate a varied experience with technology. Our descriptive study indicates a higher readiness among students in fields of engineering sciences (71%) while political science students (25%) demonstrated the lowest appetite (Table 3). This was corroborated by a previous study that evaluated the moderating effect of student's field of study on technology acceptance which showed that engineering, science and technology students were more motivated towards the adoption of new innovative technologies based on their perceived ease of use [35]. Finally, part time and full-time workers are mostly ready to use TDM now. This finding is coherent with studies in the literature. Patients who work full time or part time are now free to choose between online consultations or in-person visits and many have opted for the virtual method to save time and money, at the same time expressing their satisfaction towards these medical innovations [36].

3.4 Result Demonstrability

The statistical results suggested that, results demonstrability, i.e. "the technology has to work, so that it can be useful" –Survey Question (15, 17, 31 and 32); was a strong antecedent to perceived usefulness (PU) of mobile TDM by students with a very high level of confidence (t = 11.124) and with a very strong predictor of 67.2% (path coefficient = 0.672).

For our about half of our student cohort, TDM technology is expected to do what is supposed to do – and must give a confidence that the results are accurate (Table 5). As identified in the Modified TAM (TAM2) model [37], the factor of result demonstrability indicates the effectiveness of the TDM in the early detection of the onset of the disease, the user's trust in technology. In the literature, some studies reported that users expressed their concern regarding their privacy if the application were to be hacked; they also shared their anxiety of waiting for the final diagnosis, and their doubt about the accuracy of the image [38]. In other studies, medical practitioners expressed their concern towards overloading their system with images [29], yet among young students, 49% of informants in our study found TDM beneficial for monitoring and self-examining skin lesions to detect any suspicious lesions. About 40% of the students in our study have expressed confidence in the accuracy of the mobile application compared to face-to-face diagnosis; and only 34% believed that a suspicious mole or lesion diagnosis would be understandable (thus able to provide the value expected).

Table 5. Descriptive Analysis – Results Demonstrability.

Results Demonstrability - (Fit For Purpose)	
RD1 - Will do what is supposed to do (Q15)	49%
RD3 - Perceived accuracy (Q32)	46%
RD2 - Will trust diagnostics (Q31)	40%
RD4 - Understandble prognosis (Q17)	34%

3.5 Perceived Risk

Perceived Risk (PR) was a strong predictor in our statistical study [27]. Perceived risk (resistance to use, efficiency and technology anxiety) predict the outcome by 46.4% [27]. The informants would use TDM if it is convenient (loading factor = 0.773), and if it saves time (0.834) as long as they receive the adequate training (0.776) [27]. Research has shown that PR can be an antecedent and a moderator of user acceptance [40, 41]. Perceived risk could be due to factors of efficiency (saving time and money) [42, 43] – Our cohort agrees (74% and 71% respectively). TDM must save time and money (Table 6). On the other hand, only 44% found the technology easy to learn. Perceived risk could also be induced by technology anxiety (training, technical assistance and skill acquisition) [15], our informants also agree (71%) that they are more prone to adopt it if they receive adequate training. The presence of facilitating conditions (here shown as professional assistance with the required dermatologists support to realize the benefits from their mobile TDM APP is also a factor.

3.6 Subjective Norms

The descriptive analysis of the survey data indicated that almost half (47%) of the sampled population would be influenced by their family and friends to use TDM (Table 7).

Table 6. Descriptive Analysis – Perceived Risk.

Perceived Risk (PR) - Efficiency	
PR-EFF1 - Q25 - Save Time	74%
PR-EFF2 - Q26 - Save Money	67%
Perceived Risk (PR) - Technology Anxiety	
PR-TA1 - Q33 - If I receive adequate training	71%
PR-TA2 - Q34 - I receive technical assistance when I need it	66%
PR-TA3 - Q18 - Easy to learn	44%
Perceived Risk (PR) - Resistance to Use	
PR-RC1 - Q20 - Self examination practice	65%
PR-RC2 - Q21 - Can fit my self examination habit	63%
PR-RC3 - Q22 - May interfere with my work	18%
Perceived Risk (PR) - Facilitating Conditions	
PR-FC1 - Q35 - HCP available to help	61%

This phenomenon invokes the theory of planned behavior [43], where subjective norms (indicated here by social influence) are believed to shape an individual's behavioral intentions, here the intention to use TDM. However, the statistical findings did not indicate that Subjective norms were predictors of intention to use, whilst the influence of family and friends has indeed shown as a strong predictor of subjective norms, in the context of our study.

Table 7. Descriptive Analysis – Subjective Norms.

Subjective Norm - (Social influence)	
SI2 - Q30 - Family & Friends influence	47%
SI1 - Q29 - HealthCare Practitioner Influence	38%

3.7 Medical Factors

Medical factors are included to examine the potential significance of the existence of family cancer history in the adoption context. Family history of skin cancer, previous skin cancer removed and presence of moles larger than 2 mm were considered significant in an earlier study [39]. Therefore, we included them in the initial model, as they are contextual to the setting of TDM. Perceived usefulness of the TDM application for USJ students is unaffected by medical considerations. The use of mobile TDM as a screening tool for early skin cancer detection has seemed counter to cancer risk conditions, which is surprising (Table 8).

When we evaluated the connection between medical factors and TDM adoption, both, our statistical and descriptive analysis show a rather counterintuitive result. While other studies have determined that those who perceive being at high risk of Cancer due to family history, and skin related medical factors, are favorable to the use of TDM

Table 8. Descriptive Analysis – Medical Factors.

Medical Factors	Ready to Use Now (Q.23)	Future Intention (Q.24)
N=	89	89
No Family History	56	49
No Previous Skin cancer	55	49
Brown Eyes	37	32
No Moles Present	33	31
Medium / Dark Skin	29	26
Fair Skin	28	25
Moles > 2mm	24	20
Hazel Eyes	12	12
Green Eyes	6	6
Previous Skin cancer	2	2
Family History	1	2
Blue Eyes	1	1

[39], our survey found that students do not necessarily consider medical conditions of cancer risk in the context of TDM adoption. Although dermatologists considered TDM to be helpful for the triage and diagnosis of the majority of skin disorders treated in primary care [44], our study showed weak evidence that, in the context of the Lebanese youth, patient usage of the technology was influenced by their condition. What is more interesting that, participants with family history of cancer have low acceptance rate than the ones who don't (8). This may also be an indication that cancer is a subject that people, who have antecedent patients, avoid the subject. Cancer has a psychological effect on family members that have lived and suffered the consequences of the disease [45].

4   Summary of Findings

Our study provides a good insight into the propensity of University Students in Lebanon to use Mobile Teledermatology (TDM) (Fig. 2). Whereas, 77% of younger students (< = 20 years old) are ready to use TDM now, while students in fields of engineering sciences (71%) are the most ready and political science students (25%) demonstrated the lowest appetite – This could be attributed to the affinity of science leaning students toward technology.

Both genders are more or less equally ready to embrace TDM now, but female students showed a higher intention to use TDM in the future (8% more than males). However, younger (21 - 25 years old), married male students, are ready to use TDM now (100%) while only a third of their married female classmates of the same age, are ready to use TDM now (33%) with two- thirds (67%) stating their intent to use it in the future.

We can also conclude that whilst almost half (47%) of the sampled population would be influenced by their family and friends to use TDM, perceived usefulness of the TDM application for USJ students is unaffected by medical considerations. The use of mobile TDM as a screening tool for early skin cancer detection has seemed counter to cancer risk

77% of younger students are ready

100% young married male students

33% married female classmates

71% Students in Engineering sciences.

25% Students in Political Sciences

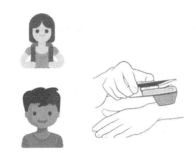

Mobile TDM Intention to Use Among Young University Students

Would use TDM because:

74% Save time

71 % Save money

44% Found the technology easy to learn

71% Adequate training required

47% Would be influenced by family and friends

Fig. 2. Our study provides a good insight into the propensity of University Students in Lebanon to use Mobile Tele Dermatology (TDM).

conditions, which is surprising. This may be an indication that cancer is a subject that people, who have antecedent patients, avoid the subject, as cancer has a psychological effect on family members that have lived and suffered the consequences of the disease.

5 Conclusion

The manuscript succeeds in tackling a fascinating subject through an empirical pilot study. However, the study is limited by the fact that the sample is made up of students from a single university. The gender distribution (83% female and 17% male) and the prevalence of medical and health students (i.e., over 50% of the sample) are two additional drawbacks. The additional observations and findings from this pilot survey should be helpful to both scholars and practitioners. To expand on this pilot and gain a greater knowledge of the variables affecting usage intention, a qualitative study is advised. This study can be extended to a larger population with a variety of age groups and occupations, providing a useful comparison of the markets that can be served and the target audience that could provide insight for manufacturers and practitioners alike.

Appendix

Survey Questions and Possible Answers

1- Gender: Male, Female
2- Age: <20 years; 21 – 25; 26 – 30; 31 – 35; 36 – 40; 41 – 45; Above 46
3- Education specialty: Business Management; Engineering & Sciences; Humanities; Medical & Health; Political Science & Law; Other
4- Work: Part time; Full time; Other or Null
5- Marital status: Single; Married

6- Skin colour: Fair; Medium; Dark

7- Eye colour: Brown; Hazel; Blue; Green; Other or Null

8- Family history of skin cancer: No; Yes

9- Previous skin cancer removed: No; Yes

10- Presence of moles larger than 2 mm: None; Less than 10; 11+

11- Mobile Teledermatology will help me examine my skin more rapidly: Strongly agree; Agree; Unsure; Disagree; Strongly disagree

12- Mobile Teledermatology will improve my self-skin examination: Strongly agree; Agree; Unsure; Disagree; Strongly disagree

13- Mobile Teledermatology is useful to diagnose moles on my skin for suspicious lesions: Strongly agree; Agree; Unsure; Disagree; Strongly disagree

14- Mobile Teledermatology will help save time: Strongly agree; Agree; Unsure; Disagree; Strongly disagree

15- Mobile Teledermatology will help detect skin cancer in early stages: Strongly agree; Agree; Unsure; Disagree; Strongly disagree

16- Mobile Teledermatology will be easy to use: Strongly agree; Agree; Unsure; Disagree; Strongly disagree

17- A suspicious mole or lesion diagnosis through Mobile Teledermatology will be understandable: Strongly agree; Agree; Unsure; Disagree; Strongly disagree

18- Mobile Teledermatology users will easily acquire the skills to preform it: Strongly agree; Agree; Unsure; Disagree; Strongly disagree

19- Mobile Teledermatology will encourage me to examine my skin thoroughly: Strongly agree; Agree; Unsure; Disagree; Strongly disagree

20- The use of Mobile Teledermatology will change my self-skin examination practice: Strongly agree; Agree; Unsure; Disagree; Strongly disagree

21- The use of Mobile Teledermatology can fit in my skin examination habit: Strongly agree; Agree; Unsure; Disagree; Strongly disagree

22- The use of Mobile Teledermatology may interfere with my work: Strongly agree; Agree; Unsure; Disagree; Strongly disagree

23- I will use Mobile Teledermatology when its offered to me: Strongly agree; Agree; Unsure; Disagree; Strongly disagree 24- I will use Mobile Teledermatology in my routine self-skin examination in the future: Strongly agree; Agree; Unsure; Disagree; Strongly disagree

24- I will use Mobile Teledermatology if it will save me time: Strongly agree; Agree; Unsure; Disagree; Strongly disagree

25- I will use Mobile Teledermatology if it will save me money: Strongly agree; Agree; Unsure; Disagree; Strongly disagree

26- Mobile Teledermatology will be useful to diagnose skin cancer in general: Strongly agree; Agree; Unsure; Disagree; Strongly disagree

27- Mobile Teledermatology will be for my best interest: Strongly agree; Agree; Unsure; Disagree; Strongly disagree

28- Health professionals (nurses, physicians…) will welcome the fact that I use Mobile Tele-dermatology: Strongly agree; Agree; Unsure; Disagree; Strongly disagree y

29- My friends and my family will welcome the fact that I use Mobile Teledermatology: Strongly agree; Agree; Unsure; Disagree; Strongly disagree

30- I will completely trust the diagnosis of the dermatologist based on a photo I've sent using Mobile Teledermatology: Strongly agree; Agree; Unsure; Disagree; Strongly disagree

31- I will rely on the Teledermatology process to supply accurate information about a mole or a spot: Strongly agree; Agree; Unsure; Disagree; Strongly disagree

32- I will use Mobile Teledermatology if I receive adequate training: Strongly agree; Agree; Unsure; Disagree; Strongly disagree

33- I will use Mobile Teledermatology if I receive technical assistance when I need it: Strongly agree; Agree; Unsure; Disagree; Strongly disagree

34- There are health professionals available who will help me with Mobile Teledermatology: Strongly agree; Agree; Unsure; Disagree; Strongly disagree

Latent Variables for Our Statistical Model from Aroutine et al. (2022)

SI: Subjective norms (Q: 29 & 30);
SDH: Social determinants (Q: 3 thru 5);
MED: Medical factors (Q: 1, 2, 6 thru 10);
RES DEM: Result demonstrability (Q: 15, 17, 31, 32);
PR: Perceived risk (Q: 18, 20 thru 22, 25, 26, 33 thru 35);
PU: Perceived usefulness (Q: 11 thru 14, 19, 27 & 28);
PEOU: Perceived ease of use (Q: 16); UI (UI1 & UI2): Intention to Use (Q: 23 & 24).

Hypotheses - Summarized from Aroutine et al. (2022)

H1: Social Determinants such as age, marital status and education specialty affect perceived usefulness of mobile TDM by students

H2: Medical factors such as family cancer history, age and gender affect perceived usefulness of mobile TDM by students

H3: Results Demonstrability (or effectiveness) indicated by the user's trust in technology performance and the perceived ability of mobile TDM to offer early detection, with accurate information and an understandable outcome affects perceived usefulness of mobile TDM by students

H4: Perceived risk, indicated by the resistance to change, efficiency and technology anxiety affects intention to use of mobile TDM by students

H5: Perceived risk, indicated by resistance to change, efficiency and technology anxiety moderates the relationship between perceived ease of use and intention to use of mobile TDM by students

H6: Perceived risk, indicated by resistance to change, efficiency and technology anxiety moderates the relationship between perceived usefulness and intention to use of mobile TDM by students

H7: Subjective norms, indicated by social influence, affects the intention to use of mobile TDM by students.

H8: Perceived usefulness, indicated by the perception that the technology will serve the best interest of the user, in a rapid, self-examination, affects intention to use of mobile TDM by students.

H9: Perceived ease of use affects intention to use of mobile TDM by students

H10: Perceived ease of use affects perceived usefulness of Mobile TDM by students.

References

1. Chou, H.M.: A smart-mutual decentralized system for long-term care. Appl. Sci. **12**(7), 3664 (2022)
2. Abbaspur-Behbahani, S., Monaghesh, E., Hajizadeh, A., Fehresti, S.: Application of mobile health to support the elderly during the COVID-19 outbreak: a systematic review. Health Policy Technol. **11**, 100595 (2022)
3. Cox, A., et al.: Cancer survivors' experience with telehealth: a systematic review and thematic synthesis. J. Med. Internet Res. **19**(1), e6575 (2017)
4. Hilty, D.M., Maheu, M.M., Drude, K.P., Hertlein, K.M.: The need to implement and evaluate telehealth competency frameworks to ensure quality care across behavioral health professions. Acad. Psychiatry **42**(6), 818–824 (2018). https://doi.org/10.1007/s40596-018-0992-5
5. Barnason, S., et al.: Influence of a symptom management telehealth intervention on older adults' early recovery outcomes after coronary artery bypass surgery. Heart Lung **38**(5), 364–376 (2009)
6. Ohinmaa, A., Chatterley, P., Nguyen, T., Jacobs, P.: Telehealth in substance abuse and addiction: review of the literature on smoking, alcohol, drug abuse and gambling (2010)
7. Lew, S.Q., Sikka, N.: Operationalizing telehealth for home dialysis patients in the United States. Am. J. Kidney Dis. **74**(1), 95–100 (2019)
8. Sung, H., et al.: Global cancer statistics 2020: GLOBOCAN estimates of incidence and mortality worldwide for 36 cancers in 185 countries. CA Cancer J Clin. **71**, 209–249 (2021)
9. Jolliffe, V.M., Harris, D.W., Whittaker, S.J.: Can we safely diagnose pigmented lesions from stored video images? A diagnostic comparison between clinical examination and stored video images of pigmented lesions removed for histology. Clin. Exp. Dermatol. **26**(1), 84–87 (2001)
10. Desai, B., McKoy, K., Kovarik, C.: Overview of international teledermatology. Pan Afr. Med. J. **6** (2010)
11. Massone, C., Maak, D., Hofmann-Wellenhof, R., Soyer, H.P., Frühauf, J.: Teledermatology for skin cancer prevention: an experience on 690 Austrian patients. J. Eur. Acad. Dermatol. Venereol. **28**(8), 1103–1108 (2014)
12. Sáenz, J.P., Novoa, M.P., Correal, D., Eapen, B.R.: On using a mobile application to support teledermatology: a case study in an underprivileged area in Colombia. Int. J. Telemed. Appl. (2018)
13. Wang, R.H., et al.: Clinical effectiveness and cost-effectiveness of teledermatology: where are we now, and what are the barriers to adoption? J. Am. Acad. Dermatol. **83**(1), 299–307 (2020)
14. McGee, J.S., Reynolds, R.V., Olbricht, S.M.: Fighting COVID-19: Early teledermatology lessons learned. J. Am. Acad. Dermatol. **83**(4), 1224–1225 (2020)
15. Mostafa, P.I.N., Hegazy, A.A.: Dermatological consultations in the COVID-19 era: is teledermatology the key to social distancing? An Egyptian experience. J. Dermatol. Treat. 1–6 (2020)
16. Koonin, L.M.: Trends in the use of telehealth during the emergence of the COVID-19 pandemic—United States, January–March 2020. MMWR (2020)
17. Cartron, A.M., Rismiller, K., Trinidad, J.C.L.: Store-and-forward teledermatology in the era of COVID-19: a pilot study. Dermatol. Therapy **33**, e13689–e13689 (2020)
18. Ha, J., Park, H.K.: Factors affecting the acceptability of technology in health care among older Korean adults with multiple chronic conditions: a cross-sectional study adopting the senior technology acceptance model. Clin. Interv. Aging **15**, 1873–1881 (2020)
19. AshaRani, P., et al.: Readiness and acceptance of ehealth services for diabetes care in the general population: cross-sectional study. J. Med. Internet Res. **23**(9), e26881 (2021)

20. Huberty, J., Green, J., Glissmann, C., Larkey, L., Puzia, M., Lee, C.: Efficacy of the mindfulness meditation mobile app "calm" to reduce stress among college students: randomized controlled trial. JMIR Mhealth Uhealth 7(6), e14273 (2019)
21. Arcury, T.A., et al.: Older adult internet use and ehealth literacy. J. Appl. Gerontol. Off. J. Southern Gerontol. Soc. 39(2), 141–150 (2020)
22. Peracca, S.B., Jackson, G.L., Weinstock, M.A., Oh, D.H.: Implementation of teledermatology: theory and practice. Curr. Dermatol. Rep. 8(2), 35–45 (2019). https://doi.org/10.1007/s13671-019-0252-2
23. Armstrong, A.W., Kwong, M.W., Chase, E.P., Ledo, L., Nesbitt, T.S., Shewry, S.L.: Teledermatology operational considerations, challenges, and benefits: the referring providers' perspective. Telemed. e-Health 18(8), 580–584 (2012)
24. Walters, L.E., Mars, M., Scott, R.E.: A review and critique of teledermatology in the South African public health sector. Stud Health Technol. Inform. 231, 143–151 (2016)
25. Coustasse, A., Sarkar, R., Abodunde, B., Metzger, B.J., Slater, C.M.: Use of teledermatology to improve dermatological access in rural areas. Telemed. e-Health 25(11), 1022–1032 (2019)
26. Gupta, R., Ibraheim, M.K., Doan, H.Q.: Teledermatology in the wake of COVID-19: advantages and challenges to continued care in a time of disarray. J. Am. Acad. Dermatol. 83(1), 168–169 (2020)
27. Aroutine, N., Badr, N.G., Yeretzian, J.: Factors influencing tele-dermatology adoption among the Lebanese youth: a pilot study at Saint Joseph University. In: HEALTHINF, pp. 15–25 (2022)
28. Venkatesh, V., Morris, M.G., Davis, G.B., et al.: User acceptance of information technology: toward a unified view. MIS Q. 27, 425–478 (2003)
29. Tao, D., Shao, F., Wang, H., Yan, M., Qu, X.: Integrating usability and social cognitive theories with the technology acceptance model to understand young users' acceptance of a health information portal. Health Informatics J. 26(2), 1347–1362 (2020)
30. Zhang, Y., et al.: Factors influencing patients' intentions to use diabetes management apps based on an extended unified theory of acceptance and use of technology model: web-based survey. J. Med. Internet Res. 21(8), e15023 (2019)
31. Rouidi, M., Elouadi, A., Hamdoune, A.: Acceptance and use of telemedicine technology by health professionals: development of a conceptual model. Digital Health 8, 20552076221081692 (2022)
32. Davis, F.D.: Perceived usefulness, perceived ease of use, and user acceptance of information technology. MIS Q. 319–340 (1989)
33. Kucuk, S., Baydas Onlu, O., Kapakin, S.: A model for medical students' behavioral intention to use mobile learning. J. Med. Educ. Curric. Dev. 7, 2382120520973222 (2020)
34. Hair, J.F., Risher, J.J., Sarstedt, M., Ringle, C.M.: When to use and how to report the results of PLS-SEM. Eur. Bus. Rev. 31(1), 2–24 (2019)
35. Rosli, M.S., Saleh, N.S.: Technology enhanced learning acceptance among university students during Covid-19: integrating the full spectrum of self-determination theory and self-efficacy into the technology acceptance model. Curr. Psychol. (New Brunswick, N.j.), 1–20 (2022) https://doi.org/10.1007/s12144-022-02996-1
36. Al Quran, H.A., Khader, Y.S., Ellauzi, Z.M., Shdaifat, A.: Effect of real-time teledermatology on diagnosis, treatment and clinical improvement. J. Telemed. Telecare 21(2), 93–99 (2015)
37. Venkatesh, V., Davis, F.: A theoretical extension of the technology acceptance model: four longitudinal field studies. Manage. Sci. 46, 186–204 (2000)
38. Abbott, L.M., et al.: Practice guidelines for teledermatology in Australia. Australas. J. Dermatol. 61, e293–e302 (2020)
39. Horsham, C., Loescher, L.J., Whiteman, D.C., Soyer, H.P., Janda, M.: Consumer acceptance of patient-performed mobile teledermoscopy for the early detection of melanoma. Br. J. Dermatol. 175(6), 1301–1310 (2016)

40. Im, I., Kim, Y., Han, H.: The effects of perceived risk and technology type on users' acceptance of technologies. Inf. Manag. **45**, 1–9 (2008)
41. Kamal, S.A., Shafiq, M., Kakria, P.: Investigating acceptance of telemedicine services through an extended technology acceptance model (TAM). Technol. Soc. **60**, 101212 (2020)
42. Yang, X., Barbieri, J.S., Kovarik, C.L.: Cost analysis of a store-and-forward teledermatology consult system in Philadelphia. J. Am. Acad. Dermatol. **81**(3), 758–764 (2019)
43. Ajzen, I.: The theory of planned behaviour: reactions and reflections. Psychol. Health **26**(9), 1113–1127 (2011)
44. Giavina Bianchi, M., Santos, A., Cordioli, E.: Dermatologists' perceptions on the utility and limitations of teledermatology after examining 55,000 lesions. J. Telemed. Telecare **27**(3), 166–173 (2021)
45. Pitceathly, C., Maguire, P.: The psychological impact of cancer on patients' partners and other key relatives: a review. Eur. J. Cancer **39**(11), 1517–1524 (2003)
46. Arcury, T.A., et al.: Older adult internet use and eHealth literacy. J. Appl. Gerontol. **39**(2), 141–150 (2020)

Predictive Alarm Prevention by Forecasting Threshold Alarms at the Intensive Care Unit

Jonas Chromik[1]([⊠])[iD], Bjarne Pfitzner[1][iD], Nina Ihde[1][iD], Marius Michaelis[1][iD],
Denise Schmidt[1][iD], Sophie Anne Ines Klopfenstein[2][iD], Akira-Sebastian Poncette[2][iD],
Felix Balzer[2][iD], and Bert Arnrich[1][iD]

[1] Hasso Plattner Institute, University of Potsdam, Potsdam, Germany
{jonas.chromik,bjarne.pfitzner,bert.arnrich}@hpi.de,
{nina.ihde,marius.michealis,denise.schmidt}@student.hpi.de
[2] Charité – Universitätsmedizin Berlin, Berlin, Germany
{sophie.klopfenstein,akira-sebastian.poncette,
felix.balzer}@charite.de
https://hpi.de/arnrich, https://medinfo.charite.de

Abstract. Patient monitors at intensive care units produce too many alarms –
most of them being unnecessary. Medical staff becomes desensitised and ignores
alarms. This phenomenon is called alarm fatigue and it negatively influences for
both patients and staff. Some alarms are due to an acute and unforeseeable events
but others are the result of a continued trend and hence foreseeable. We present a
system that forecasts alarms – at least the foreseeable share – and transforms them
into scheduled tasks. To achieve this, we use time-series models to forecast the
patient's vital parameters and check whether the forecast violates the corresponding alarm threshold. The vital parameter measurements and alarm data stem from
MIMIC-III but go through extensive preprocessing before the actual forecasting
can take place. The result is a proof of concept but unfit for productive use. Lack
of alarm data and low sampling frequencies for vital parameters impair alarm
forecasting. Our work shows that gated recurrent unit models generally perform
best for this task. A next step towards productive use is evaluating the approach
on vital parameter data with higher time-resolution.

Keywords: Patient monitoring · Medical alarms · Alarm fatigue · Time-series
forecasting

1 Introduction

Too many alarms from various devices make the intensive care unit a noisy and stressful
place for both patients and medical staff. Different studies and reviews report numbers
as high as 700 alarms per day [6] or 187 alarms per bed per day – only counting audible

This work was partially carried out within the INALO project. INALO is a cooperation project
between AICURA medical GmbH, Charité – Universitätsmedizin Berlin, idalab GmbH, and
Hasso Plattner Institute. INALO is funded by the German Federal Ministry of Education and
Research under grant 16SV8559.

A. C. A. Roque et al. (Eds.): BIOSTEC 2022, CCIS 1814, pp. 215–236, 2023.
https://doi.org/10.1007/978-3-031-38854-5_12

alarms [8]. Most of the alarms are either technically false, clinically irrelevant, or otherwise unnecessary [24,27]. This causes *alarm fatigue*: a desensitisation of clinicians by numerous alarms, many of which are either false or otherwise irrelevant [8,24]. Alarm fatigue negatively influences both for patients and medical staff [6].

The effects on medical staff are not extensively studied yet [23]. But studies indicate impaired mental efficiency and short-term memory [17] as well as stress [16] and stress-induced ailments such as burn-out [26]. A very recent study showed that false alarms are the medical staff's main concern and almost all members of the intensive care unit's staff requested a reduction in false alarms [22].

In patients, too many alarms and too much noise cause sleep deprivation [20], cardiovascular abnormalities [1,11], longer hospital stays [9], increased rehospitalisation rates [11], increased need for analgesic medication [15], delayed wound healing [28], intensive care unit syndrome (a cluster of psychological and cognitive impairments) [2], and feelings of vulnerability and fear [10].

We still do not know how to effectively reduce the alarm burden on intensive care units and no single existing solution seems to be sufficient. In this work, we address threshold alarms – the most frequent type of alarms [8]. Threshold alarms on patient monitors inform the medical staff that a vital parameter – such as heart rate or blood pressure – is either too low or too high. If we could forecast these alarms, we could spot critical conditions early – even before they pose a danger to the patient. And we could convert acute, urgent, and disruptive alarms into scheduled tasks that the medical staff can handle at their own discretion – flexibly and over an extended period of time.

To forecast threshold alarms, we try to forecast the associated vital parameter. This is a regression task that we can solve with statistical or machine learning models for time-series. We try to find in the vital parameter measurements that will result in the vital parameter crossing one of the respective alarm thresholds. We are certain that we can not forecast all alarms since some alarms are actually the result of an acute event rather than a continued trend. But some alarms are foreseeable by inspecting the vital parameter measurements – these are the alarms we try to forecast and convert into scheduled tasks. We aim for few false positives to avoid increasing the staff's workload any further. But we are willing to accept many false negatives since not every alarm is foreseeable from the vital parameter trend.

This is an extended version of a conference paper [4]. We include content that we could not report in the conference paper due to page limitations, especially regarding data set preparation. The rest of this work is structured as follows: In Sect. 2 we describe the data we use, why we chose this data set, and how we have to prepare it before usage. In Sect. 3 we describe the methods we use for alarm forecasting. In Sect. 4 we show results on how well alarm forecasting works and which methods appear to be the most promising. Finally, in Sect. 5 we discuss our results including limitations and directions for future work.

2   Data Preparation

We surveyed the variety of medical data sets and found several large intensive care unit data sets. We assessed the 3rd version of the Medical Information Mart for Intensive

Care (MIMIC-III) [14], the eICU Collaborative Research Database (eICU CRD) [21], the High Time Resolution ICU Data Set (HiRID) [13], and the Amsterdam University Medical Centers Database (AmsterdamUMCdb) [25] and found that none of these data sets records patient monitor alarms. In fact, eICU CRD, HiRID, and AmsterdamUMCdb contain no alarm system information at all. MIMIC-III does not record alarm *events* but at least alarm *thresholds* and changes to these thresholds. Using thresholds and vital parameter measurements, we can reconstruct when alarms went off although the data set does not explicitly record these alarm events.

Other data sets record vital parameters with a higher temporal resolution (for example up to $f_s = 5\,\text{min}^{-1}$ for eICU CRD) and might allow for better results in the regression task described in Sect. 3. But we definitely need the alarm threshold information – which are unique to MIMIC-III – to determine when an alarm goes off.

In the remainder of this section we describe how we reconstructed alarm events from the data provided in MIMIC-III. We used the methods described in [3] and we reproduce parts of these methods here.

2.1   Data Slicing

Data set preparation starts with reducing the data set to a subset of relevant information. MIMIC-III contains many table with various information such as diagnoses, lab values, and medications. But we are only interested in a single table: The CHARTEVENTS table records so called "charted events" – among them vital parameter measurements and alarm threshold updates. In CHARTEVENTS, all charted events are coded as data items with a unique ITEMID that identified the type of event, measurement, or value. The D_ITEMS table resolves the different ITEMIDs. We are only interested in the data items representing measurements for heart rate (HR), non-invasively measured systolic blood pressure (NBP_s), and peripheral blood oxygen saturation (SpO_2) – and their respective alarm thresholds. We selected these three vital parameters because they have the highest temporal resolution within MIMIC-III. Table 1 shows a complete list of used data items.

2.2   Data Cleaning

Vital parameters cannot assume arbitrary values but are limited to certain physiologically possible ranges. For example, SpO_2 can not exceed 100% and HRs above 350 bpm are rare and unsustainable. MIMIC-III contains some instances of unrealistically high or low values for the vital parameter measurements or the alarm thresholds. We consider these extreme values to be erroneous or to have a special but undocumented meaning. Either way, we can not interpret these values. From a contextual inquiry at an intensive care unit we learned that keyboards at the intensive care unit might have a rubber cover to stop germs from accumulating in and on the keyboard. But this causes the keyboard's keys to be sticky which impairs data entry and causes documentation errors. To deal with unrealistically high or low values, we remove all vital parameter measurements and alarm thresholds that we consider to be invalid from the data set. Table 2 lists lower and upper limits for each parameter type. We retain values within

Table 1. Adapted from [3]: ITEMIDs retained while filtering CHARTEVENTS.

ITEMID	Label
220045	HR
220046	HR Alarm - High
220047	HR Alarm - Low
220179	NBP_s
223751	NBP_s Alarm - High
223752	NBP_s Alarm - Low
220277	SpO_2
223769	SpO_2 Alarm - High
223770	SpO_2 Alarm - Low

this range and discard values beyond this range. Figure 1 shows the distribution of measurements and thresholds before cleaning as boxplots. Many extreme outlier force the interquartile range to be a single line at the leftmost corner of the plot. A histogram would be completely unintelligible. Figure 2 shows the distributions of measurements and thresholds after cleaning as boxplots and histograms. This distribution is much more reasonable. The measurement histogram exhibits a bell-shaped distribution that is only slightly positively skewed.

Table 2. Adapted from [12]: Physiologically possible ranges for the vital parameters considered in this work.

Parameter	Lower Limit	Upper Limit
HR	0 bpm	350 bpm
NBP_s	0 mmHg	375 mmHg
SpO_2	0%	100%

For thresholds one condition must always hold true: The low threshold must always be lower than the high threshold. This is an invariant for all vital parameters. If this condition is not met, every measurement of the vital parameter – regardless of its value – will trigger an alarm event; which defies the purpose of alarms altogether. MIMIC-III violates this invariant occasionally: Although high and low thresholds are always recorded simultaneously, the high threshold is sometimes lower than the low threshold. We address this problem in two ways:

Exact Threshold Swaps. When thresholds are exactly swapped, the low threshold takes the value of the high threshold and vice versa. We correct this by swapping the set of thresholds back to normal (Fig. 3).

Threshold Overlaps. When thresholds overlap but we cannot identify an exact swap, we just remove the erroneous threshold value and carry over the previously active threshold (Fig. 4).

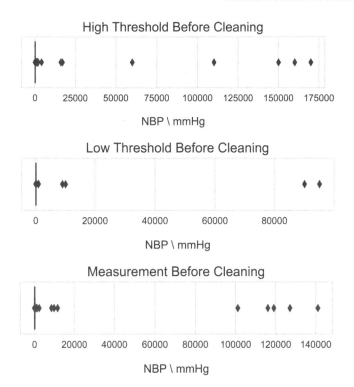

Fig. 1. Adapted from [3]: Boxplots showing the distribution of NBP$_s$ high alarm thresholds, low alarm thresholds, and measurements before cleaning. The distribution is vastly skewed with the valid range barely visible at the far left corner and a wide range of outliers.

2.3   Extracting Alarm Events

Now that we addressed all data quality issues, we can extract alarm events. We do this by using Algorithm 1 on MIMIC-III's CHARTEVENTS table. First, we split the CHARTEVENTS table by ICUSTAY – a patient's single stay at the intensive care unit (one patient might be at the same intensive care unit multiple times throughout his or her life). Then, we compare each of the patient's vital parameter measurements to the high and low thresholds active at the time of measurement. If the measurement exceeds the high threshold or is below the low thresholds, the algorithm yields and alarm event. A major drawback of this methods is that the sampling frequency of the measurements influences the number of alarms: HR and SpO$_2$ are measured and recorded more often than NBP$_s$, hence more alarms are extracted by the algorithm. But this does not show that the patient actually spend more *time* with unhealthy NBP$_s$ as compared to unhealthy HR or SpO$_2$.

2.4   Resampling Vital Parameters

By extracting the alarm events, we created the labels for our forecasting system. Now we still have to prepare the vital parameter time series to be used as input for the sta-

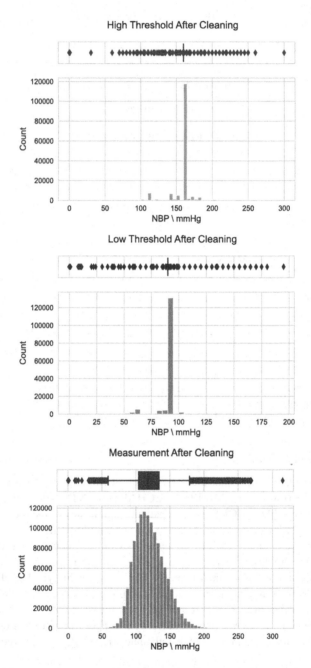

Fig. 2. Adapted from [3]: Boxplots and histograms showing the distribution of NBP$_s$ high alarm thresholds, low alarm thresholds, and measurements after cleaning. With outliers removed, the distribution looks much more reasonable and especially the measurement values are almost normally distributed with only a slight positive skew.

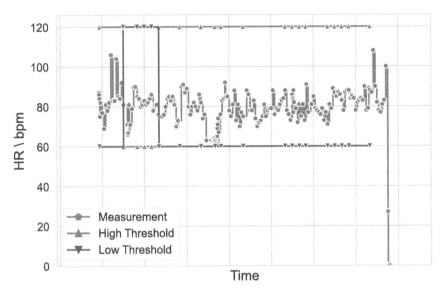

(a) Exactly swapped low and high thresholds before correction. Every measurement in the time period where the thresholds are swapped will produce an alarm.

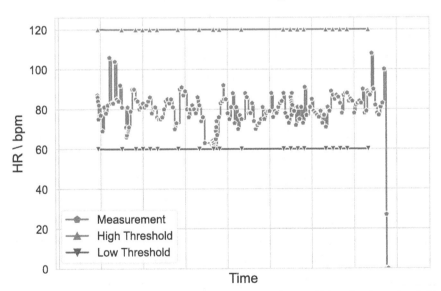

(b) A data cleaning step removes the exact threshold swap thus rectifying the alarm thresholds. Now we will not recognise any alarm events in the respective time period.

Fig. 3. Adapted from [3]: Example for an exact threshold swap correction.

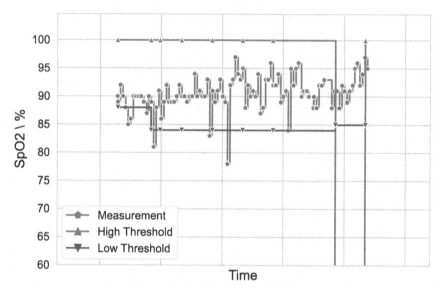

(a) In this case, the thresholds overlap without being exactly swapped. Here, the unreasonable low value for the high threshold would result in all measurements in the respective period of time triggering a high threshold alarm.

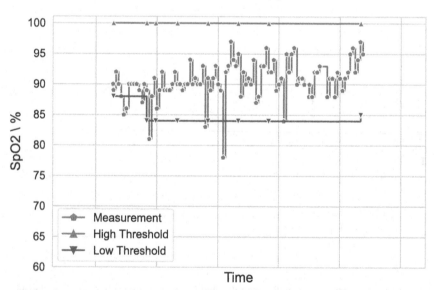

(b) Threshold overlap was corrected by removing the responsible alarm threshold settings. After correction, the measurements do not trigger any high alarms in the respective period of time.

Fig. 4. Adapted from [3]: Example for threshold overlap correction.

tistical and machine learning models described in Sect. 3. The input data preparation involves two steps: resampling and chunking. Our approach is that we want to use time-series models to forecast on the patient's vital parameter measurements – as a regression task. Time-series models rely on constant sampling frequencies in the time series. But unlike eICU CRD with its vitalPeriodic table, MIMIC-III's CHARTEVENTS table does not record measurements with a constant sampling frequency but reports all charted events and data (incl. measurements) only sporadically. We first have to establish constant sampling frequencies for all vital parameter measurements so that time-series models can work with them. Whenever possible, we resample to $f_s = 1h^{-1}$ since this is approximately equal to the median sampling frequency of the measurements. To do this, we employ three different resampling methods: minimum, maximum, and median resampling. Later-on, we will compare how the different resampling methods influence the forecasting performance.

Algorithm 1. Taken from [3]: Algorithm for extracting alarm events from measurements and thresholds.

Data: MIMIC-III CHARTEVENTS
Result: List of Alarm Events
foreach *ICUSTAY* **do**
    foreach *Parameter* **do**
        msmts := measurements for Parameter and ICUSTAY;
        highs := high threshold settings for Parameter and ICUSTAY;
        lows := low threshold settings for Parameter and ICUSTAY;
        foreach *high in highs* **do**
            foreach *msmt in msmts* **do**
                if *time(high) <= time(msmt) < time(high+1)* **then**
                    if *value(msmt) > value(high)* **then**
                        Return a high alarm event at msmt;
                    end
                end
            end
        end
        foreach *low in lows* **do**
            foreach *msmt in msmts* **do**
                if *time(low) <= time(msmt) < time(low+1* **then**
                    if *value(msmt) < value(low)* **then**
                        Return a low alarm event at msmt;
                    end
                end
            end
        end
    end
end

2.5 Chunking to Avoid Data Gaps

Occasionally, there are larger gaps in the vital parameter measurements. We assume that this is because the patient is not at the intensive care unit but in the operation theatre or some other ward. In these cases we do not attempt resampling but revert to chunking: We subdivide the patient's time-series data along the data gaps and treat these gaps separately as if they would belong to different ICUSTAYs for the same patient. This chunking procedure has the disadvantage that the model has to re-learn every time a data gap occurs and cannot provide alarm forecasts for some hours. We argue that our chunking methods makes sense anyway since the patient might be in a completely different state after surgery then before.

3 Alarm Forecasting

We want to forecast threshold alarms. To do this, we use time-series models to forecast the vital parameters measurements as a regression task. Then we use the forecast vital parameters to check whether they will be above the high threshold or below the low threshold in the near future. For the time-series models we compare two different model paradigms: Statistical models that do not need a separate set of training data and machine learning models that we first train on a dedicated training data set (a part of the original data set). We frame the problem as a regression task to ensure comparability between the model paradigms since the statistical models cannot perform classification right away. Also, all models are provided with the same set of features: Although we could improve machine learning models by adding more features we refrained from doing so. With all the data set issues listed in Sect. 2, superb model performance is not the goal of this work. We rather want to provide a proof of concept and compare different model paradigms using the same data.

Experiment Setup. The basic setup is the same for both model paradigms: We provide the model with either 12 or 30 timesteps (lags) of vital parameter. This is equivalent to 12 h or 30 h of intensive care unit stay data as input. We expect a vital parameter forecast for the 13th or 31st lag. If the vital parameter forecast is above the high threshold, a high alarm is forecast. If the vital parameter forecast is below the low threshold, a low alarm is forecast. Otherwise, no alarm is forecast. Finally, we compare the forecast with the actual alarm situation as established in Sect. 2.3.

Evaluation. For evaluation, we face a similar problem as Clifford et al. when they posed the 2015 PhysioNet/Computing in Cardiology Challenge which aims at reducing false arrhythmia alarms in the intensive care unit [5]. For Clifford et al., false negatives were much worse than false positives since no arrhythmia should pass unnoticed. They developed a metric that accounts for this imbalance and penalised false negatives five times more heavily than false positives (Eq. 1). For us the situation is vice versa: We already noticed in Sect. 1 that some alarms cannot be forecast because they are the result of an acute event and not a continued trend – false negatives are to be expected. But we absolutely want to avoid increasing the workload for medical staff, hence we want to avoid false positives. We adapted the evaluation score from Clifford et al. to fit our problem (Eq. 2). We also removed the true negatives from the equation since we are not interested in no-alarm situations where there is neither an alarm not a forecast for an alarm.

$$\text{Clifford's evaluation score} = \frac{TP + TN}{TP + TN + FP + 5 \cdot FN} \tag{1}$$

$$\text{our evaluation score} = \frac{TP}{TP + 5 \cdot FP + FN} \tag{2}$$

Statistical Models. Statistical time-series models forecast without training on other time-series in advance and thus without prior knowledge through similar-time series. We use the autoregressive integrated moving average (ARIMA) model and the autoregressive integrated moving average with exogenous variables (ARIMAX) model. ARIMA uses only one time-series as input: the *endogenous* series. For ARIMA, we compare median resampling with either minimum resampling for low alarms or maximum resampling for high alarms. ARIMAX has another time-series – the *exogenous* series – in addition to the endogenous series. For ARIMAX, we use minimum resampling for low alarms and maximum resampling for high alarms as endogenous series. As exogenous series, we use the median-resampled vital parameter series for both high and low alarms. Additionally, we modulate the input size resulting in six different model configurations (Table 3).

Table 3. Adapted from [4]: ARIMA and ARIMAX models.

Model ID	Input Size	Model Type	Endog
A_01_12	12	ARIMA	Median
A_02_12	12	ARIMA	Min/Max
A_03_12	12	ARIMAX	Min/Max
A_01_30	30	ARIMA	Median
A_02_30	30	ARIMA	Min/Max
A_03_30	30	ARIMAX	Min/Max

Machine Learning Models. Unlike statistical model, machine learning models undergo a separate training phase before they can make predictions. We use the class of recurrent neural networks (RNNs), since these are usually used on time-series [7, 18, 19]. Specifically, we compare vanilla RNNs, gated recurrent units (GRUs), and long short-term memory neural networks (LSTMs). With all model types, we use 80% of each chunk as training data and 20% as test data for assessing model performance. Otherwise, we use the same setup as for the statistical models: 12 or 30 lags as input and the 13th or 31st lag to be forecast and then checked against the alarm threshold. We then repeat this to cover the whole chunk. Additionally, we also want to test if and how scaling the input data influences the model's performance. We compare:

1. no scaling (suffix n)
2. standard scaling: $x_{scaled} = \frac{x-\mu}{\sigma}$ (suffix s1)
3. min-max scaling: $x_{scaled} = \frac{x-min}{max-min}$ (suffix s2)

Table 4 lists a machine learning model configurations.

Table 4. Adapted from [4]: Machine learning (ML) models. Standard scaling is indicated by the suffix "s1". Min-max scaling by the suffix "s2". If no scaling is performed, the suffix is "n" for "non-scaled".

Model ID	Scaling	Model Type	Endog
LS_01_s1	Standard	LSTM	Median
LS_02_s1	Standard	LSTM	Min/Max
GR_01_s1	Standard	GRU	Median
GR_02_s1	Standard	GRU	Min/Max
RN_01_s1	Standard	RNN	Median
RN_02_s1	Standard	RNN	Min/Max
LS_01_s2	Min-Max	LSTM	Median
LS_02_s2	Min-Max	LSTM	Min/Max
GR_01_s2	Min-Max	GRU	Median
GR_02_s2	Min-Max	GRU	Min/Max
RN_01_s2	Min-Max	RNN	Median
RN_02_s2	Min-Max	RNN	Min/Max
LS_01_n	None	LSTM	Median
LS_02_n	None	LSTM	Min/Max
GR_01_n	None	GRU	Median
GR_02_n	None	GRU	Min/Max
RN_01_n	None	RNN	Median
RN_02_n	None	RNN	Min/Max

4   Results

In this section, we present the individual model performances. We first compare the statistical models among each other. Then, we compare the ML models among each other. Finally, we compare both model paradigms to each other.

Figure 5 compares how the input size influences the models performance across statistical models. As expected, longer input sequences usually yield better model performance. This suggests that predictions will improve the longer the patient stays at the intensive care unit. To get better predictions earlier, we need to increase the sampling frequency. This is not possible with MIMIC-III but eICU CRD might be promising as long as we find a way to add alarm data.

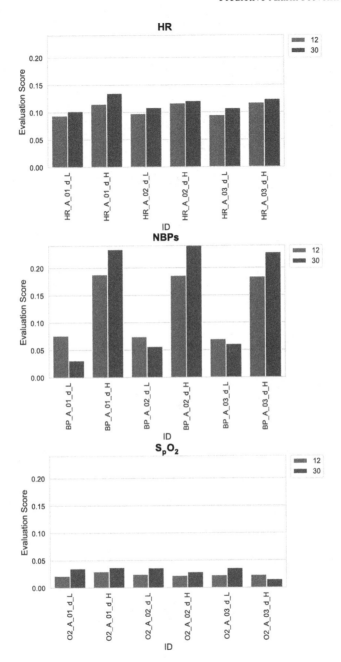

Fig. 5. Comparison of train sizes for statistical models (ARIMA and ARIMAX). For all parameters and model we compare a train size of 12 lags with a train size of 30 lags both for high alarms (suffix _H) and low alarms (suffix _L).

Figure 6 compares the best statistical models among each other, contrasting high and low alarms for different vital parameters separately. We highlighted the best performing model for each alarm type in a more saturated colour. The performance varies greatly

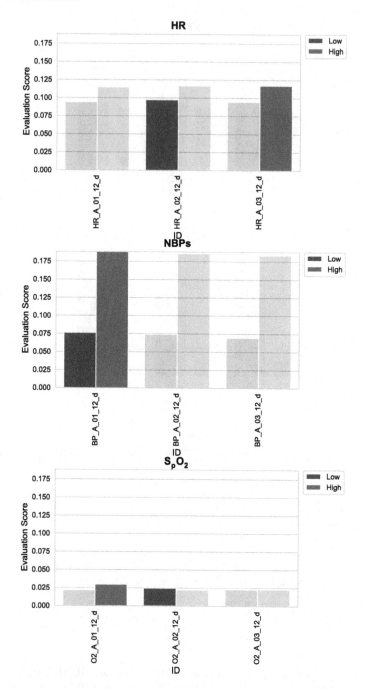

Fig. 6. Comparison of alarm types (high alarm and low alarm) for statistical models across all vital parameters.

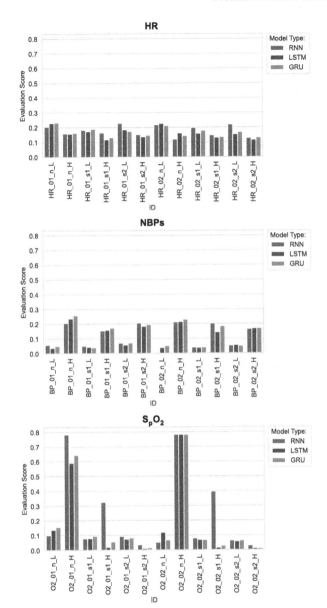

Fig. 7. Comparison of ML model types vanilla RNN, LSTM and GRU with different configurations across vital parameters and alarm types (suffix _H for high alarms and suffix _L for low alarms).

with alarm type. High alarms are generally more foreseeable, at least for HR and NBP$_s$. Peak performance for high and low alarms is not necessarily achieved with the same model, for example in HR and SpO2. For future work it might be best to consider high and low alarms as completely different endpoints and not trying to build one model for multiple alarm types.

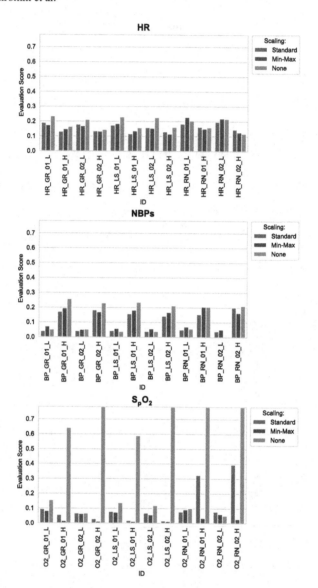

Fig. 8. Comparison of ML models executed with different scaling methods applied (Standard, Min-Max) or without scaling (None) across vital parameters and alarm types (suffix _H for high alarms and suffix _L for low alarms).

Figure 7 compares all machine learning models among each other, contrasting model type. No single model type stands out as alarm type, vital parameter, and scaling obviously influence the performance of all models. But it seems that scaling has a clearly negative effect on the models' performance. This calls for further investigation in the next figures.

Figure 8 compares the effect of different scaling methods on machine learning models. The figure confirms that scaling negatively influences the models' performance. The

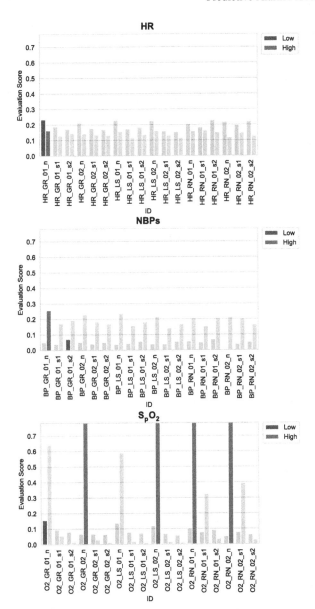

Fig. 9. Selection of best ML models. Models with model type GRU and median resampled chunks as endogenous input variable always perform best (except for high alarm forecasting of SpO_2).

negative influence is most obvious in SpO_2 models. As with statistical models (Fig. 6), alarm type influences the performance, but differently. For HR, low alarms are more foreseeable. For NBP_s, high alarms are more foreseeable. For SpO_2, the influence of scaling is serve and obscures differences between high and low alarms. But looking at SpO_2 models with no scaling, high alarms are more foreseeable as per this model.

Figure 9 compares all machine learning models and contrasts performances for high and low alarms. Again, we highlighted the best performing models for each alarm type

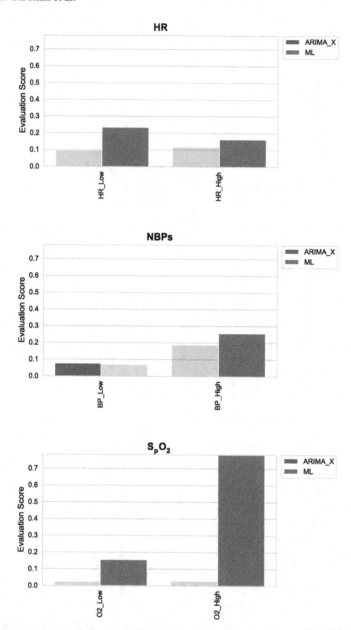

Fig. 10. Comparison of best performing statistical models to best performing ML models.

in a more saturated colour. Multiple models exhibit the same peak performance for SpO₂ high alarms. Otherwise, this figure clearly shows that GRU models with median resampling show an overall superior performance. This is an important direction for future research.

Finally, Fig. 10 compares the best performing statistical models with the best performing machine learning models. Mostly, machine learning models outperform

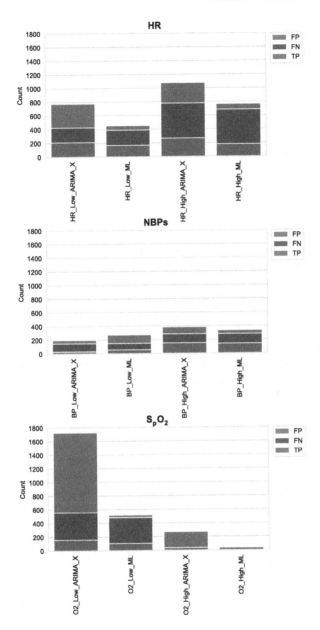

Fig. 11. Comparison of confusion matrix values (false positives, false negatives, and true positives; not showing true negatives) of best performing statistical models to best performing ML models.

statistical models, especially in the SpO_2 use case. Figure 11 shows why this is the case: The confusion matrix reveals that machine learning models are much better at avoiding false positives. Since false positives are penalised five times more heavily as per our evaluation metrics, this is a major advantage for the model in this specific scenario. Machine learning models – with their prior knowledge through training – do not tend to forecast extreme values as much as statistical model that do not have prior knowledge on the domain. As extreme vital parameter forecasts cause alarms forecasts, this prior knowledge helps avoiding false positive alarms and improves evaluation scores.

5   Discussion

We have shown a method to forecast threshold alarms. This, however, is limited to the share of alarms that can be forecast because of a continued trend. Acute events – for example sudden onset of cardiac arrhythmia – cannot be foreseen by our method. With our method, we can transform a share of the alarms into scheduled tasks. Thus removing the urgency from the situation and reducing the alarm load. Also, forecasting alarms buys staff more time to treat critical conditions which also benefits patients. This way, patients can get treatment even before their conditions becomes overly critical.

Alarm fatigue is a well-known problem in medicine with many detrimental effects on patients and staff. From existing research on alarm fatigue, it is perfectly clear that we must reduce the number of alarms. But we do not know yet how we can reduce the number of alarms without risking to overlook a critical condition and sacrificing patient safety. Paine et al. systematically reviewed existing literature on alarm fatigue and compiled a list of alternative approach to reduce the alarm load: Widening alarm thresholds and introducing alarm delays can reduce the total number of alarms but might have adverse safety outcomes. Using disposable electrocardiographic lead wires and changing electrodes daily will reduce measurement errors and reduce technically false alarms without endangering patients but increases staff workload and monitoring costs. Finally, for some interventions the safety outcomes are yet unclear, for example changing alarm sounds and presentation, personal alarming through pagers or mobile phones, and focusing monitoring on high-risk patients while relaxing monitoring on low-risk patients. Our forecasting approach does not endanger patients, produces no additional cost, and – by emphasising low false positive rates – does not increase staff workload.

The method we proposed in this work is only a proof of concept. We showed that the approach works in principle and we found important indications for future work. The methods, however, is not yet ready for productive use. The most striking limitation is a data set issue. As we already mentioned in Sect. 2, MIMIC-III is the only clinical data set that contains alarm data. But its low temporal resolution regarding vital parameter measurements vastly limits MIMIC-III's usability. With unsteady sampling frequencies of $f_s \approx 1\,h^{-1}$, forecasting is difficult and limited. Other clinical data sets feature higher and steady sampling frequencies – for example eICU CRD with steady $f_s \approx 12\,h^{-1}$ – but lack alarm data altogether. For this work, we chose MIMIC-III and tried to cope with the low temporal resolution. To circumvent the low sampling frequency issue, future work can focus on vital parameter forecasting using eICU CRD, omitting the actual alarm event forecasting or using simulated alarm thresholds. Another approach for future work could be framing the problem as a classification task rather than a regression task. Through this work, we already know that machine learning models outperform statistical models. A possible next step can be to remove the indirection of forecasting the vital parameter measurement and forecast the alarm right away.

Reducing the number of false alarms at the intensive care unit and counteracting alarm fatigue is very much necessary according to domain experts. The models we proposed are far from providing perfect alarm forecasts. This is mostly due to the data set issues described above. But there is huge potential for this approach to alleviate alarm fatigue in the future with better data sets featuring high temporal vital parameter resolution and precise alarm data.

References

1. Baker, C.F., Garvin, B.J., Kennedy, C.W., Polivka, B.J.: The effect of environmental sound and communication on CCU patients' heart rate and blood pressure. Res. Nurs. Health 16(6), 415–421 (1993). https://doi.org/10.1002/nur.4770160605
2. Bennun, I.: Intensive care unit syndrome: a consideration of psychological interventions. Br. J. Med. Psychol. 74(3), 369–377 (2001). https://doi.org/10.1348/000711201161046
3. Chromik, J., et al.: Extracting alarm events from the MIMIC-III clinical database. In: 15th International Conference on Health Informatics, pp. 328–335 (2022). https://doi.org/10.5220/0010767200003123
4. Chromik, J., et al.: Forecasting thresholds alarms in medical patient monitors using time series models. In: 15th International Conference on Health Informatics, pp. 26–34 (2022). https://doi.org/10.5220/0010767300003123
5. Clifford, G.D., et al.: The PhysioNet/computing in cardiology challenge 2015: reducing false arrhythmia alarms in the ICU. In: 2015 Computing in Cardiology Conference (CinC), pp. 273–276. IEEE, Nice (2015). https://doi.org/10.1109/CIC.2015.7408639
6. Cvach, M.: Monitor alarm fatigue: an integrative review. Biomed. Instrum. Technol. 46(4), 268–277 (2012). https://doi.org/10.2345/0899-8205-46.4.268
7. Dai, X., Liu, J., Li, Y.: A recurrent neural network using historical data to predict time series indoor PM2.5 concentrations for residential buildings. Indoor Air 31(4), 1228–1237 (2021). https://doi.org/10.1111/ina.12794
8. Drew, B.J., et al.: Insights into the problem of alarm fatigue with physiologic monitor devices: a comprehensive observational study of consecutive intensive care unit patients. PLoS ONE 9(10), e110274 (2014). https://doi.org/10.1371/journal.pone.0110274
9. Fife, D., Rappaport, E.: Noise and hospital stay. Am. J. Public Health 66(7), 680–681 (1976). https://doi.org/10.2105/ajph.66.7.680
10. Granberg, A., Bergbom Engberg, I., Lundberg, D.: Patients' experience of being critically ill or severely injured and cared for in an intensive care unit in relation to the ICU syndrome. Part I. Intensive Crit. Care Nurs. 14(6), 294–307 (1998). https://doi.org/10.1016/S0964-3397(98)80691-5
11. Hagerman, I., Rasmanis, G., Blomkvist, V., Ulrich, R., Eriksen, C.A., Theorell, T.: Influence of intensive coronary care acoustics on the quality of care and physiological state of patients. Int. J. Cardiol. 98(2), 267–270 (2005). https://doi.org/10.1016/j.ijcard.2003.11.006
12. Harutyunyan, H., Khachatrian, H., Kale, D.C., Ver Steeg, G., Galstyan, A.: Multitask learning and benchmarking with clinical time series data. Sci. Data 6(1), 96 (2019). https://doi.org/10.1038/s41597-019-0103-9
13. Hyland, S.L., et al.: Early prediction of circulatory failure in the intensive care unit using machine learning. Nat. Med. 26(3), 364–373 (2020). https://doi.org/10.1038/s41591-020-0789-4
14. Johnson, A.E.W., et al.: MIMIC-III, a freely accessible critical care database. Sci. Data 3, 160035 (2016). https://doi.org/10.1038/sdata.2016.35

15. Minckley, B.B.: A study of noise and its relationship to patient discomfort in the recovery room. Nurs. Res. **17**(3), 247–250 (1968)
16. Morrison, W.E., Haas, E.C., Shaffner, D.H., Garrett, E.S., Fackler, J.C.: Noise, stress, and annoyance in a pediatric intensive care unit. Crit. Care Med. **31**(1), 113–119 (2003). https://doi.org/10.1097/00003246-200301000-00018
17. Murthy, V.S., Malhotra, S.K., Bala, I., Raghunathan, M.: Detrimental effects of noise on anaesthetists. Can. J. Anaesthesia = J. Can. D'anesthesie **42**(7), 608–611 (1995). https://doi.org/10.1007/BF03011878
18. Mussumeci, E., Codeço Coelho, F.: Large-scale multivariate forecasting models for Dengue - LSTM versus random forest regression. Spat. Spatio-Temp. Epidemiol. **35**, 100372 (2020). https://doi.org/10.1016/j.sste.2020.100372
19. Pathan, R.K., Biswas, M., Khandaker, M.U.: Time series prediction of COVID-19 by mutation rate analysis using recurrent neural network-based LSTM model. Chaos, Solitons Fractals **138**, 110018 (2020). https://doi.org/10.1016/j.chaos.2020.110018
20. Pisani, M.A., Friese, R.S., Gehlbach, B.K., Schwab, R.J., Weinhouse, G.L., Jones, S.F.: Sleep in the intensive care unit. Am. J. Respir. Crit. Care Med. **191**(7), 731–738 (2015). https://doi.org/10.1164/rccm.201411-2099CI
21. Pollard, T.J., Johnson, A.E.W., Raffa, J.D., Celi, L.A., Mark, R.G., Badawi, O.: The eICU collaborative research database, a freely available multi-center database for critical care research. Sci. Data **5**, 180178 (2018). https://doi.org/10.1038/sdata.2018.178
22. Poncette, A.S., et al.: Improvements in Patient Monitoring in the Intensive Care Unit: Survey Study. J. Med. Internet Res. **22**(6), e19091 (2020). https://doi.org/10.2196/19091
23. Ryherd, E.E., Waye, K.P., Ljungkvist, L.: Characterizing noise and perceived work environment in a neurological intensive care unit. J. Acoust. Soc. Am. **123**(2), 747–756 (2008). https://doi.org/10.1121/1.2822661
24. Schmid, F., Goepfert, M.S., Kuhnt, D., Eichhorn, V., Diedrichs, S., Reichenspurner, H., Goetz, A.E., Reuter, D.A.: The wolf is crying in the operating room: patient monitor and anesthesia workstation alarming patterns during cardiac surgery. Anesthesia Analgesia **112**(1), 78–83 (2011). https://doi.org/10.1213/ANE.0b013e3181fcc504
25. Thoral, P.J., et al.: Sharing ICU patient data responsibly under the society of critical care medicine/european society of intensive care medicine joint data science collaboration: the Amsterdam university medical centers database (AmsterdamUMCdb) Example*. Crit. Care Med. **49**(6), e563–e577 (2021). https://doi.org/10.1097/CCM.0000000000004916
26. Topf, M., Dillon, E.: Noise-induced stress as a predictor of burnout in critical care nurses. Heart Lung: J. Crit. Care **17**(5), 567–574 (1988)
27. Wilken, M., Hüske-Kraus, D., Klausen, A., Koch, C., Schlauch, W., Röhrig, R.: Alarm fatigue: causes and effects. Stud. Health Technol. Inform. **243**, 107–111 (2017)
28. Wysocki, A.B.: The effect of intermittent noise exposure on wound healing. Adv. Wound Care: J. Prevent. Heal. **9**(1), 35–39 (1996)

ST-Segment Anomalies Detection from Compressed Sensing Based ECG Data by Means of Machine Learning

Giovanni Rosa[1], Marco Russodivito[1], Gennaro Laudato[1(✉)], Angela Rita Colavita[2], Luca De Vito[4], Francesco Picariello[4], Simone Scalabrino[1,3], Ioan Tudosa[4], and Rocco Oliveto[1,3]

[1] STAKE Lab – University of Molise, Pesche, IS, Italy
{giovanni.rosa,marco.russodivito,gennaro.laudato,
simone.scalabrino,rocco.oliveto}@unimol.it
[2] ASREM, Campobasso, CB, Italy
angelarita.colavita@asrem.org
[3] Datasound srl, Pesche, IS, Italy
{simone,rocco}@datasound.it
[4] Department of Engineering, University of Sannio, Benevento, BN, Italy
{devito,fpicariello,ioan.tudosa}@unisannio.it

Abstract. Telemedicine allows to constantly monitor patients without the need of hospitalization. Such a practice is enabled by IoMT (Internet of Medical Things) devices, which acquire signals, and by AI (Artificial Intelligence)-based algorithms, able to automatize the analysis carried out on many patients. The large quantity of data produced every minute by IoMT devices, however, makes the use of compression fundamental to reduce the bandwith used to transmit those data and the memory required to acquire them, and lossy compression (specifically, Compressed Sensing) has shown to be the most effective technique to use for the task. Previous work introduced AI-based approaches for automatically detecting hearth-related anomalies based on the electrocardiographic (ECG) signal. However, most of them assume the presence of the complete raw ECG signal. In this paper, we extend our previous work in which we introduced RAST, an approach for detecting ST segment-related anomalies. We present $RAST^C$, an approach able at identifying the same abnormalities but on a highly compressed ECG signal. The results of our experiment, carried out on the Physionet European ST-T Database, shows that $RAST^C$ is capable of discriminating Normal ECG from ST-depression and ST-elevation with classification metrics around 90%, even with the highest compression ratio experimented, *i.e.,* with an ECG signal compressed by a factor of 16.

Keywords: Machine learning · Compressed sensing · Automatic detection · ECG signal · ST-segment · Anomalies

1 Introduction

Due to the growing popularity of wearable devices applied in the medical field, the Internet of Medical Things (IoMT) paradigm is experiencing rapid growth from the sci-

A. C. A. Roque et al. (Eds.): BIOSTEC 2022, CCIS 1814, pp. 237–255, 2023.
https://doi.org/10.1007/978-3-031-38854-5_13

entific perspective of Research and Development (R&D). Basically, an IoMT network comprises numerous smart medical devices connected to each other over the internet. Modern telemedicine relies on an IoT-based smart healthcare system [42]. A smart healthcare system built upon the IoMT paradigm is composed of many stages. First, by using smart sensors built into wearable (or implanted) devices that are linked by a Wireless Body Sensor Network (WBSN), medical data will be gathered from the patient's body [33,46]. Next, the component handling the prediction and analysis step will get this data through internet transmission. After obtaining the medical data, an analysis may be carried out using an Artificial Intelligence (AI)-based data transformation and interpretation approach, [35]. Based on them, the system can decide how to act based on the urgency of the possibly detected issue, *e.g.,* contacting a physician in case of critical conditions [36].

Telemedicine is another name for the process of employing IoMT tools to remotely monitor patients while they're at home. When a patient receives this type of care, they are spared from visiting a hospital or doctor's office every time they have a medical inquiry or a change in their condition. The greatest advantage of telemedicine, however, is having continuous monitoring of the health parameters of the caregivers. Recent telemedicine systems proposed in the literature include ATTICUS [2,26]. ATTICUS grew out of the development of a prototype hardware and software system based on advanced artificial intelligence techniques, capable of constantly monitoring an individual and reporting anomalies affecting both his or her health status, detected through the automatic measurement and analysis of biological parameters, and in his or her behavior, detected through the monitoring and analysis of the movements the person makes in the normal course of his or her activities. The system consists of one key element: a "smart wearable" device [11]. This consists of a T-shirt made of innovative fabrics, which integrates a data acquisition system (integrated into the T-shirt fabric) capable of measuring the person's vital parameters, such as electrocardiogram tracing, temperature, respiratory behaviors, etc. [2,26].

Among the many signals that can be considered in IoMT devices (and, particularly, in ATTICUS), the electrocardiographic signal acquired through the Electrocardiogram (ECG) is of paramount importance for identifying possible hearth-related issues. Specifically, within the ATTICUS project, several detectors where designed aimed at automatically analysing pathological features derived from the ECG. These detectors allow to automatically identify (i) Atrial Fibrillation (AF) episodes [21,23,25], (ii) arrhythmia related conditions [37], and (iii) Congestive Heart Failure [39]. Most of such detectors assume the presence of a raw ECG signal to run their analyses and provide predictions. However, the electronic core components in a wearable device (such as those that capture real-time multi-lead ECG signals) create and transmit large amount of data, which make the adoption of compression techniques necessary to save memory and bandwidth. Specifically, lossy compression techniques based on Compressed Sensing (CS), particularly digital CS techniques, can be adopted to reduce the local power consumption and to reduce memory size [3]. In this context, it is necessary to adapt existing AI-based detection approaches to make them work with the compressed signal [22,24].

In our previous work [38], we introduced RAST, a detector for ST segment-related anomalies. RAST, however, relies on the uncompressed ECG signal. In this paper, we extend our previous work, and we introduce $RAST^C$, an innovative detector of ST segment-related anomalies that directly relies on a compressed version of a single lead digital ECG. The results show that $RAST^C$ is capable of achieving results comparable with the state-of-the-art, by obtaining classification metrics above 90% even with Compression Ratios up to 16.

Specifically, the contributions of this paper can be summarized as follows:

- We introduce $RAST^C$, which is provided in two versions: BINARY-$RAST^C$, based on identification of only ST abnormality from Normal ECG and TERNARY-$RAST^C$, based on discrimination between ST-depression, ST-elevation and Normal ECG. To increase the information component, which is compromised by the compression process, we present 4 newly defined features. These features are measures derived from the ϕ matrix of the Bernoulli compression algorithm application case;
- We present a study aimed at testing whether an approach based on detection of cardiac pathologies derived from ST-segment analysis can be dropped into a context of compressed ECG signal analysis. In order to conduct a comprehensive study, two compression techniques were analyzed: one deterministic (DBBD) and one random (Bernoulli).

This paper is structured as follows: in Sect. 2 a report on the incidence of ST-segmnent anomalies is offered together with a (i) review of the recent state-of-the-art dedicated to the automatic analysis of ST-segment and (ii) a description of the compressed sensing algorithm. Section 3 describes the workflow of the approach, that includes details on the preprocessing, compression, calculation of the features and the classification. Section 4 proposes details on the design of the study and the results. Finally, Sect. 5 concludes the paper.

2   Background and Related Work

In this section an overview on the incidence of ST-segment anomalies on the general population. This enhances the importance of provindig fast and reliable detection of anomalies. After this, an updated review of the state-of-the-art related to recent works dedicated to the detection of ST-segment anomalies.

2.1   ST-Related Conditions

An electrically neutral region of the complex between ventricular depolarization (QRS complex) and repolarization (T wave) can be represented by the ST segment on an electrocardiogram [41]. It can, however, adopt a variety of waveform morphologies that could point to a benign or clinically severe myocardial infarction or insult. For clinical management since it might affect treatment, it is essential to comprehend the differential diagnosis for alterations in the ST segment [4].

As already described in the introduction, morphological variants for the ST-segment can happen in the form of ST elevation and depression (Fig. 1).

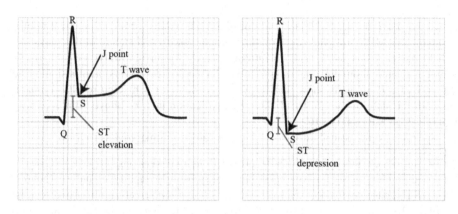

Fig. 1. St depression and elevation phenomena on the left and on the right part of the figure respectively. The amount of depression or elevation can be measured in terms of boxes (or mm).

ST elevation is frequently caused by three factors. The first situation is when ST elevation is only a common variety. Early repolarization is a common term used to describe this. In these situations, the J-point is often elevated and the ST section has a normal or quickly ascending slope. Acute ischemia or ventricular dyskinesis damage currents are the second prevalent cause. The third is brought on by pericarditis-related damage currents [18].

When the J point is relocated below baseline, ST depression happens. ST depression is linked to a variety of illnesses. Some of these include heart ischemia, hypokalemia, and drugs like digitalis. ST depression might also result in T wave alterations [18].

Despite not being common, ST-segment elevation problems, often known as STEMI, Even in young people, ST-segment elevation acute myocardial infarction (STEMI) is common. In fact, 6% of STEMI incidents included relatively young persons under the age of 35 [19].

Here, we report some clinical relevance data about the incidence of ST-related pathological conditions [15]:

– Acutely blocked coronary arteries are present in 80% of individuals with typical STEMI;
– acutely occluded coronary arteries were seen in 10% of individuals with ST segment elevation in the electrocardiographic augmented vector right (aVR) lead.

Also, a recent study was conducted to identify any anomalies in the ECG that would indicate cerebral vascular disease [17]. Within 24 to 48 h, a computed tomography (CT) scan of the brain was obtained, evaluated, and patients were divided into three groups: those with cerebral infarction, intracranial hemorrhage, and subarachnoid hemorrhage (SAH). In patients with cerebral hemorrhage (CH), ST segment alterations were the most typical anomaly seen. More specifically, following cerebral hemorrhage, ST segment alterations were most frequently observed. ST depression is present in 33% of infarction patients. 50% of individuals with CH had ST elevation [17].

In addition, the COVID-19 outbreak may have increased the incidence of st problems, particularly st depression problems. Indeed, separation and limiting people's movement during the COVID-19 pandemic appeared to impair physical activity and dietary consumption of fresh fruit and vegetables, which may have an impact on long-term cardiovascular results. On the other hand, melancholy, rage, and ongoing stress brought on by separation, mobility restrictions, a lack of supplies and knowledge, financial loss, and a fear of getting sick might have short-term consequences on the cardiovascular system [30]. Numerous studies have revealed connections between vascular health and psychological factors [44]. It has been shown that people with depressive disorders have a higher chance of developing coronary artery disease, increased blood clotting, reduced fibrinolysis, and cardiac death [6, 13, 20, 40]. The COVID-19 pandemic's psychological stress may have contributed to the greater rates of ST-segment depression and aberrant Q waves. These seem the results over a brief observation period [44].

2.2   Automatic Detection of ST-Related Conditions

Several works have been proposed in the literature for the detection of ST-related anomalies.

Meglaveras *et al.* [29] proposed an approach for real-time detection of ischemia episodes using an adaptive Backpropagation Neural Network. In detail, their method is based on the processing of the whole ST pattern, by evaluating the ST segments of the first 10 successive heartbeats. Their results show a sensitivity of 88.62% and 72.22% for detection and duration of ischemia episodes.

Bulusu *et al.* [7] proposed an approach using the Support Vector Machine (SVM) algorithm for the automatic recognition of ST-segment anomalies. In detail, it uses morphological features from ECG, including ST-segment information for the diagnosis of myocardial ischemia and cardiac arrhythmia. Their results report an accuracy of 93.3% for the European ST-T Database. Also, they achieved an accuracy value of 96.4% for the classification of cardiac arrhythmia episodes from the MIT-BIH Arrhythmia Database.

Xiao *et al.* [47] proposed an approach based on image analysis using deep learning techniques for the detection of ischemic ST change for ECGs. In detail, they build a Convolutional Neural Network (CNN) using transfer learning and training it on a dataset, extracted from the Long Term ST database [16], composed of 10 s image samples regarding signals having significant ST changes and control samples (no significant changes). Their results show an average ROC AUC score of 89.6%, while selecting an optimum cutoff level they achieve an average sensitivity of 84.4%.

Wang *et al.* [45] proposed a beat-to-beat classification method for ST segment changes using the Random Forest algorithm. They use, for the classification, the morphological features and Poincaré characteristics of the ST segments. The approach was trained and tested on the European ST-D Database, achieving an average sensitivity of 85.2% for normal ST segments, 86.9% for ST depression, and 88.8% for ST elevation.

Moreover, Harun-Ar-Rashid [15] proposed a technique for the automatic classification of ST segments based on cross-correlation for five ST categories (*i.e.,* concave, Convex, Up slope, Down slope, and Horizontal). In detail, after the first denoising preprocessing phase, it follows a two-step ECG annotation starting with (i) R wave identification, and (ii) the annotation of S and T waves, along with J point. The last step is the identification of ST change categories by performing a cross-correlation with the supervised ST change data, to measure the similarity between the ST segment and the corresponding ST change category. Their approach achieved an accuracy value of 88.2% for the MIT-BIH ST change database, and 96.2% for the European ST-T change database.

All the above-mentioned works process an ECG trace as it is acquired, without any loss of information. To the best of our knowledge, this paper represents the first attempt to define an approach for the detection of ST-segment-related abnormalities from a highly compressed ECG.

2.3   The Compressed Sensing Algorithm

Compressed Sensing (CS) is a technique widely adopted in ECG monitoring with wireless-connected wearable devices [3]. CS allows for reducing the amount of wirelessly transmitted data to the host (e.g., smartphone, tablet, server) and requires a low computational load for the data compression.

In the literature, the CS-based techniques for ECG signals are classified into (i) randomly-based, and (ii) deterministic-based. In the former case, random distributions (e.g., Bernoulli and Gaussian) are adopted for data compression, while, in the latter case, a deterministic number sequence is utilized. According to the CS theory, the data compression is modeled as:

$$\mathbf{y} = \boldsymbol{\Phi} \cdot \mathbf{x} \tag{1}$$

where, $\mathbf{x}$ is a vector of N ECG samples acquired in a certain time window, at Nyquist rate, $\mathbf{y}$ is the M-size vector of the compressed samples, where $M < N$ and $\boldsymbol{\Phi}$ is an $M \times N$ matrix called sensing matrix. In randomly-based techniques the matrix $\boldsymbol{\Phi}$ is randomly built according to a probability distribution, such as Gaussian and Bernoulli. On the other hand, in the deterministic-based techniques the matrix $\boldsymbol{\Phi}$ is built according to a well-defined sequence of numbers. For example, in [12], the Authors implemented Toeplitz, Circulant, and Triangular structured sensing matrices, which do not require the generation of random numbers and therefore are easier to be implemented on wearable devices. In [34], a Deterministic Binary Block Diagonal matrix (DBBD) is adopted as sensing matrix. In this case, each row of $\boldsymbol{\Phi}$ consists of a sequence of one and zero according to the imposed compression ratio (i.e., $CR = N/M$).

The compressed samples need to be processed to obtain an estimation of the original vector $\mathbf{x}$. The estimation of $\mathbf{x}$ (i.e., the reconstruction step) requires the definition of a dictionary matrix $\boldsymbol{\Psi}$ selected according to the domain where the signal can be represented by few K non-zero coefficients. According to $\boldsymbol{\Psi}$ and $\boldsymbol{\Phi}$, the coefficients θ, representing $\mathbf{x}$ in the selected domain, are estimated by solving:

$$\hat{\theta} = \arg\min_{\theta} ||\theta||_1, \quad \text{subject to:} \quad \mathbf{y} = \boldsymbol{\Phi}\boldsymbol{\Psi}\theta \tag{2}$$

where, $||\cdot||_1$ indicates the l_1 norm operator. $\hat{\mathbf{x}}$ is estimated from $\hat{\theta}$ as follows:

$$\hat{\mathbf{x}} = \boldsymbol{\Psi} \cdot \hat{\theta} \tag{3}$$

In terms of reconstruction quality, among the randomly-based techniques, the best results are obtained with the Bernoulli sensing matrix and the two scales Mexican hat-based dictionary matrix, [9]. However, it was demonstrated the deterministic-based technique performances outperform the randomly-based, [32]. In [34], the DBBD with Discrete Cosine Transform (DCT) as a dictionary matrix obtained the best results in terms of reconstruction quality. However, in the literature, more complex deterministic-based techniques are proposed to outperform the performance of DBBD with DCT [10].

All the above-mentioned results require solving of Eq. 2 by means of Orthogonal Matching Pursuit (OMP) algorithm that exhibits a computational complexity $\mathcal{O}((N + M)S)$, where $S < N$ is the number of iterations. Thus, the reconstruction step limits the use of CS when the application requires the implementation of real-time monitoring and early-warning systems.

3 Automatically Detecting ST-Related Conditions from Compressed ECG: Workflow of the Approach

In this section we describe the workflow of the original RAST [38], an approach for the automatic detection of ST-related conditions on digital uncompressed ECG signals. In Fig. 2 we report the workflow of RAST. Firstly, RAST takes as input a digital ECG signal containing at least K successive heartbeats (*i.e.*, at least K R peaks detected). After the preprocessing of the ECG segment, it follows the extraction of the feature vector and then the classification of the ECG segment. The parameter K in Fig. 2 indicates that in our previous study [38], a study was conducted to determine the best temporal window in terms of successive heartbeats within two cross-validation schemes experimented. The result showed that 4 successive heartbeats are enough to obtain good classification performances in the 80–20 cross validation). The first phase is the processing of the input ECG signal. The Pan-Tomphkins algorithm [31] is applied to detect the number of R peaks in the input ECG signal. The ECG is buffered until it reaches the required size of K successive heartbeats. This to allow the extraction of the features and then the detection of ST-related anomalies. Next, a detrend operation is applied to the ECG segment to improve the extraction of the features. There are two versions of RAST: BINARY-RAST (RAST$_{bin}$), which classifies the ECG segment as Normal or ST-anomaly, and TERNARY-RAST (RAST$_{ter}$), which supports the detection of ST depression, ST elevation, and Normal.

After a brief description of the original RAST, we describe in the following subsections the detailed workflow phases of the study proposed in this paper, which led to the definition of RAST^C.

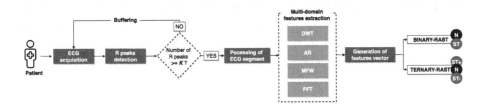

Fig. 2. The workflow of RAST [38].

3.1 Introducing RAST^C: Uncompressed vs Compressed Domain

With the term "uncompressed domain" we refer to the initial version of RAST, in which the features were evaluated directly on the input ECG segments extracted from the signal. On the other hand, with "compressed domain" we refer to the ECG signal compressed using one of the two compression algorithms (*i.e.,* CA$_{DBBD}$ and CA$_{Bernoulli}$).

As those compression algorithms used in our study permit the use of integer CRs, the sensing matrix Φ cannot be defined (see (4)). For convenience, the CRs in this work are chosen in powers of 2 to experiment with the maximum number of CRs, *i.e.,* for a total of four.

Specifically, in our experiment, we want to compare the classification performances of RAST in the compressed domain, evaluating the compression ratios in the set 2, 4, 8, 16 for both compression algorithms.

3.2 ECG Signal Compression

In the considered analysis, two CS algorithms have been implemented, one based on a deterministic approach, i.e., DBBD [34], and the other based on a random approach according to the Bernoulli distribution [9].

- In the case of DBBD, the compressed vector **y** of M elements is obtained according to (1) where the sensing matrix Φ is defined as:

$$\Phi = \begin{bmatrix} 1_{CR} & 0_{CR} & \cdots & 0_{CR} \\ 0_{CR} & 1_{CR} & \cdots & 0_{CR} \\ \vdots & \cdots & \ddots & \vdots \\ 0_{CR} & \cdots & 0_{CR} & 1_{CR} \end{bmatrix} \tag{4}$$

where, $CR = N/M$ is the compression ratio, 1_{CR} and 0_{CR} are row vectors of CR one and zero, respectively, where CR must be an integer value.

- In the case of Bernoulli, the sensing matrix Φ is defined as a matrix of $M \times N$ elements of −1 and 1 according to a Bernoulli distribution. In particular, the probability of occurring -1 is equal to the probability of 1.

  Both methods have been implemented in MATLAB and the data have been compressed by considering CRs of 2, 4, 8, and 16.

3.3 Features Evaluated on the Compressed ECG Information

A set of multi-domain features are extracted from each preprocessed and compressed ECG segment composed of successive R peaks. We selected a set of state-of-the-art features from the literature, also evaluated in a previous study about the detection of ECG anomalies [37]. The selected features for RAST are described as follows.

- *Autoregressive Model (AR) coefficients.* We perform the computation of the Autoregressive (AR) Model Coefficients of order 4 to obtain the temporal structures of ECG waveforms, as evaluated in the study performed by Zhao and Zhang [48].

– *Energy of Maximal Overlap Discrete Wavelet Transform (MODWT).* We perform a decomposition of the input signal applying the Maximal Overlap Discrete Wavelet Transform (MODWT). The extraction procedure is partially based on the one performed by Li *et al.* [28]. In detail, to extract the coefficient required for our analysis, (i) a wavelet function W and the decomposition level L are selected, then follows (ii) the decomposition of an input segment according to the specified W and L coefficients, and finally there is the computation of the energy, in the last level L, for each of the coefficients. We used *db2* Daubechies as wavelet function (W), and three levels of decomposition (L).
– *Fast Fourier Transform (FFT).* We compute the Fast Fourier Transform, provided by the Cooley-Turkey algorithm [8], on the input ECG segment.
– *Multifractal Wavelet (MFW) leader.* We involved the multifractal analysis to estimate the log-cumulants of the scaling exponents of the input ECG segment [27]. The *db3* Daubechies is used as a wavelet function.

When applying the Bernoulli compression algorithm to the ECG segment, we opted for calcualting 4 additional features to enrich the knowledge of the classifier. These latter are based on metrics evaluated on the Φ Matrix:

– $\mathbf{tot_1}$: the total number of 1s embedded in the matrix;
– $\mathbf{perc_1}$: total number of 1s divided by the total number of elements in the matrix;
– $\mathbf{tot_{not1}}$: total number of not-1s divided by the total number of elements in the matrix;
– **sequences**: length measures of 1s sequence.

3.4   Beat Classification

The last phase of RAST is the classification of the ST segment observed on the processed ECG segment provided by a Machine Learning (ML) model. There are no constraints related to a specific ML algorithm. As reported in our previous study, the Random Forest algorithm [5] performs better compared to the others evaluated. RAST is proposed in two variations based on the type of detected ST-related anomaly. We define the first as BINARY-RAST, which provides a more high-level classification as it classifies the input ECG segment as Normal or ST Sloping. The latter is TERNARY-RAST, which provides a more specific classification with the capability to identify the ECG segment as Normal, ST Elevation and Depression. In this way, our evaluation is twofold concerning the application context. BINARY-RAST works well in a context where is required a rapid screening for anomalies, while TERNARY-RAST suits better when there are medical constraints requiring more detailed information on the category of the ST-related conditions.

4   The Study

This section provides a full description of the study, including the experimental design, the context of the study and the final results.

4.1   Study Design

The main goal of our study is to evaluate the effectiveness of both $RAST_{bin}$ and $RAST_{ter}$ in the compressed domain.

In particular, we want to answer the following research questions:

RQ_1: *Which ECG compression algorithm provides the best classification performances of* RAST*?* With the second research question, we want to compare two different algorithms for ECG compression, namely DBBD (CA_{DBBD}) [34] and Bernoulli compression ($CA_{Bernoulli}$) [9], using different compression ratios (CRs).

RQ_2: *What are the classification performances of* RAST *when dealing with compressed ECG signals?* We want to evaluate the applicability of RAST in a context where we have compressed ECG signals, using the same features applied for uncompressed ECGs in the previous study [38].

In Fig. 3 we report a comparison between uncompressed and compressed ECG using CA_{DBBD} (fig. a) and $CA_{Bernoulli}$ (fig. b) compression.

Context of the Study. The context of our study is the Physionet European ST-T Database [14,43], a state-of-the-art dataset to support the analysis of ST segment and T-wave morphology. This database is made up of 90 ambulatory two-hour ECG signals with annotations from 79 distinct individuals that were collected at a sample rate 250 Hz and a resolution of 12 bits. Additionally, the information includes 401 events of T-wave transition and 367 instances of ST segment change. ranging from 30 s to several minutes in length. Two cardiologists defined such labels after working separately, beat by beat, and discussing any instances of label discrepancies at the conclusion.

In our study, We considered only 3 categories of annotations, related to ST segment changes, namely *NSR, ST+* and *ST-*. For the binary variant of RAST, we merged the two *ST* annotations obtaining only two types of heartbeats, *i.e., NSR* and *ST*. The distribution of the heartbeats reporting that labels is described in Fig. 4 for both $RAST_{bin}$ (left) and $RAST_{ter}$ (right). It is worth saying that we did not use the MIT-BIH ST Change DB [1] as it does not include ST change annotations.

Experimental Workflow. In Fig. 5 we represent the experimental procedure to answer our RQs. In summary, the experimental procedure is the following:

1. An input ECG trace is extracted and buffered according to the minimum number of R peaks required for the classification (*i.e.,* 4);
2. Follow a preprocessing step where the signal is filtered and prepared for the feature extraction by dividing the input ECG in 4-beats segments;
3. At this point, we have the features extraction phase. Here, we (i) extract the features used by RAST on both compressed and uncompressed domains, and (ii) compare the two compression algorithm previously described (CA_{DBBD} and $CA_{Bernoulli}$), selecting the best compression ratio;
4. The last step is the training of the classifier and the detection of ST-related anomalies on both compressed and uncompressed signals for both $RAST_{bin}$ and $RAST_{ter}$.

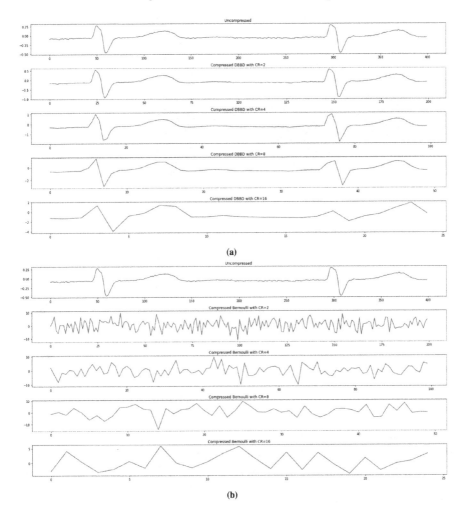

Fig. 3. Comparison between uncompressed and compressed ECG signal using CA_{DBBD} (fig. a), and $CA_{Bernoulli}$ (fig. b) at different values of CR.

For this last step, we use the same validation scheme used in the previous study [38], and the settings which achieved the best results. In detail, we have (i) a TWHO (Temporal Window for the Heartbeat Observation) of 4, (ii) the SMOTE sampling technique applied on the training set, and (iii) the Random Forest classifier as machine learning model. We adopt the same validation scheme, *i.e.*, we perform a 80–20 random split cross validation, repeated 1000 times to avoid any bias due to convenient split. We apply it, in the two RQs, for the uncompressed and the compressed ECG signal using both CA_{DBBD} and $CA_{Bernoulli}$ compression algorithms using 4 different CRs.

For convenience, We use $RAST^C$ to identify the modified version of RAST where the compression procedure is applied, with its two variants $RAST_{bin}^C$ and $RAST_{ter}^C$.

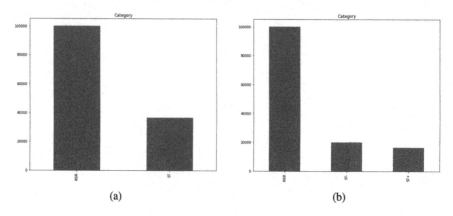

Fig. 4. Count of selected heartbeat from the European ST-T Database [43] used for $RAST_{bin}$ (left) and $RAST_{ter}$ (right)

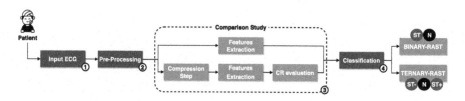

Fig. 5. The experimental workflow conducted in this study.

Thus, we apply the described procedure to answer both RQs. To answer the first RQ, we evaluate the classification performance for $RAST^C$ by comparing the two compression algorithms (*i.e.,* CA_{DBBD} and $CA_{Bernoulli}$) with different CRs. To answer the second, we compare the overall classification performance between RAST and $RAST^C$ having the best performing combination of compression algorithm and CR. In our study, we evaluate both *binary* and *ternary* variants for RAST and $RAST^C$.

Moreover, we measure the classification performance for both RQs using the following class-level metrics:

- **Accuracy:** the number of correctly categorized instances divided by the total number of instances. $\dfrac{TP + TN}{TP + TN + FP + FN}$
- **Precision:** the number of correctly categorized positive instances divided by the total number of positive instances. $\dfrac{TP}{TP + FP}$
- **Specificity:** the number of correctly categorized negative instances divided by the total number of correctly classified negative instances and incorrectly classified positive instances. $\dfrac{TN}{TN + FP}$

– **Recall:** the number of correctly categorized positive instances divided by the total number of correctly categorized positive instances and incorrectly classified negative instances. $\dfrac{TP}{TP + FN}$

– **F1 Score:** the harmonic mean of precision and recall. $\dfrac{2 * TP}{(2 * TP) + TN + FP}$

4.2 Study Results

In this section we report the results of our empirical study.

RQ$_1$: Best ECG Compression Algorithm. To answer RQ$_1$, we compare the overall classification performance between CA$_{DBBD}$ and CA$_{Bernoulli}$ for both RAST$^C_{bin}$ and RAST$^C_{ter}$. CA$_{DBBD}$ exhibit an overall better classification performance compared to CA$_{Bernoulli}$. Also, the achieved results for the first are slightly more stable than the latter, which decreases as CR increases. Those results are the same for both settings of RAST^C, *i.e.,* RAST$^C_{bin}$, and RAST$^C_{ter}$. While CA$_{DBBD}$ achieves similar results for both settings, CA$_{Bernoulli}$ works better overall in RAST$^C_{bin}$. For RAST$^C_{ter}$, it achieves good performance only in terms of *specificity* and *accuracy*, which are also higher than the RAST$^C_{bin}$ setting. This means that Bernoulli's features are more effective to identify the absence of ST anomaly, *i.e.,* achieving few false positive results. Thus, it is

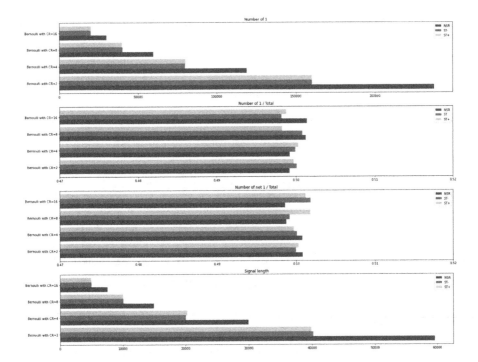

Fig. 6. Bernoulli's features evaluated for an ECG signal compressed using CA$_{Bernoulli}$ with different CRs.

more useful to distinguish between Normal and ST anomalous ECG segments, than to classify Normal, ST Depression, or ST Elevation.

It is observed better in Fig. 8, where, for each of the newly introduced Bernoulli's features (*i.e.,* the ones evaluated on the ϕ matrix, we report their value for NSR, ST elevation, and ST depression classes, calculated for different values of compression ratios. Their effectiveness for the NSR class is far higher compared to the others. Indeed, the binary discrimination between normal ECG and ST abnormality can be easily obtained thanks to these new attributes. For this particular case, it is evident that **tot$_1$** and **sequences** are the most suited for the binary scenario. For the ternary scenario, these attributes provide less information. In this case, **perc$_1$** and **tot$_{not1}$** seem the most appropriate.

We computed the boxplots for the values of the accuracy metric collected following our validation scheme (1,000 iterations performing 80–20 random splits). In detail, in Fig. 7 we describe the distribution of the *accuracy* values gathered from the experimental procedure of $RAST^C_{bin}$ using CA_{DBBD} (Fig. 6 a), and $CA_{Bernoulli}$ (Fig. 6 b). The same is reported in Fig. 8. We have a larger number of outliers when applying CA_{DBBD}, while for $CA_{Bernoulli}$ we obtain more stable results among all the CRs in terms of *accuracy* at a price of a lower score overall.

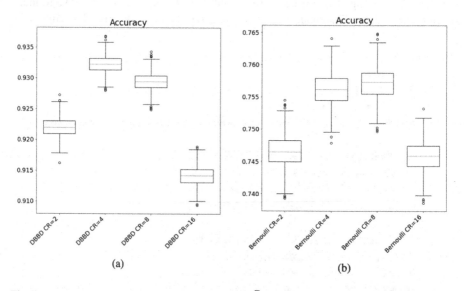

Fig. 7. Comparison of the accuracy values for $RAST^C_{bin}$ using CA_{DBBD} (fig. a), and $CA_{Bernoulli}$ (fig. b) with different CRs.

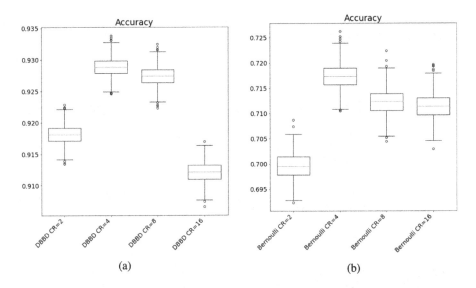

(a)   (b)

Fig. 8. Comparison of the accuracy values for $RAST_{ter}^{C}$ using CA_{DBBD} (fig. a), and $CA_{Bernoulli}$ (fig. b) with different CRs.

Table 1. Classification metrics for $RAST_{bin}$ in compressed and uncompressed domain. $RAST_{bin}^{C}$ indicates the variant using CA_{DBBD}.

Approach	Accuracy	Precision	Specificity	Recall	F1 Score
$RAST_{bin}$	93.05	93.03	88.78	93.05	93.04
$RAST_{bin}^{C}$ (CR=2)	92.20	92.40	**89.81**	92.20	92.27
$RAST_{bin}^{C}$ (CR=4)	**93.23**	**93.23**	89.53	**93.23**	**93.23**
$RAST_{bin}^{C}$ (CR=8)	92.94	92.99	89.76	92.94	92.97
$RAST_{bin}^{C}$ (CR=16)	91.42	91.48	87.29	91.42	91.44

RQ₂: Classification Performances of RAST. To answer RQ_2, we compare the overall classification performance between uncompressed vs. compressed domains for RAST. We reported the overall results for $RAST_{bin}$ and $RAST_{bin}^{C}$ in Table 1, and for $RAST_{ter}$ and $RAST_{ter}^{C}$ in Table 2. For $RAST^C$ we reported the results achieved using the best compression algorithm resulting from the previous RQ, *i.e.*, CA_{DBBD}. In the first table it can be observed that $RAST_{bin}^{C}$ offers similar or slightly better performance to the uncompressed version ($RAST_{bin}$), particularly with a compression rate of 4. For the second, $RAST_{ter}$ shows higher performance than $RAST_{ter}^{C}$ for almost all classification metrics, except for *specificity*, which is better for $RAST_{ter}^{C}$ with a CR of 2. As seen for the *binary* version, $RAST_{ter}^{C}$ achieves the best performance overall with a CR of 4 for the compressed domain.

In summary, the performance of RAST in both uncompressed and compressed domains are comparable, where the latter works at best using a compression ratio of 4.

Table 2. Classification metrics for $RAST_{ter}$ in compressed and uncompressed domain. $RAST_{ter}^C$ indicates the variant using CA_{DBBD} .

Approach	Accuracy	Precision	Specificity	Recall	F1 Score
$RAST_{ter}$	**93.07**	**93.14**	91.20	**93.07**	**93.09**
$RAST_{ter}^C$ (CR=2)	91.82	92.22	**91.87**	91.82	91.94
$RAST_{ter}^C$ (CR=4)	92.88	92.99	91.23	92.88	92.92
$RAST_{ter}^C$ (CR=8)	92.74	92.88	91.26	92.74	92.79
$RAST_{ter}^C$ (CR=16)	91.21	91.35	88.92	91.21	91.26

5   Conclusion and Future Works

In this paper, we have proposed a new version of RAST, i.e. the approach proposed in our previous work [38]. The new approach, called $RAST^C$, has the big difference of working with a compressed ECG compared to a full ECG trace, i.e. without any loss of information. Performing detection directly on compressed signals allows IoMT devices to preserve battery life and to offer accurate detection with algorithms at a lower computational cost. To this end, in this paper we experimented with two different signal compression techniques: DBBD and Bernoulli. As the latter is a random compression technique, we introduced 4 new features—calculated on the ϕ matrix—to increase the information potential in the latter case. Furthermore, we evaluated the compression factor in the set $[2,4,8,16]$ to observe the performance of $RAST^C$ even at very high CRs. And finally, we evaluated two classification versions: (i) a binary one, where the objective is simply the discrimination between normal ECG and an ST-abnormality and (ii) a ternary one where the objective of the classification model is to identify normal ECG, ST-depression and ST-elevation. The first major result obtained in this study is that a deterministic DBBD technique is preferable to a random one. Thus, by applying a compression with a DBBD algorithm, it is possible to obtain—both in the binary and ternary case—average results above 90% even with a CR of 16. Consequently, this paper aims to confidently promote efforts dedicated to the detection of clinical features, such as ST-segment abnormalities, from the analysis of highly compressed ECG signals.

Future works will be dedicated to the study of more compression techniques, in order to achieve comparable results with higher compression ratios.

References

1. Albrecht, P.: ST segment characterization for long term automated ECG analysis [dissertation]. Massachusetts Institute of Technology, Department of Electrical Engineering and Computer Science: Massachusetts Institute of Technology, no. 378 (1983)
2. Balestrieri, E., et al.: The architecture of an innovative smart t-shirt based on the internet of medical things paradigm. In: 2019 IEEE International Symposium on Medical Measurements and Applications (MeMeA), pp. 1–6. IEEE (2019)
3. Balestrieri, E., Daponte, P., De Vito, L., Picariello, F., Rapuano, S., Tudosa, I.: A Wi-Fi Internet-of-Things prototype for ECG monitoring by exploiting a novel compressed sensing method. Acta IMEKO 9(2), 38–45 (2020)

4. Bhattarai, S., Chhabra, L., Hashmi, M.F., Willoughby, C.: Anteroseptal myocardial infarction (2022). http://europepmc.org/books/NBK540996
5. Breiman, L.: Random forests. Mach. Learn. **45**(1), 5–32 (2001)
6. Brunner, E., Marmot, M., Canner, R., Beksinska, M., Smith, G.D., O'Brien, J.: Childhood social circumstances and psychosocial and behavioural factors as determinants of plasma fibrinogen. Lancet **347**(9007), 1008–1013 (1996)
7. Bulusu, S.C., Faezipour, M., Ng, V., Nourani, M., Tamil, L.S., Banerjee, S.: Transient ST-segment episode detection for ECG beat classification. In: 2011 IEEE/NIH Life Science Systems and Applications Workshop (LiSSA), pp. 121–124. IEEE (2011)
8. Cooley, J.W., Tukey, J.W.: An algorithm for the machine calculation of complex fourier series. Math. Comput. **19**(90), 297–301 (1965)
9. Craven, D., McGinley, B., Kilmartin, L., Glavin, M., Jones, E.: Compressed sensing for bioelectric signals: a review. IEEE J. Biomed. Health Inform. **19**(2), 529–540 (2015)
10. De Vito, L., Picariello, E., Picariello, F., Rapuano, S., Tudosa, I.: A dictionary optimization method for reconstruction of ECG signals after compressed sensing. Sensors **21**(16) (2021)
11. De Vito, L., et al.: An undershirt for monitoring of multi-lead ECG and respiration wave signals. In: 2021 IEEE International Workshop on Metrology for Industry 4.0 & IoT (MetroInd4. 0&IoT), pp. 550–555. IEEE (2021)
12. Dixon, A.M.R., Allstot, E.G., Gangopadhyay, D., Allstot, D.J.: Compressed sensing system considerations for ECG and EMG wireless biosensors. IEEE Trans. Biomed. Circuits Syst. **6**(2), 156–166 (2012)
13. Ghiadoni, L., et al.: Mental stress induces transient endothelial dysfunction in humans. Circulation **102**(20), 2473–2478 (2000)
14. Goldberger, A.L., et al.: Physiobank, physiotoolkit, and physionet: components of a new research resource for complex physiologic signals. Circulation **101**(23), e215–e220 (2000)
15. Harhash, A.A., et al.: aVR ST segment elevation: acute STEMI or not? Incidence of an acute coronary occlusion. Am. J. Med. **132**(5), 622–630 (2019)
16. Jager, F., et al.: Long-term ST database: a reference for the development and evaluation of automated ischaemia detectors and for the study of the dynamics of myocardial ischaemia. Med. Biol. Eng. Comput. **41**(2), 172–182 (2003)
17. Kandala, V.K., Vadaparthi, J.K.: Study of incidence and pattern of ECG changes in cerebrovascular accidents. Radiology **3**(1), 107–109 (2018)
18. Kashou, A.H., Basit, H., Malik, A.: St segment. In: StatPearls [Internet]. StatPearls Publishing (2021)
19. Khoury, S., et al.: Incidence, characteristics and outcomes in very young patients with ST segment elevation myocardial infarction. Coronary Artery Dis. **31**(2), 103–108 (2020)
20. Kop, W.J., et al.: Effects of mental stress on coronary epicardial vasomotion and flow velocity in coronary artery disease: relationship with hemodynamic stress responses. J. Am. Coll. Cardiol. **37**(5), 1359–1366 (2001)
21. Laudato, G., et al.: Combining rhythmic and morphological ECG features for automatic detection of atrial fibrillation. In: 13th International Conference on Health Informatics, pp. 156–165 (2020)
22. Laudato, G., Picariello, F., Scalabrino, S., Tudosa, I., de Vito, L., Oliveto, R.: Morphological classification of heartbeats in compressed ECG. In: 14th International Conference on Health Informatics, HEALTHINF 2021-Part of the 14th International Joint Conference on Biomedical Engineering Systems and Technologies, BIOSTEC 2021, pp. 386–393. SciTePress (2021)
23. Laudato, G., et al.: Combining rhythmic and morphological ECG features for automatic detection of atrial fibrillation: local and global prediction models. In: Ye, X., et al. (eds.) BIOSTEC 2020. CCIS, vol. 1400, pp. 425–441. Springer, Cham (2021). https://doi.org/10.1007/978-3-030-72379-8_21

24. Laudato, G., et al.: Identification of r-peak occurrences in compressed ECG signals. In: 2020 IEEE International Symposium on Medical Measurements and Applications (MeMeA), pp. 1–6. IEEE (2020)

25. Laudato, G., et al.: Simulating the doctor's behaviour: a preliminary study on the identification of atrial fibrillation through combined analysis of heart rate and beat morphology, pp. 446–453 (2022). https://doi.org/10.5220/0010823900003123

26. Laudato, G., et al.: Atticus: ambient-intelligent tele-monitoring and telemetry for incepting and catering over human sustainability. Front. Hum. Dyn. 19 (2021)

27. Leonarduzzi, R.F., Schlotthauer, G., Torres, M.E.: Wavelet leader based multifractal analysis of heart rate variability during myocardial ischaemia. In: 2010 Annual International Conference of the IEEE Engineering in Medicine and Biology, pp. 110–113. IEEE (2010)

28. Li, T., Zhou, M.: ECG classification using wavelet packet entropy and random forests. Entropy 18(8), 285 (2016)

29. Maglaveras, N., Stamkopoulos, T., Pappas, C., Strintzis, M.G.: An adaptive backpropagation neural network for real-time ischemia episodes detection: development and performance analysis using the European ST-T database. IEEE Trans. Biomed. Eng. 45(7), 805–813 (1998)

30. Mattioli, A.V., Nasi, M., Cocchi, C., Farinetti, A.: COVID-19 outbreak: impact of the quarantine-induced stress on cardiovascular disease risk burden (2020)

31. Pan, J., Tompkins, W.J.: A real-time QRS detection algorithm. IEEE Trans. Biomed. Eng. 3, 230–236 (1985)

32. Picariello, F., Iadarola, G., Balestrieri, E., Tudosa, I., De Vito, L.: A novel compressive sampling method for ECG wearable measurement systems. Measurement 167, 108259 (2021)

33. Quwaider, M., Biswas, S.: On-body packet routing algorithms for body sensor networks. In: 2009 First International Conference on Networks & Communications, pp. 171–177. IEEE (2009)

34. Ravelomanantsoa, A., Rabah, H., Rouane, A.: Compressed sensing: a simple deterministic measurement matrix and a fast recovery algorithm. IEEE Trans. Instrum. Meas. 64(12), 3405–3413 (2015)

35. Rehman, A., Saba, T., Haseeb, K., Larabi Marie-Sainte, S., Lloret, J.: Energy-efficient IoT e-health using artificial intelligence model with homomorphic secret sharing. Energies 14(19), 6414 (2021)

36. Rghioui, A., Lloret, J., Harane, M., Oumnad, A.: A smart glucose monitoring system for diabetic patient. Electronics 9(4), 678 (2020)

37. Rosa, G., Laudato, G., Colavita, A.R., Scalabrino, S., Oliveto, R.: Automatic real-time beat-to-beat detection of arrhythmia conditions. In: HEALTHINF, pp. 212–222 (2021)

38. Rosa, G., Russodivito, M., Laudato, G., Colavita, A.R., Scalabrino, S., Oliveto, R.: A robust approach for a real-time accurate screening of ST segment anomalies. In: HEALTHINF, pp. 69–80 (2022)

39. Rosa, G., Russodivito, M., Laudato, G., Scalabrino, S., Colavita, A.R., Oliveto, R.: A multiclass approach for the automatic detection of congestive heart failure in windowed ECG. Stud. Health Technol. Inform. 290, 650–654 (2022)

40. Rosengren, A., et al.: Association of psychosocial risk factors with risk of acute myocardial infarction in 11 119 cases and 13 648 controls from 52 countries (the INTERHEART study): case-control study. Lancet 364(9438), 953–962 (2004)

41. Ryu, K.S., Bae, J.W., Jeong, M.H., Cho, M.C., Ryu, K.H., Investigators, K.A.M.I.R., et al.: Risk scoring system for prognosis estimation of multivessel disease among patients with ST-segment elevation myocardial infarction. Int. Heart J. 60(3), 708–714 (2019)

42. Srivastava, J., Routray, S., Ahmad, S., Waris, M.M.: Internet of medical things (iomt)-based smart healthcare system: trends and progress. Comput. Intell. Neurosci. 2022 (2022)

43. Taddei, A., et al.: The European ST-T database: standard for evaluating systems for the analysis of ST-T changes in ambulatory electrocardiography. Eur. Heart J. **13**(9), 1164–1172 (1992)
44. Tsuji, H., Shiojima, I.: Increased incidence of ECG abnormalities in the general population during the COVID-19 pandemic. Int. Heart J. **63**(4), 678–682 (2022)
45. Wang, H., et al.: ST segment change classification based on multiple feature extraction using ECG. In: 2018 Computing in Cardiology Conference (CinC), vol. 45, pp. 1–4. IEEE (2018)
46. Wei, W., Qi, Y.: Information potential fields navigation in wireless ad-hoc sensor networks. Sensors **11**, 4794–4807 (2011)
47. Xiao, R., Xu, Y., Pelter, M.M., Mortara, D.W., Hu, X.: A deep learning approach to examine ischemic ST changes in ambulatory ECG recordings. AMIA Summits Transl. Sci. Proc. **2018**, 256 (2018)
48. Zhao, Q., Zhang, L.: ECG feature extraction and classification using wavelet transform and support vector machines. In: 2005 International Conference on Neural Networks and Brain, vol. 2, pp. 1089–1092. IEEE (2005)

A Proof-of-Concept Implementation Based on the Framework of AI-Enabled Proactive mHealth: Health Promotion with Motivation

Muhammad Sulaiman[✉], Anne Håkansson, and Randi Karlsen

Department of Computer Science, UiT The Arctic University of Norway, Tromsø, Norway
{muhammad.sulaiman,anne.hakansson,randi.karlsen}@uit.no

Abstract. Digital health with mHealth contributes to health promotion by empowering the user with a holistic view of their health. Proactive mHealth is to predict and prevent a situation beforehand, promptly. Most health decisions are taken by the user pervasively. They have a short or long-term impact. Being proactive requires support as ubiquitous decision-making is prone to sudden changes. Changes in users' internal and contextual states require adaptive systems with timeliness. Personalized health information needs analysis to support user-level decision-making. The goal is to automate processes and augment healthy behaviour. Data from wearables, together with the context, requires automated decision-making with AI modelling, for predicting intervention values. Prediction and prevention mechanism in implementation requires timely interventions, triggered with a supportive action. The health information (wearables + context) can provide information about the states (current, future, and goal). AI-enabled proactive mHealth framework accentuates abstraction by presenting modules with rules of user-level decision-making, tools for automated decision-making, design with P5 principles, and the architecture of Just-in-time adaptive interventions. In this paper, a proof-of-concept (POC) for health promotion with physical activity is implemented based on the framework. The goal is to promote health with motivation. The paper also categorizes intervention with type, properties, and principles. Components of intervention and behaviour change are also listed. POC includes parameters of context and user profile. The paper provides a step-by-step approach to implementing the system on the framework, from input/output mapping to modelling. The outcome is a POC that alters and augments behaviour change for health promotion with physical activity.

Keywords: Proactive health · mHealth · Digital health · Health interventions · Just-in-time adaptive intervention · Machine learning · Artificial intelligence · Wearables · Automated decision-making · Physical activity

1 Introduction

Digital health is a fundamental component of smart cities [1]. The Future of healthcare depends on digital health transformations in complementing core health services to improve well-being. The goal is to shift the focus from a one-size-fits-all approach to

A. C. A. Roque et al. (Eds.): BIOSTEC 2022, CCIS 1814, pp. 256–287, 2023.
https://doi.org/10.1007/978-3-031-38854-5_14

individual outcomes. The ultimate objective [2] of digital health is to provide health services with the principles of when, where, and whom.

Many different health definitions are available that complement the need for digital health transformation, for instance, the definition by the Center for disease control and prevention (CDC) [3]. "The science and art of preventing disease, prolonging life, and promoting health through the organized efforts and informed choices of society, organizations, public and private communities, and individuals". This definition supports the need for health promotion for the individual through tools that provide a holistic view. This accentuates that individual health promotion is directly proportional to individual increased control of health [4].

Health promotion is also more important as current health systems around the globe are facing many challenges, one major challenge is longevity [5] which is a crucial factor for multiple chronic diseases e.g., In Norway, around 80000−100000 people suffer from dementia [6]. The increase in life expectancy also supplements the development of multiple chronic diseases e.g., cardiovascular disease, stroke, cancer, osteoarthritis, and dementia. This group of people is extending and needs care tailored to their conditions. WHO estimates that half of the health burden is due to chronic diseases [7].

Digital health can be a vital component in supporting healthcare systems globally. Healthcare also has to deal with public health crisis or situations that affect communities globally. An example is a recent pandemic [8] that affected everyone globally. When a public health crisis is in place it is important to use digital means to provide healthcare at a distance to those who are in need. This brought digital health into the spotlight again.

The data-driven connected "smart" cities would provide means to implement interoperability and integration between different health system components [1]. Digital health is not a new phenomenon in healthcare, it has been around for the last two decades, but the availability of devices and the introduction of mobile health (mHealth) sparked the need for it. A definition of digital health that complements self-empowerment is "Digital health connects and empowers people and populations to manage health and wellness, augmented by accessible and supportive provider teams working within flexible, integrated, interoperable and digitally enabled care environments that strategically leverage digital tools, technologies and services to transform care delivery" [9].

A subset of digital health is mobile health (mHealth) which empowers people to manage their health to improve their well-being. mHealth is defined as "medical and public health practice supported by mobile devices, such as mobile phones, patient monitoring devices, personal digital assistants (PDAs), and other wireless devices" [10]. The availability of devices that individuals carry on the fly makes mHealth ubiquitous. This ubiquitousness powers mHealth to deal with impediments of health delivery like location, time, and cost. A booming increase in data and new insights from these devices made mHealth a key component in the data-driven future. The role of mHealth is not limited to providing tools for health care delivery at a distance but to having more insight into the data collected from these devices. The future of mHealth and wearable is growing and estimated to reach 149.3 billion USD by 2028 [11].

mHealth is a major contributor to self-empowerment and health promotion. It holds the key to providing a holistic view to the user about all the body signals, to make them aware and conscious of their health. mHealth applications are targeted toward the user, by following the user-centric design which empowers the user and can provide new insights from the health data collected from the wearable sensors. Another aspect is the continuous measurement of the health information that is real-time and is needed for user-level decision-making.

Current healthcare system design is not targeted at individual uniqueness [12]. The current healthcare system is also reactive [12], which is "react when symptoms appear then take action, an example of crisis management" [13]. This reactive approach works in many health situations but nullifies the principles of health promotion and risk prevention.

On the contrary, Proactive health is to predict and prevent a situation beforehand, targeted towards the general population to make them aware promptly, so they do not become sick [14]. Proactive mHealth is to use mHealth tools to empower the user, and to establish proactiveness.

The goal of proactive mHealth is to provide timely awareness to the user. Different health risks and concerns are around the user [15]. Some of them have a direct impact on the health of the user. That can be short-term or long-term, for example, air pollution can have a bad long-term impact. Factors can be categorized as environmental, but are associated with lifestyle and user characteristics also. The context of the user is of utmost significance when proactive mHealth systems are implemented. The context by definition is "anything that is around a user, the condition in which something exists" [16]. The context of the user can be a resource for collecting information but also a factor when providing intervention choices to the user for motivation.

Decision-making in healthcare is divided into two main paradigms: clinical decision-making and user-level decision-making [17]. Clinical decision-making requires health professionals to provide decisions for the user in the hospital setting. User-level decisions are taken by the user away from the hospital setting. These decisions have an immediate effect on the health of the user. Wearables with mHealth have many sensors that provide new data points, patterns from the collected data can be a key to making accurate predictions. AI can be an important player for proactive mHealth to automate processes and augment healthy behaviour in the user.

Artificial intelligence (AI) is contributing to healthcare by providing predictive modelling and analytics. One of the definitions of AI that complements our use-case of proactive mHealth is "artificial intelligence is a field, which combines computer science and robust datasets, to enable problem-solving. It also encompasses sub-fields of machine learning and deep learning, which are frequently mentioned in conjunction with artificial intelligence. These disciplines are comprised of AI algorithms which seek to create [...] systems which make predictions or classifications based on input data" [18]. AI can provide automated decision-making by analysing the available health information of the user. These automated decisions are health interventions tailored for the user. Interventions motivate the user promptly to make better health choices. The prediction and prevention mechanism of proactive mHealth depends on AI to provide automated decisions. To develop proactive mHealth with the principles of prediction, prevention, and ubiquitous health Artificial Intelligence (AI) with mHealth can play a pivotal role.

The healthy behaviour of an individual is an essential component of health promotion. A proactive mHealth system considers the uniqueness of a user when implementing user-level decision-making. Many factors influence decision-making and behaviour change for health promotion, i.e., personalization, motivation, and persuasiveness. Implementation of a proactive mHealth system requires health interventions that are personalized, adaptive, and prompt. Health interventions, therefore, must be categorized with properties and principles for proactive mHealth.

The implementation of a proactive mHealth system with the ability to predict and prevent a situation in a timely manner by considering personalization is challenging. Different contributors to a proactive mHealth system: AI, mHealth, user context, user characteristics, and user preferences must operate concurrently. The collected data from wearables, sensors, and other resources need to be processed by an AI-powered engine to provide predictions. The system must follow a set design and architecture framework to compile all the components together.

This paper is an extended version of a paper published earlier [19] that introduced the framework of AI-enabled proactive mHealth. It builds upon the introduced framework by dividing the framework into modules and providing categorization of interventions. The paper also provides multiple scenarios based on the mechanism of prediction and prevention with personalization. Finally, it implements a proof-of-concept for health promotion with motivation. This proof-of-concept is based on the framework of AI-enabled proactive mHealth. The proof-of-concept is targeted at improving physical activity in users through health intervention. The result is a proactive mHealth system that can be the basis for further development of AI-enabled proactive mHealth with more parameters.

2   Related Work

Proactiveness when it comes to health promotion is very asymmetrical. A proactive system must follow a mechanism of prediction and prevention. Many mHealth applications [20] use machine learning to provide the basic level of proactiveness that is to manage the disease. This level of proactiveness is comprehensive. Some studies [21–23] are targeted at particular disease management for chronic patients proactively. The high level of proactiveness would be to follow the mechanism of prediction and prevention with personalization.

A review [14] presented that there is no existing research found for proactive mHealth that enables health promotion with motivation. Keeping in view the user's context and the data from wearables. The review also concluded that previous studies do not include the prediction and prevention mechanism for a user to provide health interventions before becoming sick.

A study [24] illustrated a health map of users with states but for emphasising the need for proactive health only.

A few studies [25, 26] used wearables as a data source but for activity only. Activity data can be useful for health promotion but when it comes to altering behaviour the prediction mechanism needs more parameters from the user context. A study [23] concludes wearables as a key to ubiquitous health. Another study [27] spotlights decision-making with mHealth.

Smartphone usage has increased in the last decade, statistics show about half of the mobile phone owners search the internet for health-related information [28]. This need is met by the increasing availability of mHealth applications, for instance, statistic [29] shows that more than 350,000 health applications are available on app stores. AI is also contributing to this growing market; an estimation indicates that 80% of mHealth applications will use AI by 2025 [29].

There are major concerns about the trustworthiness of these mHealth applications and will be a debate in the future as well. Some use cases where AI in mHealth prediction models can be, personalized treatments, early detection, recommender systems, screening, and triage, and chatbots.

Related work emphasizes the need of being proactive but at the level of managing a certain health condition. No prior research was found for health promotion with motivation. That is targeted for the user with personalization and considers user uniqueness. The existing research also does not provide a mechanism for prediction and prevention before becoming sick. The system which follows an intervention architecture of just-in-time to provide timely adaptive interventions. Such a system must consider multiple factors of the state of the user, and the context of the user. The analysis shows that many different existing systems did use wearables as a data source but just to the extent to add new data points and not providing a holistic view to alter or augment users' behaviour. Related work concludes that AI in mHealth is growing but the focus is on monitoring and self-management. This languishes proactive mHealth principle of prediction and prevention for health promotion for a user with personalized timely health interventions.

3 The Framework of AI-Enabled Proactive mHealth with Modules

The framework of AI-enabled proactive mHealth [19] was presented that provided the basis for the development of proactive mHealth systems. The framework renders abstraction to build efficient proactive mHealth systems. The framework also provided a comprehensive guide to the implementation of systems. The framework included tools for automated decision-making, design goals of the system, and architecture for implementing interventions.

This paper complements the framework introduced earlier by dividing it into modules and building upon the framework to provide five modules.

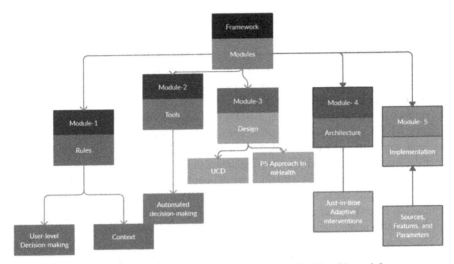

Fig. 1. The framework of AI-enabled proactive mHealth with modules.

Figure 1 presents the overview of modules of the framework. Now each of the modules is presented with use-cases and examples. The modules also serve each component, for instance, the first module decides rules.

3.1 Module-1 -Rules- Decision-Making and Context-Awareness

The first module presented here provides rules that are necessary for building the framework. An important component of this module is decision-making. In this section decision-making importance in healthcare is highlighted by presenting the type of decision-making. Furthermore, an explanation of user-level decision-making for proactive mHealth with different stakeholders.

Decision-making is an essential component which requires information, choices, and previous experience [30]. The outcome of a decision can be a critical aspect which can have either a positive or negative impact. This impact can be further categorized as long-term or short-term. By definition, decision-making is "the process of making choices by identifying a decision, gathering information, and assessing alternative resolutions" [31].

Besides, it also demands time and effort to process the knowledge at hand. Numerous factors influence decision-making, and there is a need to have a set of rules (approaches) to effective decision-making. A strategy introduced [31] for effective decision-making proposes 7-steps to effective decision-making; to identify, collect information, alternatives, and evidence at hand, choose options, take actions, and finally review the outcome.

In the healthcare decision-making model, multiple stakeholders are involved; the patient, the doctor, and the evidence [32]. Traditionally, the decision-making process has been in anticipation as decision-making was influenced by gut feeling, intuition, and instinct. But with the introduction of evidence-based decision-making (EBDM), the goal is to make decisions based on the available evidence, relying on the data and facts. EBDM provides three stages of action: gathering evidence, interpreting evidence, and applying what you have learned [32]. EBDM is beneficial but requires more evidence to interpret, which is neither cost-effective nor time [33]. Some health decision lies in the grey area; that is the area with no clear right or wrong answer [34]. It is crucial to make better decisions with a positive impact on the health of individuals.

mHealth can contribute by providing more insights into the user's health, continuous measurement, and access to multiple parameters. The user-centric design of mHealth applications treats the user as a data source which can be the key to improving decisions.

Most health-related decisions are taken by the user on the go away from the hospital. These decisions are categorized as user-level decisions. User-level decision-making requires information, along with a motivation for the user for health promotion or risk prevention. These decisions are informed choices that the user take in their daily life. The decisions can have a positive or negative impact on their health.

The contributors to these decisions are the mHealth application, the data patterns, sources, and the context. Table 1 presents some user-level decisions, with the contributors and the type of impact they have with intensity.

Table 1. User-level decision-making with contributors [Extended from previous table [19].

User-level decisions	Contributors	Impact
Air-quality trigger- The air quality tomorrow is predicted to be lunhealthyl, user-profile = COPD, Decision = wear a mask when outside	API's metrological data or sensors, User-profile for identification, Mobile phone for location and intervention	Risk prevention, requires personalization
Inactivity trigger- The user is lnot activel, from the step-count and profile, Decision: Based on the step data, you are sedentary, the weather is predicted to be nice in the next 2 h. A walk to the city center will be 5000 steps	Wearables, Weather API, user-profile, and mobile	Health promotion, requires personalization
Warning trigger – Storm warning in the area- User-location from wearables: Based on your current location, you are in the storm warning zone	API's metrological data, Mobile, location data	Risk prevention, only location

User-level decision-making is a necessary aspect of the framework. When developing proactive mHealth applications, elements of user level and contributors must be evaluated.

The second component of this module is of utmost importance. The context is "the interrelated conditions in which something exists or occurs" [16]. The attribute which is pivotal for the context is the nature that it is very dynamic. This ever-changing ability also encloses challenges when implementing context awareness. With proactive mHealth, the context is anything that can have an impact on the health of the user. It is also critical to emphasize the context as it provides parameters e.g., the environment, the surroundings and the user profiling.

The context also accentuates personalization to highlight, let us consider an example of a user who is allergic to pollen. For that user, the parameter of the environment, in particular, pollen is of critical importance. The context is a collection of attributes measurable that collectively forms the parameters, for example, the surrounding, environment, and internal and external states of the user.

For a system to be context-aware it must be adaptive to its surroundings and states. It is also essential to identify the target to form parameters which are needed to build the context. Information from the context combined with other data from wearables can be beneficial for decision-making.

In proactive mHealth systems, the context is also a data source that provides parameters of surroundings. It can also be used for motivation to the user to promote health. A user's context is dynamic, it includes states, and environment. Based on the target of a health intervention, the context is categorized as personalized or generic. An example is a fire in the surrounding that can affect everyone and thus does not need personalization, but if a person is in a risk group for an infectious disease it must be more personalized.

Following the prediction and prevention mechanism of proactive mHealth, the context provides health promotion and risk prevention. The limitation comes with what is measurable and considered a parameter. The context can include anything, even things that are not visible. To understand the complication, let us consider an example of User-A taking a walk from point A to point B. The wearables provide health information about the user that is current state, the profile of user-A states that she has asthma caused by an inflammatory reaction- so for her, air pollution between point A and point B is vital. The walking conditions correspond to another attribute of a context. In addition, a driver driving a car between the points on the road suffering from a heart problem or epilepsy can be a threat. The example shows that context is very comprehensive, but it all comes down to what is measurable from the sensors and available resources.

The dynamic nature of the context requires adaptiveness of the build systems. A proactive mHealth system must consider the following user parameters to build the context. Table 2 presents the context with the user profile, characteristics, and states. Only measurable parameters are considered.

Table 2. The context of the user.

Context	User		
Environment/Surroundings	profile	Characteristics	States
Sensors: Environmental sensors, Indoor and outdoor weather stations	Physical attributes: BMI, Allergies	Daily patterns Schedule	Current state from wearables: location data, heart rate, and health information
	History: Family and disease or disability		
Warnings, threats, weather data, air-quality data, and outbreaks	Goal and behavior component setting	Preferences of the user	From wearables and mobile

3.2 Module-2 - Tools-AI Capabilities with Automated Decision-Making and Predictive Analytics

A decision is not merely a choice architecture, but a process that includes steps; collecting information, determining the need, identifying the options, and providing an optimal action [35].

In module 1, an extensive explanation is given about user-level decision-making. Although those decisions are for the user to take, but require automated decision-making (ADM) to augment user behaviour for health promotion. The goal of ADM is to provide decisions to the user with technical means [36]. ADM complements the user-level decision-making by analysing patterns and combining factors from the user's data to provide a decision that is valid for the user. ADM processes the data from wearables and context, models it with the user profile, and finally provides a decision to the user.

ADM is being used by many sectors already, in the financial sector it is used for automated credit applications [37], and in healthcare, it is being used to triage the patients to classify [38] who needs care first. The benefits of using ADM are speed and scalability [39].

The core of ADM is to power the AI-engine with machine learning techniques such as random forest (RF), decision trees (DT), regression models, and artificial neural networks (ANN). An AI engine then accounts for multiple inputs to provide a decision with- a prediction (a future state) and prevention (to avoid the future state) mechanism for ADM.

In proactive mHealth, it is very crucial to account for changing contexts, by adaptiveness. Also, sudden changes and the user profile is an important aspect. ADM corresponds to that by applying techniques that establish the timeliness of the system by providing decisions when needed, for example, if a user is not active; a timely intervention which is powered by ADM with inactivity and information to have a walk. Similarly, when it comes to risk prevention; A decision from ADM for the user is "Is it safe to go out?". ADM must incorporate multiple input parameters, sudden changes, and the user profile to provide timely decisions.

The outcome of the ADM is a decision, which can be categorized as an intervention based on the intensity and information. The architecture of ADM is a combination of algorithms that power the AI engine for making predictions. Since ADM needs continuous data, it needs persistent monitoring from the parameters together, for instance, data from wearable, context, and user profile.

In the framework of AI-enabled proactive mHealth, ADM is the core part as it provides the tools to power the engine of a proactive mHealth system which is predictive and preventive. The increase in the availability of data from wearables and context makes it more achievable, but a big challenge is the quality of data that feeds the tools. Another challenge is to choose between machine learning algorithms: which depends on the use case and data.

An example Table 3 shows some machine learning techniques for ADM with use cases.

Table 3. ADM tools, techniques, and use-cases.

Automated decision-making	Tools	Use-cases	Purpose
Machine learning	TensorFlow. Scikit-learn and Keras	Data automation, model tracking, performance monitoring, and model retraining	Classification, Perception, Understanding, Discovering, Prediction and Creation
Techniques/Algorithms	Regression (linear, logistic), Naïve Bayes, K-nearest Neighbors (KNN), Learning Vector Quantization (LVQ), SVM, Random Forest, Boosting, AdaBoost		

3.3 Module-3 Design with P5 Approach to Mhealth

When it comes to the design of mHealth applications, User-centric design (UCD) is the ultimate choice [40]. The goal of UCD is to improve the usability of the designed system by increasing user-engagement. The life cycle of the whole system involves the end-user at each step.

Since UCD is comprehensive when defining a proactive framework. The design of mHealth applications must follow principles of design and implementation. A P4 spectrum [41] which is a basis for personalized medicine complements the UCD by providing design principles. The objective of following the design principles is to develop applications that are: vigilant, adaptive and can understand the uniqueness of the user. P4 spectrum of medicine is defined as predictive, personalized, preventive, and participatory.

A P5 approach to mHealth extends the P4 medicine spectrum by adding another principle of Psycho-cognitive [42]. This approach can be the standard for designing mHealth systems. The current mHealth application designs are becoming user-centric but focus on getting input from the user. Many fundamental deficiencies in current mHealth systems complement the use P5 approach to mHealth. Some examples:

- Data from wearables with health information that is real-time and needs processing for better outcomes.
- The context of the user as a source.
- The ability of the systems to forecast trends in health information and future states can have a good or bad impact.
- Need of having the user in the loop for modifications and feedback to learn from.
- The uniqueness of the user when it comes to daily patterns and characteristics.
- The behaviour of the user towards health promotion.

As a design module of the framework of AI-enabled proactive mHealth, the P5 approach to mHealth is the absolute choice. It increases precision and allows for implementing systems that are predictive and preventive with personalization. The design also allows users to be in the loop. Finally, to alter or augment user behaviour for health promotion. The Table 4 explains each of the principles with an example.

Table 4. Principles of P5 with use-cases.

Principle of P5	Explanation	The use-case
Predictive	Allowing perdition about a future sate from the input: current state	A mobile application that predicts air-quality
Preventive	An action that prevents the future state, measure to be taken	An intervention to prevent the future state: wear a mask
Personalized	Understanding the uniqueness of the user by design	User health profile as input: Knowing location of the user
Participatory	User as an active decision-maker	Throughout the process, user involvement
Psycho-cognitive	Improving ability and behavior of the user	Motivation and adaption

3.4 Module-4 the Architecture with Just-in-Time Adaptive Interventions

An intervention is an event, with a set of information that is triggered for a reason [43]. Digital health interventions aim to provide health information at a particular time to the user. This information must be beneficial and acceptable to the user.

In proactive mHealth, the mechanism of prediction and prevention depends on the architecture of health interventions. The objective is to provide support at the right time by understanding the gravity of the changing internal and contextual state. This proffers that a specific architecture is required for the framework.

This module explains the architecture of the framework. The architecture is built on the properties of intervention; timeliness and adaptiveness. Just-in-time adaptive interventions (JITAI) are an ideal choice architecture for the framework. It implements timeliness by providing support at the right time, to the user with information. JITAI also accounts for the changing user states when providing interventions. JITAI requires a start state and a goal state of the user.

– Start state: The current state
– Goal state: Future state

JITAI provides three principles for implementing intervention architecture [44]. The three W's corresponds to:

– When: When to intervene
– What: With what information
– Whom: To whom

The principles are also an implementation challenge for the system (Figs. 2 and 8). The graph below shows the need for JITAI as an architecture of proactive mHealth for User A.

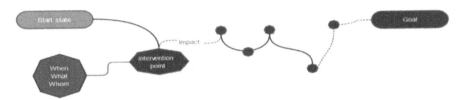

Fig. 2. JITAI with user health-map.

3.5 Module-5- Implementation with Components, Parameters, Factors, and Features: Sources, Wearables, Data Points and APIS

This module provides extensive information about implementation details, requirements and available gear to support the framework. After the identification of parameters from defined factors, the next step is to determine the sources. Most of the sources provide multiple features, that harmonise with the requirements of having multiple parameters as input. Table 5 provides sources and resources associated with the user for input, and the second column features in alignment with the factors. Finally, the table also presents the purpose of the features in comparison to the sources.

Table 5. Sources with available features and purpose.

Sources	Features	Purpose
Wearables	Health information: Activity data, location data, heart rate, SpO2, body temperature, readiness score, sleep, active minutes, and calories burned	Holistic view, States and user-profiling, user-characteristics
Sensors	Weather station, indoor outdoor air quality, humidity, temperature, CO2, Noise, and sound meter	Context information and user states
Resources	Weather, warnings, threats, outbreaks, air-quality, ice-map, and Met-alerts	Context information and user states

The Table 5 illustrates different components, each component is a layer above the other in terms of implementation. The first component is the factor which forms the parameters that are required for the input.

Factors.

- User profile: It is the key to personalization by collecting information that is unique to the user. A profile in proactive mHealth corresponds to health information, collected implicitly or explicitly from the user. The user profile also furnishes information about the user's state and goals. Some examples of the parameters of the user profile are shown in the Fig. 3.

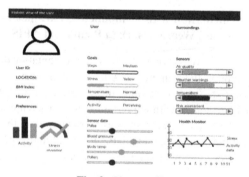

Fig. 3. User-profile.

Some examples of the parameters of the user profile are shown in the Fig. 3.

- User context: The context of the user holds information about the surroundings/environment of the user along with anything that is measurable, and can have a good or bad impact on the user.

- User characteristics: User characteristics have a salient contribution towards personalization. It accounts for user behaviour along with daily patterns.

The factors as a component dispense multiple parameters, for a proactive mHealth framework. These parameters are also vital for considering the states of the user before implementing JITAI. The next component is the sources and resources for the parameters.

Sources.
The section presents available sources and resources for collecting data following the parameters of the user.

Wearables:
Wearables are devices with a combination of sensors e.g., altimeter, accelerometer, and temperature sensors that the user wears. They provide portability and data which can be processed as useful information [45]. The fact that these devices are ubiquitous and can collect data all the time makes them very useful for continuous monitoring. In healthcare, there are many available wearables [46], for instance, fitness trackers, biosensors, smartwatches and health rings. The goal of all of them is to provide continuous measurement of biosignals. The list of available biosignals is expanding, depending on vendors. A comparison is drawn below that shows what can be measured using these wearable devices.

– List of features: Activity, GPS, Heart rate, breathing, SpO2, temperature, and sleep.

For a proactive mHealth framework, wearables are essential as they provide health information about the user characteristics e.g., daily patterns, user profile e.g., location. Wearables are also necessary for real-time data collection for sudden changes and historical data for predictive modelling.

Different vendors have provided APIs to integrate, but still, the data produced by the wearables need a good collection mechanism. There is a compatibility problem between vendors that makes it a challenge. Another challenge is the raw data collected from the sensors which need proper treatment before analysis. The abundance of real-time data can be very critical for proactive mHealth, but a challenge to process and analyse. For mHealth applications, it is important to choose the right vendor for connecting to your application. Most of the devices have overlapping features, but the accuracy is very different.

For the framework of proactive mHealth, it is important to choose the right wearable depending on which biosignals are to be measured, system integration, and ultimately access to real-time data.

Sensors:
Another source is the availability of sensors that provide information about the context. Many different sensors are available, some provide raw data but need a microcontroller to get access. A challenge is then to create a system by combining those sensors. Some examples are:
MQ-135, BME-180, and PM 2.5. They require a microcontroller for use. Another available system that also provides an API is the NETATMO weather station [47]. Which

serves well for the context information in our use case. Here is a brief detail of the data it can provide with features:

- NETATMO weather station features (Real-time Indoor and outdoor information) temperature, CO_2, humidity, air quality, sound meter, and barometric pressure.

Resources:
The framework of proactive mHealth also requires context information from a metrological institute. For example, the proactive mHealth system does not need to handle weather forecasting, but it can collect that information from available APIs. Some other APIs provide historical weather data along with pollen counts. APIs can be integrated when building a proactive mHealth system. Here is an example of an available resource with contextual data it provides.

- YR.no: air quality, met-alerts, weather forecast, ice-map, and ocean-forecast.

The sources and resources furnish the required information for the holistic view of the user. Which is formed by incorporating multiple parameters. This holistic view is important when providing intervention to the user. The Fig. 3 shows an example of the holistic view. User states are also another factor that is measurable but needs continuous measurement. The current state and future state complement the mechanism of prediction and prevention. An example of a scenario and the use of sources is given in Table 6.

Table 6. Sources with available features and purpose.

Scenario	Sources
lLow activity—user will not be able to complete activity goall prediction lMotivating the user for a walk- to complete the remaining stepsl prevention lUser-current state and future state from the available health informationl personalization	Health information: Activity data, location data, Current state from wearables

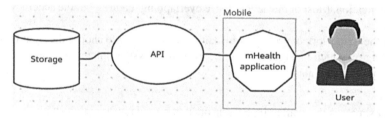

Fig. 4. Architecture of a mHealth application.

Figure 4 presents an architecture of a mHealth application. The back-end of the application depends on the server that provides the functionality of request/response through API. A dynamic end-point API. The storage is the resource that collect input data from sensors and other resources.

4   Health Interventions with Categorization and Properties

Altering or augmenting behaviour is complicated. Behavioural interventions influence users' actions concerning their health [48]. Implementation of behavioural interventions can have different levels, depending on the purpose of the intervention. Therefore, behaviour change depends on the decision environment and the choice architecture of the user [49].

Users can behave differently, not aligned to their intentions, establishing that the decision-making has flaws and biases [50]. Altering or augmenting behaviour requires the classification of interventions, which depends on the goal of the intervention.

In behavioural science, health interventions are classified as nudges, boosts, and recommendations [51]. A nudge is a subtle behavioural intervention that helps users make better health choices [52]. It works predictably without mandating or forbidding the user. Nudges are also cheaper and easier to accept with beneficial information for the user. The goal of a nudge is to design the context of decision-making, in a way that promotes behaviour, considering the interest of the user and society. An effective nudge must follow a two-step approach: Starting from identifying the target and then designing the context with the choice architecture of the user [50].

With the availability of digital resources, a new term smart-nudging is introduced "where the guidance of user behaviour is presented through digital nudges tailored to be relevant to the current situation of each user" [53]. The objective of a smart nudge is to provide an intervention with useful information that motivates the user to alter or augment behaviour. A smart nudge is personalized based on the user profile, it also accounts for the changing context to provide timely intervention to the user.

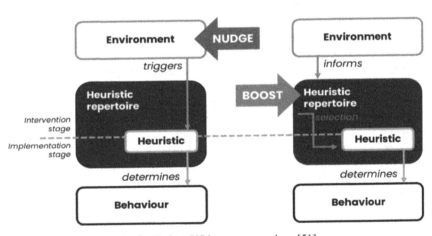

Fig. 5. Nudges VS boosts comparison [51].

Boosts, contrastingly target the user's ability of decision-making [51]. The goal is to improve the competence of the user. The Fig. 5 presents a comparison between the mechanism of nudges and boosts. It shows that the nudge targets the choice architecture, whereas a boost works with the set architecture of choices and improves the user's ability.

After identifying the type of interventions, the next step is to explain the level of interventions. Interventions are of different levels: First is the individual user level that requires more personalization. The goal of these interventions is to promote the health of the user. The second level corresponds to managing a certain disease, the level of intervention requires the personalization of a group of people. Finally, the third level is of a community, the interventions are based on location. An example is a storm or an infectious disease that has an equal impact on everyone. It is to be noted that some interventions on a community level are for the user as well e.g., a threat in a nearby environment based on the location. So, this level of intervention also forms the need for personalization.

After explaining the level of intervention; the explanation continues with the properties of intervention. These properties also form a relationship with type: Each type of intervention holds certain properties.

Properties of Intervention. Intensity, adaptive, timeliness, cost, impact, transparency, persuasiveness, to alter behaviour, and augment the behaviour.

- **Intensity:** An intervention must specify the attention required: an example is a sensor that predicts fire that will have a higher magnitude, than low physical activity.
- **Timeliness:** Timely intervention has significance. The ideal time for an intervention is before the event, with enough time so the user can react. The whole prediction is dependent on timely prevention.
- **Adaptiveness:** The states and context are dynamic, and interventions must be adaptive to consider sudden changes.
- **Cost:** Is the intervention cheaper to accept for the user?
- **Long and Short-term Impact:** An intervention can have a long or short-term impact. Low physical activity and sedentary behaviour can lead to long-term consequences. Also, a high-intensity intervention needs a short-term effect, feedback can provide information about the repercussions.
- **Transparency:** An intervention can either be transparent or opaque, more information it carries about the impact, more transparent it will be.
- **Impact:** An impact of a prediction can be positive or negative. Therefore, an intervention must furnish details to the user for the impact; if the weather and user preference correlate, the activity will help to promote health.
- **Level of Personalization:** Personalization is dependent on the target and the parameters required. Physical activity requires more parameters (steps, preferences), in contrast, a threat in the surroundings requires only location.
- **Persuasive:** An intervention must be convincing so the user can accept it, for example, providing an activity with the calories target and the map or distance location if it is for skiing.
- **Alter Behaviour:** Most of the interventions alter behaviour positively. A key component for altering behaviour is motivation.
- **Augment Behaviour:** An intervention can augment behaviour, for instance, if the user is already physically active but can be nudged to do some extra steps for health promotion.

Table 7. Intensity w.r.t health promotion and risk prevention.

Table 8. Types of interventions with properties, goal, and parameters.

Type of decision-type	Properties									Goal	Parameters
	Intensity	adaptive	Impact	timeliness	cost	behavior	personalized	persuasive	Transparent		
Air-quality trigger- The air quality tomorrow is predicted to be lunhealthyl, user-profile = COPD, Decision = wear a mask when outside	high	✓	Short-term	✓	high	alter	✓	✓	✓	Risk prevention	API's metrological data or sensors, User-profile for identification, Mobile phone for location and intervention
Inactivity trigger- The user is lnot activel, from the step-count and profile, Decision: Based on the step data, you are sedentary, the weather is predicted to be nice in the next 2 h. A walk to the city center will be 5000 steps	low	✓	Long-term	✓	cheap	augment	✓	✓	✓	Health promotion	Wearables, Weather API, user-profile, and mobile

The Table 8 presents properties in comparison to the type of intervention. Parameters also differ based on a property, so the table also shows the required parameters for these properties e.g., a low level of personalization requires a few parameters. The Table 7 above draws a comparison between intensity and health promotion or risk prevention with a graph.

Moving forward the next segment corresponds to the principle of intervention. The principles of interventions are When, What, and Whom.

– When: When to intervene is one of the principles of intervention; in automated interventions. This is a trigger point of intervention.

- What: What information does an intervention possess? The intervention design must have useful (trustworthy) information for the user. This information must be motivating for the user.
- Whom: Whom is this information for? The target of an intervention is also the key to personalization.

These principles of the intervention are also challenging when it comes to the implementation of interventions.

To highlight the intervention mechanism and architecture, let's consider a scenario. The Fig. 6 presents an example of an intervention for a user who is allergic to pollen. The weather forecast is a prediction from the system that triggers an intervention by combining the user profile. The second part is a prevention mechanism that possesses information useful for the user. The user profile information provides personalized information for the user. The example also accentuates the principles of intervention.

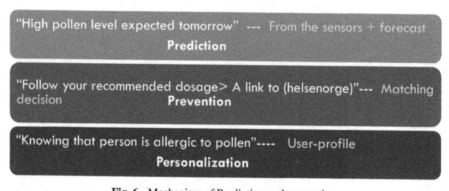

Fig. 6. Mechanism of Prediction and prevention.

The intervention must also be precise and consider the whole time of the intervention into account. The right time to intervene depends on different factors and must be within the frame of action, so the user has enough time to adapt to the prevention mechanism.

Another significant perspective is the states: The start state, goal state, current state, and future state.

- Start state: The position where the system starts collecting users' data, the baseline.
- Goal State: A state that the user intends to achieve: it is to be set by the user profile.
- Current state: State of the user in real-time, a position where the user is.
- Future state: Predicted from the system based on historical data.

Ultimately after principles, the components of intervention must be presented. These components are drawn from the architecture of JITAI [44].

- **Intervention Points:** An intervention point is when the system predicts a future state that needs to be changed by a possible action. to identify an intervention point the system must have a continuous assessment. the point is also when the user is most likely to accept the intervention.

- **Decision Options:** It is the choice architecture, that includes possible actions needed for prevention. An automated decision, that can prevent the future state. These are very prompt and require the attention of the user.
- **Decision Values (Variables):** These are the values that decide when an intervention is due e.g., the location of a threat or the pollen count. They are predicted from the system and are the first step in the mechanism of proactive mHealth.
- **Decision Rules:** It combines decision options with decision values to specify which decision to offer to the user. Decision rules are also modelled to work with the principles of intervention: when, what, and whom.

Apart from components of interventions, there are components of behavioural interventions. These components harmonise with motivation for the user. Components of behaviour change are impressionistic and can include: goal setting, the users' context and others.

5 Proof-of-Concept Implementation

Physical activity is defined as "any bodily movement produced by skeletal muscles that require energy expenditure" [54]. An activity is any movement of the user from one point to another e.g., transport, leisure, and daily work. Some examples of activities are walking, cycling, running, and sports. This definition accentuates that physical activity is the body movement that results in energy expenditure. The cited explanation is a more orthodox illustration of physical activity and does serve most of the use cases. Another definition by Piggins [55] provides a holistic view of physical activity: "People moving, acting and performing within specific spaces and context, influenced by interests, emotions, ideas, instructions, and relationships". The holistic approach verifies that physical activity is not a mere bodily movement, but can be influenced by several factors.

Statistics show that 80% or more of the world's population does not fulfil the physical activity recommendation [54]. Physical activity helps prevent noncommunicable diseases, for instance, stroke, dementia, high blood pressure, cancer, and diabetes [54]. The physical activity enables health benefits beyond disease management, allowing betters sleep, and improving cognitive abilities of thinking and learning [56]. It also contributes by reducing anxiety and depression [56]. So, physical activity improves overall well-being, but globally the proportion of people meeting the recommended physical activity standard is far lower.

CDC [57] recommends 150 min of moderate-intensity physical activity for adults. The recommendation is for healthy adults, WHO [54] provides detailed suggestions for different age groups, and people in certain groups. The guidance is to reduce the risks of diseases by enhancing physical activity. The intensity of physical activity is another factor that requires explanation: A standard unit MET (metabolic equivalent of task) [58] is a popular way of understanding intensity. MET is the ratio of energy expenditure per unit of time. The relative measurement is set at 1 MET, the energy exerted while resting. Thus, any activity that requires more energy will be more intense. The human body creates energy by using oxygen, an approximate 3.5 millilitres of oxygen consumption/kg of body weight in a minute.

This energy usage is also very impressionistic and depends on the user's health, age and fitness. Hence better fitness level one has, the more energy expenditure reduces. Likewise, the recommendation of 150 min of physical activity every week is equal to approximately 500 METs [58]. The Table 9 shows activity intensity with respect to METs.

Table 9. Intensity of activities with METs [58].

Intensity level	METs
Sedentary	< 1.5 METs
Light	1.6–2.9 METs
Moderate	3.0–5.9METs
Vigorous	> 6.0 METs

Another method of measurement is the daily step counts, it is easier to measure with the availability of wearables. Daily step count can contribute to reducing certain health conditions and the risk of diseases as advised. The number of daily steps can improve health and contribute to the requirement of physical activity (150 min).

Wearables can help measure step counts and activities continuously. A study [59] presented that healthy adults can take 4000 to 18000 steps/day, but depends on their goals and other circumstances. The users' step count can also be a vital factor in classifying activity, Table 10 shows the activity as very low (inactivity), low, moderate, and very active. Another study [60] uncovered that 8000 steps a day reduce the risk of dying by 51%. Recent research shows a mere two weeks of inactivity can cause a reduction in muscles and increase the risk of chronic diseases.

Table 10. Activity levels with daily step count [60].

Steps activity level	Steps per day
Inactive	< 1000
Low activity	1000–4000
Moderate activity (less then recommended)	4001–7000
Active zone	7000–10000
Very active	> 10000

The more steps taken by the user can positively impact promoting health. Doing some activity is better than no activity. The daily step goal is vital, and it depends on personalization, for instance, some people can take several steps during work or commuting. An average adult in America takes 3000–4000 steps a day [61]. The intensity of these steps may not be in line with the recommendation, but it does count towards health promotion. Additionally, walking can be another activity that can help increase step count.

It is essential to understand the user's current state to implement a system to increase step count. Besides, interventions must be adaptive: a user in an inactive zone (taking less than 1000 steps) cannot be nudged to complete 10000 steps/ day. A realistic goal must be established, which is adaptive and can enhance health promotion. The current step average of the user can be used as a baseline. Most wearables by default, are set to 10000 steps a day, the user profile can be an important factor to learn from. Daily patterns of the user can be taken as a baseline by a system.

The proof-of-concept (POC) implements a proactive mHealth system for health promotion by physical activity. The POC is based on the framework of AI-enabled proactive mHealth. POC implements a system to promote physical activity by behaviour change. The component of behaviour change for this POC is "motivation by context". The goal is to promote physical activity through health intervention; the system uses wearables and other resources for timely interventions. The design is based on the framework and principle of UCD. Physical activity alone as a vital sign is insufficient for prediction and prevention mechanisms. The system must account for the context and user profile as a parameter. The automated decision for the user must be based on their preferences. So, the system must consider multiple parameters.

1. Implementation Table:
The Table 11 shows the implementation of the POC based on the framework of AI-enabled proactive mHealth.

Table 11. POC implementation table based on the framework.

Framework modules	Proof-of-concept implementation
Module-1 ---- Rules Decision-making and context	User-level decision-making, Context = good or bad
Module-2 ---Tools Automated decision-making	AI-model----generic or personalized for predicting low activity and perfect match
Module-3 ---- Design P5 approach to mHealth	Predictive- low activity Preventive- with intervention Personalized- wearable step counts Participatory- user involvement at each step Psycho-cognitive - alter user behavior with motivation
Module-4 ---- Architecture JITAI	Following principle of JITAI of when, what, and whom Components of interventions: point, options, values, decision Adaptive and timely
Module-5 Implementation, sources, and resources	Fitbit charge-5 as wearable YR.no API for weather data mHealth application for notifications and collecting feedback

The table furnishes requirements for implementing POC based on the framework. In front of each module of the framework, a layer of implementation is drawn. The table also presents the parameters required for developing the POC.

2. Scenario Formation:

After the implementation table, the next step is to form scenarios. These scenarios accentuate the prediction and prevention mechanism. In addition, it presents the capability of the system and requirements for input/output mapping.

- Scenario-1: "low physical activity"

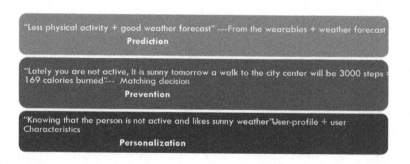

- Scenario-2: "perfect match"

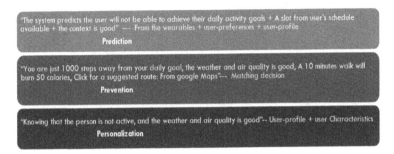

Both scenarios are for health promotion by physical activity, the first step from the system is to trigger a need for intervention: for instance, "low physical activity", combine it with the context information, and ultimately by finding user preference.

The second scenario alters user behaviour by context. The system identifies good context and matches it with the user profile. The scenarios also show that the prediction and prevention mechanism needs personalization of the user.

3. Categorization of the POC:
This section categorizes the POC by specifying the type and properties of the intervention. The intervention type is classified as a "nudge", the properties of the intervention are adaptive, personalized, timely, alter and augment behaviour, low intensity, persuasive, have a long-term impact, and cheaper to accept. The component of behaviour change used for the POC is the **"goal setting"** and **"context"**.

4. Input/Output Mapping:

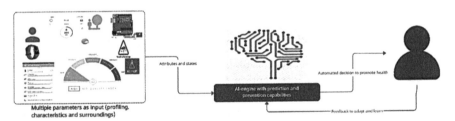

Fig. 7. Input/output mapping of the POC.

The Fig. 7 explains input/output mapping for the POC, for input sensors that include wearable data, user-profile information, states, and the context. The POC also learns from user preference for providing interventions. The centre of the whole architecture is the mHealth application that triggers timely intervention with useful information. The mHealth application is also meant to collect feedback from the user.

5. Implementation Logic:
The implementation is based on an iterative approach, starting with some parameters and then adding more parameters. In this first iteration, POC uses the context information

of the user, based on the scenario, for now, it is the weather forecast. User preference in terms of schedule availability is taken into consideration, and the health information that classifies low activity.

The pseudo-code explains the components of the intervention that forms the decision.

```
If current accumulated step count <P AND Context == Good
AND User preferences == green
  [Recommend activity]
  [Collect Feedback]
[Run in background]

If low activity == triggered AND Context == Good AND User
preferences == green
  [Recommend activity]
  [Collect Feedback]
  [Run in background]

If low activity == triggered AND Context == Bad AND User
preferences == green
  [No intervention]
  [Run in background]

If low activity == triggered AND Context == Good AND User
preferences == red
  [No intervention]
  [Run in background]

If activity == on-track AND Context == Ideal AND User
preferences == green
  [Recommend a small activity for perfect match]
  [Collect Feedback]
  [Run in background]
```

6. Components of Intervention for our Use Case from the Pseudo-code:

In the above scenarios, the components of the interventions are considered from Sect. 4. The recommendation is **an intervention point** that combines all the requirements. **Intervention options** are the activity information.
Intervention values are the conditions that are predicted or forecasted by the system. Finally, **the decision rule** combines intervention options and values.

7. Implementation Tools:

- For the implementation of the POC, each parameter is explained in detail.
- Fitbit charge-5: Used as a wearable for the POC, it provides health information in real-time: step counts, heart rate, location, distance, active minutes, and calories burned.
- Fitbit API allows usability and can be integrated to collect health information and store it for processing. An example of a Fitbit dataset is provided that shows most of the parameters over a set period.

A	B	C	D	E	F	G	H	I	J	K	L	M	N	O
Id	ActivityDa	TotalSteps	TotalDista	TrackerDis	LoggedAct	VeryActive	Moderate	LightActiv	Sedentary	VeryActive	FairlyActiv	LightlyActi	Sedentary	Calories
1.5E+09	########	11004	7.11	7.11	0	2.57	0.46	4.07	0	33	12	205	804	1819
1.5E+09	########	17609	11.55	11.55	0	6.92	0.73	3.91	0	89	17	274	588	2154
1.5E+09	########	12736	8.53	8.53	0	4.66	0.16	3.71	0	56	5	268	605	1944
1.5E+09	########	13231	8.93	8.93	0	3.19	0.79	4.95	0	39	20	224	1080	1932
1.5E+09	########	12041	7.85	7.85	0	2.16	1.09	4.61	0	28	28	243	763	1886
1.5E+09	########	10970	7.16	7.16	0	2.36	0.51	4.29	0	30	13	223	1174	1820

Fig. 8. Fitbit dataset.

The context in the POC is the weather API from YR.no that is classified as good or bad. The context information is collected for the whole period of activity and provided to the user. Classifying good or bad weather is very personalized: some people like walking in rain and some only like sunny weather. The right approach would be to have an ideal tab matching the user-profile setting for weather and making good or bad weather based on the risk or warnings.

The next element is the user-profiling, Fitbit provides a user-profile setting. The POC requires a user profile for step goal-setting. User-profile is vital for personalization. Any data related to the user is stored in the profile, for instance, if the user is allergic to pollen.

User preferences for the POC are limited to time alternatives: green or red. This feature allows the user to set the time of the day to accept an intervention. This must be adaptive but for now, it's manually set by the user.

The POC must run in the background to collect sudden changes and states. This allows the continuous measurement and enhances personalization.

8. AI-Engine for Modelling:

The AI engine is the core part of the POC, it provides the prediction and prevention mechanism. It also established adaptiveness and timeliness through automated decision-making. AI engine is powered by machine-learning algorithms, to predict from the user's data. The prediction of intervention values, for example, is based on the user's previous week's step data, and if the user will be able to complete the goal. The user-current state is considered the baseline. The model classifies, low activity triggers as a prediction from the system. This establishes that based on historical data, the user will not be able to complete the step goal.

The model also predicts, when the user is most likely to accept an intervention. The user preference is combined with the context to provide a perfect-match prediction from the system. Ultimately, the model must also learn from the feedback of the user to adapt.

- **Challenges:** The health information is very personalized, for instance, some users take steps during the night. Also, activities and the state of the user are other aspects that enhance the personalization. To model the AI engine, it is crucial to consider the uniqueness of the user. This is a challenge when it comes to prediction mechanisms. It requires further experimentation and a comparison between a generic model versus a personalized model.
- **Generic:** Adding another attribute (one-hot vector) for personalization--Cluster the user into a few clusters, then build a classifier to predict which cluster each user is in...one model per cluster.

- **If Using a Personalized Model:** Requires more data, features must be known that provide supplemental information useful for the predictive model. it is vital to distinguish between a variable and a feature, for instance, c is a variable that denotes the context of the user. C = good and C = bad, both are distinct features, at a certain time there must be only one feature for variable c. a personalized model is specialized to the features of a user to make precise predictions and ensure adaptiveness.

For modelling another challenge is the change in data due to circumstances, a user completing 8000 steps/day is sick, and the step count shows 1000 steps. It can be treated as missing data. Another change can be a certain peak, for instance, a user takes 6000 steps a day but while travelling at the airport the step count is at 16000. The type of peak identifies as the outlier.

9. mHealth Application:

The mHealth application is the tool for providing interventions to the user and collecting feedback. The mHealth application maintains a user profile and integrates with the Fitbit API. The intervention is presented as a push notification to the user with information about the nudge along with the context.

The mHealth application also maintains a history of interventions. Some screens of the mHealth application are presented with explanations. The mHealth application runs as a background process for collecting feedback. The feedback loop of the mHealth application provides feedback in both implicit and explicit forms.

Screen-1:The login screen connects to the Fitbit profile.
Screen-2:The user-profile setting shows the functionality: goal setting, preference, snooze period, and location update.
Screen-3:Provides an intervention as a push notification to the user.

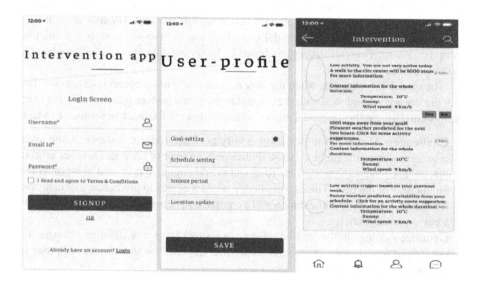

10. POC Architecture of the System:

The Fig. 9 shows the POC architecture of the system, with the input and output mapping. The architecture shows Fitbit API, YR API, and the user profile as input. The mHealth application uses Rest API to connect to the backend server for sending requests and getting a response. The application runs in the background and provides push notifications to the user. The feedback loop provides information when the user accepts the intervention.

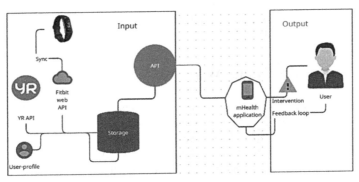

Fig. 9. POC architecture diagram.

6 Discussion

The POC provides extensive information on implementing systems based on the framework of AI-enabled proactive mHealth. The categorization of interventions complements proactive mHealth with the prediction and prevention mechanism. The inclusion of more parameters as input will increase proactiveness. The POC implements the principles of intervention for health promotion but the question is if an adaptive system must also prevent risks for the user while health promotion.

This demonstrates that health promotion and risk prevention work together for well-being. The difference is with the intensity of interventions. The more intense the intervention is, it will be more risk prevention.

Let us consider a user, who is nudged for a walk to a certain place, and the system did not consider the storm warning in that area or a fire warning. Although the goal of the intervention was to promote health it ended up more catastrophic for the user. So, a proactive mHealth system must be aware of all the aspects related to the user when providing interventions. It also manifests that for proactive health systems, both health promotion and risk preventions are essential.

A system can allow the user to ask about the context, at any time by collecting information around the user, for example, is it safe to go outside? or is it safe to run from point A to point B?

Another challenge is the explainability of the decisions provided to the user. The intervention must be more explainable, to increase transparency, so the user is most likely to accept it. Explainable AI (XAI) can be significant to enhance transparency and accuracy [62].

The framework provides abstraction and a guide to developing systems. It is essential to categorize interventions before implementing a system.

7 Limitation

POC implementation only uses some parameters, the goal and user preferences are set manually by the user and are not adaptive. The intervention values are also taken manually. Ultimately, the system is not adaptive to the full extent and in its current form does not take implicit feedback.

8 Conclusions and Future Work

The paper implements a proof-of-concept on the framework of AI-enabled proactive mHealth. It correspondingly categorizes interventions with respect to properties and types. The primary contribution is to present a proactive mHealth system based on the framework. The POC is physical activity intervention with the behavioural change component of "goal-setting" and "context". The context together with preference and profiling forms the parameters for proactiveness. Wearables are a prime source for continuous measurement of health information and the state of the user.

The paper also provides intervention components: intervention point, values, options and the decision in line with the framework implementation for building interventions. Intervention values are predicted by the AI engine combined with other inputs to trigger an automated decision. It concludes that the inclusion of more parameters is required for enhancing proactiveness. Additionally, the adaptiveness and prediction capabilities depend on the AI model. The POC also provides implementation details by mapping input/output and differentiating between generic and personalized models. The mHealth application emphasizes the need for the user profile and real-time data from wearables. The paper contributes to the development of AI-enabled proactive mHealth.

In future, the system must include more parameters e.g., health information (heart rate, body temperature), contextual data like warnings and pollution from sensors and APIs, and user profiling. The system will be more adaptive by the AI model to predict low activity; from the user's personalized data of the previous week, along with user preference.

The system will also provide a mechanism to include active minutes, to establish the intensity of an activity. Fitbit active minutes can be a substantial source to combine step counts with the heart rate of the user.

References

1. Smart cities, smarter public health. https://www2.deloitte.com/us/en/insights/focus/smart-city/building-a-smart-city-with-smart-digital-health.html
2. Global Observatory for eHealth. https://www.who.int/observatories/global-observatory-for-ehealth

3. Winslow, C.: https://www.cdc.gov/training/publichealth101/public-health.html
4. Health Promotion. https://www.who.int/westernpacific/about/how-we-work/programmes/health-promotion
5. Global Health Estimates: Life expectancy. https://www.who.int/data/gho/data/themes/mortality-and-global-health-estimates
6. Dementia in Norway. https://www.fhi.no/en/op/hin/health-disease/dementia-in-norway/
7. Hacker, K., Briss, P., Richardson, L., Wright, J., Petersen, R.: COVID-19 and Chronic Disease: The Impact Now and in the Future
8. Koronavirus. https://www.fhi.no/sv/smittsomme-sykdommer/corona/
9. Digital Health Transformation. https://www.himss.org/what-we-do-solutions/digital-health-transformation
10. Edirippulige, S., Senanayake, B.: Professional practices for digital healthcare. Opportunities and Challenges in Digital Healthcare Innovation, pp. 97–112 (2020)
11. GrandView. https://www.grandviewresearch.com/press-release/
12. Amir, M.: https://blackcreek.io/insights/the-shift-from-reactive-to-proactive-healthcare
13. Waldman, S., Terzic, A.: Health care evolves from reactive to proactive. Clin. Pharmacol. Ther. 105, 10–13 (2018)
14. Sulaiman, M., Håkansson, A., Karlsen, R.: AI-Enabled proactive mhealth: a review, pp. 94–108. ICT for Health, Accessibility and Wellbeing (2021)
15. CDC. https://www.cdc.gov/nceh/tracking/tracking-intro.html
16. Merriam-Webster. https://www.merriam-webster.com/dictionary/context
17. Berman, S.: Clinical decision making. Berman's Pediatric Decision Making, pp. 1–6 (2011)
18. Education, I.: What is Artificial Intelligence (AI)? https://www.ibm.com/cloud/learn/what-is-artificial-intelligence
19. Sulaiman, M., Håkansson, A., Karlsen, R.: A framework for AI-enabled proactive mHealth with automated decision-making for a user's context. In: Proceedings of the 15th International Joint Conference on Biomedical Engineering Systems and Technologies (2022)
20. Istepanian, R., Al-Anzi, T.: m-Health 2.0: New perspectives on mobile health, machine learning and big data analytics. Methods. 151, 34–40 (2018)
21. McConnell, M., Turakhia, M., Harrington, R., King, A., Ashley, E.: Mobile health advances in physical activity, fitness, and atrial fibrillation. J. Am. Coll. Cardiol. 71, 2691–2701 (2018)
22. Aguilera, A., Figueroa, C.: mHealth app using machine learning to increase physical activity in diabetes and depression: clinical trial protocol for the DIAMANTE Study. BMJ Open 10, e034723 (2020)
23. Baig, M.: Early detection and self-management of long-term conditions using wearable technologies (2022)
24. Nag, N., Pandey, V., Jain, R.: Health multimedia. In: Proceedings of the 2017 ACM on International Conference on Multimedia Retrieval (2017)
25. Shei, R., Holder, I., Oumsang, A., Paris, B.: Wearable trackers–advanced technology or advanced marketing? Eur. J. Appl. Physiol. 122, 1975–1990 (2022)
26. Correction to Lancet Respir Med 2021; published online April 9. The Lancet Respiratory Medicine, vol. 9, p. e55 (2021). https://doi.org/10.1016/S2213-2600(21)00171-5.
27. Menictas, M., Rabbi, M., Klasnja, P., Murphy, S.: Artificial intelligence decision-making in mobile health. Biochemist 41, 20–24 (2019)
28. U.S. Smartphone Use in 2015. https://www.pewresearch.org/internet
29. How Digital Health Apps are Empowering Patients. https://www2.deloitte.com/us/en/blog/health-care-blog/2021
30. Simon, H.: The New Science of Management Decision. University of Michigan (2008)
31. Decision-making process. https://www.umassd.edu/fycm/decision-making
32. Heathfield, S.M.: Evidence-based decision making (EBDM). https://www.thebalancemoney.com/evidence-based-decision-making-4799980

33. Evidence-based decision-making (EBDM). National Institute of Corrections (2017)
34. Abbasgholizadeh Rahimi, S., Menear, M., Robitaille, H., Légaré, F.: Are mobile health applications useful for supporting shared decision making in diagnostic and treatment decisions? Glob. Health Action **10**, 1332259 (2017)
35. Wang, Y., Ruhe, G.: The cognitive process of decision making. Int. J. Cogn. Inf. Nat. Intell. **1**, 73–85 (2007)
36. Guidelines on Automated individual decision-making and Profiling for the purposes of Regulation 2016/679 (wp251rev.01). https://ec.europa.eu/newsroom/article29/items/612053
37. Sachan, S., Yang, J.: An explainable AI decision-support-system to automate loan underwriting. Expert Syst. Appl. **144**, 113100 (2020)
38. Kim, C., Choi, J., Jiao, Z.: An automated COVID-19 triage pipeline using artificial intelligence based on chest radiographs and clinical data. NPJ Digit. Med. **5** (2022)
39. Woo, W.: Future trends in I&M: Human-machine co-creation in the rise of AI. IEEE Instrum. Meas. Mag. **23**, 71–73 (2020)
40. Triberti, S., Brivio, E.: User-centered design approaches and methods for P5 eHealth. P5 eHealth: An Agenda for the Health Technologies of the Future, pp. 155–171 (2019)
41. Sagner, M., McNeil, A.: The P4 Health spectrum – a predictive, preventive, personalized and participatory continuum for promoting healthspan. Prog. Cardiovasc. Dis. **59**, 506–521 (2017)
42. Gorini, A., Mazzocco, K.: A P5 approach to m-Health: Design suggestions for advanced mobile health technology. Front. Psychol. **9** (2018)
43. International Classification of Functioning, and Health (ICF). https://www.who.int/standards/classifications/international-classification-of-health-interventions
44. Nahum-Shani, I., et al.: Just-in-time adaptive interventions (JITAIs) in mobile health: key components and design principles for ongoing health behavior support. Annals Behav. Med. **52**(6), 446–462 (2017). https://doi.org/10.1007/s12160-016-9830-8
45. Wu, M.: Wearable technology applications in healthcare: A literature review. Online J. Nurs. Inform. Contributors (2022)
46. Loucks, J., Stewart, D.: Wearable technology in health care: Getting better all the time. https://www2.deloitte.com/xe/en/insights/industry/technology/technology-media-and-telecom-predictions/2022/wearable-technology-healthcare.html
47. Smart Weather Station Indoor Outdoor | Netatmo. https://www.netatmo.com/en-gb/weather/weatherstation
48. Araújo-Soares, V., Hankonen, N.: Developing behavior change interventions for self-management in chronic illness. Eur. Psychol. **24**, 7–25 (2019)
49. Cutler, D.: 17, Behavioral Health Interventions: What Works and Why?. Critical Perspectives on Racial and Ethnic Differences in Health in Late Life (2022)
50. Roekel, H.: https://behavioralscientist.org/building-the-behavior-change-toolkit-designing-and-testing-a-nudge-and-a-boost/
51. Hertwig, R., Ryall, M.: Nudge versus boost: Agency dynamics under libertarian paternalism. Econ. J. **130**, 1384–1415 (2019)
52. Siemer, R.: An Overview of the Various Types of Nudges — Museum Membership Innovation. https://www.membershipinnovation.com/insights-and-ideas
53. Karlsen, R., Andersen, A.: Recommendations with a Nudge. . Technologies. **7**, 45 (2019)
54. Physical activity. https://www.who.int/news-room/fact-sheets/detail/physical-activity
55. Piggin, J.: What is physical activity? A holistic definition for teachers, researchers and policy makers. Front. Sports Active Living **2**, 72 (2020)
56. American Heart Association Recommendations for Physical Activity in Adults and Kids. https://www.heart.org/en/healthy-living/fitness/fitness-basics
57. CDC. https://www.cdc.gov/physicalactivity/basics/adults/index.htm

58. Roland, J.: What Are METs, and How Are They Calculated? https://www.healthline.com/health/what-are-mets
59. Tudor-Locke, C., Craig, C.: How many steps/day are enough? for adults. Int. J. Behav. Nutr. Phys. Act. **8**, 79 (2011)
60. CDC. https://www.cdc.gov/media/releases/2020/p0324-daily-step-count.html
61. Rieck, T.: https://www.mayoclinic.org/healthy-lifestyle/fitness/in-depth
62. Explainable AI. https://www.ibm.com/watson/explainable-ai

Improved Blood Vessels Segmentation of Infant Retinal Image

Vijay Kumar[1]([✉]), Het Patel[2], Shorya Azad[3], and Kolin Paul[1,2]

[1] Khosla School of Information Technology, Indian Institute of Technology Delhi, Delhi, India
vijay.kumar@sit.iitd.ac.in
[2] Department of Computer Science and Engineering, Indian Institute of Technology Delhi, Delhi, India
[3] Dr. Rajendra Prasad Centre for Ophthalmic Sciences, All India Institute of Medical Sciences Delhi, Delhi, India

Abstract. Retinopathy of prematurity (ROP), is the most common cause of blindness in premature infants. ROP is measured by looking at the width, curvature, and length of the blood vessels map on a retina. So, the quality of the segmented blood vessel map affects how well the quantitative method works. Current vessel segmentation algorithms work well on images of the retina of adults, but they cannot tell the difference between structures of vessels that have not yet grown in images of the fundus of infant. Also, the lack of a dataset of infant fundus images has made it harder to develop data-driven techniques for separating blood vessels. This study shows how to use a Deep Convolutional Neural Network (DCNN)-based vessel segmentation system to determine if a infant has ROP. The proposed method uses a DCNN, Generative Adversarial Network (GAN) Pix2Pix, or U-Net to segment vessels. We trained the proposed system with datasets of fundus images that were available to the public, and we tested it with images of premature infants' eyes from a nearby hospital. Experimental results show that the proposed method is more robust to noise and inter-class variation. It has a dice coefficient between 0.60 and 0.64 and an average accuracy of 96.69% for vessel segmentation. We have also examined its potential use in the treatment of ROP and Plus disease.

Keywords: Fundus image · Retinopathy of prematurity (ROP) · Plus disease · Computer aided diagnosis (CAD) · Generative adversarial network (GAN) · U-Net · Blood vessels segmentation · Deep convolutional neural network (DCNN)

1 Introduction

Retinopathy of prematurity (ROP) is the leading cause of blindness in premature babies worldwide [36]. ROP is caused by the abnormal growth of blood vessels in the retina of a preterm, low-weight infant [9]. The International Classification

A. C. A. Roque et al. (Eds.): BIOSTEC 2022, CCIS 1814, pp. 288–314, 2023.
https://doi.org/10.1007/978-3-031-38854-5_15

of ROP (ICROP) classifies the severity of ROP disease based on vascular structure, anatomical variation, and extent [27]. One such vascular activity is known as Plus disease, which is characterised by alterations in the structural characteristics of blood vessels, including vessel dilatation and tortuosity [36]. Therefore, examination of retinal vessels has significant potential to contribute to the early detection and treatment of disorders associated with ROP and Plus. It is also beneficial to monitor disease improvement and severity [9]. So, by analysing the networks of vessels in the retina, one can get accurate information about the ROP disease conditions. During the treatment of ROP, it is crucial for the ophthalmologist to evaluate the width and tortuosity of the retinal vessels using computer-assisted diagnosis (CAD) software so that he or she can effectively comprehend and choose the treatment course [7,9].

Therefore, it is necessary to develop an automated method for classifying and segmenting vessels in fundus pictures. However, the shape and color of vessels are very dynamic, dependent on variables such as the retinal imaging technique, the subject's surroundings, and the subject's ocular health. Thus, it has proven difficult for the image processing and computer vision groups to establish a precise and practical approach for segmenting blood vessels. The fundus images utilised for infant eye examination are affected by artifacts and noise due to patient movements, uneven lighting (underexposure), poor contrast, ocular media opacities, iris refraction and reflection, and device misalignment [7]. Image processing, computer vision, and machine learning (ML)-based blood vessel segmentation techniques have shown promising results on retinal scans of adults. In recent years, computer vision tasks, including object identification, classification, segmentation, and tracking, have been greatly improved by data-driven Deep Convolutional Neural Networks (DCNN) to the point that they now beat human experts in several datasets [9]. DCNN models, including Generative Adversarial Networks (GAN), U-Net, and its variations, show considerably high performance on publicly accessible datasets of young adults for vascular segmentation tasks [13,47].

However, these DCNN models are unable to distinguish and identify the small, weak, and dilated blood vessel branches. In premature infants, the retina includes small, thinner, dilated blood vessels that are not fully developed. Therefore, existing technologies cannot effectively detect and segment the blood vessels in an infant's retina. Like other data-driven technologies, DCNN or deep learning (DL) models also require a large quantity of data for training, testing, and validation. However, there are no publicly available retinal imaging datasets of an appropriate size for premature infants.

In our earlier work [28], we presented a DL-based approach for segmenting retinal vessels during ROP examination utilising the current DCNN, GAN, and U-Net models. These models are trained and optimised using publically available image datasets of patients with diabetic retinopathy (DR), glaucoma, and age-related macular degeneration (AMD). The trained model is evaluated on manually annotated infant retinal images collected from a local hospital. Furthermore, our DL-based segmentation approach for ROP screening can be used in works like [27] for vascular segmentation to improve diagnosis accuracy.

This is an extended version of the conference paper [28], titled "Improved Blood Vessel Segmentation of Retinal Image of Infants", which was presented at the 15th International Joint Conference on Biomedical Engineering Systems and Technologies - HEALTHINF. This edition has more up-to-date information on the related works in Sect. 2 and a complete look at the models used for collecting retinal data, processing it, and separating the blood vessels in Sect. 3. The effectiveness of preprocessing was not evaluated in our previous study. Instead, we based our estimations of its quality only on subjective evaluations. However, in this edition, we have objectively and statistically evaluated their performance. Additionally, ROP zoning and Plus disease screening are included as additional applications of blood vessel segmentation in this work. Moreover, we examined the effect of the preprocessing phase on the image quality of the infant's fundus during the preprocessing phase to improve image quality.

To summarise, the contribution of this work is as follows:

- Using images captured by the infant fundus camera RetCam, a test dataset and ground truth were generated to verify the proposed segmentation method and show its relevance.
- We have proposed a novel DL-based segmentation approach for the separation of blood vessels required for diagnosing and monitoring ROP and PLUS disease, which can be trained and validated on a minimal number of ROP images.
- Due to the restricted availability of infant ROP fundus images, the proposed approach trains the DL-model using a publically accessible young individual fundus dataset, while the created model is compared, evaluated, and validated using the ROP image dataset.

The remainder of the paper is structured as follows: Recent work on segmenting blood vessels is presented in Sect. 2. Section 3 provides design specifications for the proposed DL-based vessel segmentation approach. Section 4 presents findings from different stages of the proposed technique's pipeline. Section 5 outlines the technique's shortcomings and needed research.

2   Related Work

Over the past several years, ophthalmologists have used retinal vessels to examine and classify retinal diseases. In this case, the ophthalmologist looks at the disease's symptoms to make a picture of the retinal blood vessels. There are two types of methods used to look into it. One is manual screening. This procedure is very biased and stressful.

Table 1. Works related to blood vessel segmentation of retinal images using DNN.

Method	Dataset (Accuracy)	Work
RV-GAN	DRIVE (0.9790), CHASE_DB1 (0.9914), STARE (0.9887)	[22]
U-Net	DRIVE (0.9712)	[43]
SA-UNet	DRIVE (0.9698), CHASE_DB1 (0.9905)	[12]
EAR-NET	DRIVE (0.9633), STARE (0.9690)	[45]
Model-Specific Alignment Networks (MSAN)	CHASEDE1 (0.9728), STARE (0.9612), DRIVE (0.9582)	[39]
Pixel-wise adaptive filters	DRIVE (0.9843), CHASE_DB1 (0.9835), STARE (0.9843)	[31]
Mobile-RetinaNet	DRIVE (0.968) and CHASE (0.985)	[24]
DR-VNet	DRIVE (0.9682), CHASE DB (0.9694), STARE (0.9744)	[23]
MTPA_Unet	DRIVE (0.9718), CHASE DB1 (0.9762), STARE (0.9773)	[20]
AADG framework	STARE (0.9475), HRF (0.9049), DRIVE (0.9241), CHASE_DB1 (0.9384)	[33]
Modified U-Net (U-Net, AG U-Net, SE-U-Net)	HVDROPDB-BV (dice score 0.686, 0.667 and 0.674 for U-Net, AG U-Net and SE U-Net)	[1]
Improved U-Net (NoL-UNet)	DRIVE (0.9697), CHASE_DB1 (0.9826) and HRF (0.9732)	[15]
MCPANet	DRIVE (0.9705) , CHASE (0.9758), STARE (0.9768)	[21]
IterNet	DRIVE (0.9816), CHASE_DB1 (0.9851)	[30]
IterMiUnet	DRIVE (0.9568), STARE (0.9649), CHASE DB1 (0.9591)	[26]

In order to overcome these constraints, ophthalmologists and researchers have adopted CAD approaches for medical diagnostic applications that identify and monitor the structure of retinal blood vessels. CAD-based approaches use image processing, computer vision, and machine learning-based algorithms to study retinal blood vessels and detect eye disorders. The CAD-based techniques are categorised into two subgroups: the rule-based CAD system and the data-driven CAD system. Rule-based systems applications have been built for the standard protocols and procedures formulated by specialists, focusing mostly on vessel enhancement and segmentation. As mentioned in [27,34], typical rule-based approaches are model-based adaptive thresholding, vessel tracking, matched filter responses, morphological operation, entropy filtering, Gabor wavelet

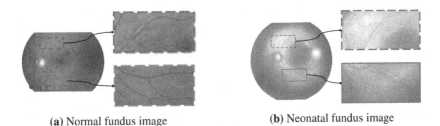

(a) Normal fundus image   (b) Neonatal fundus image

Fig. 1. Analysis of retinal vessels segmentation problem [28]. (a) Retinal images of elderly person and the enlarge patches. (b) Neonatal fundus image and the enlarge patches.

transform, etc. On the other hand, rule-based screening methods need a manual and labor-intensive system-wide update if there is even a minor change or update to the CAD system.

In the past few years, many data-driven techniques for medical applications have been developed, especially for identifying, segmenting, and monitoring retinal blood vessels. In many medical applications, machine learning (ML) and deep learning (DL) are data-driven algorithms that work well at image segmentation, object detection, and object tracking. DL-based systems perform better than conventional CAD applications [5,14,42,49]. The DL-based screening method provides the flexibility and adaptability the rule-based system lacks. Researchers have recently developed many vessel segmentation techniques based on DCNN, which are listed in Table 1. Retinal vessel segmentation has been done successfully using DL approaches for Diabetic Retinopathy (DR) on public datasets using machine learning and other methods such as mathematical morphology, multi-scale approaches, vessel tracking, model-based approaches, and matched filtering. However, the ROP dataset has not yet been released and is not accessible for testing by a large audience. These vessel-segmentation methods work well on publicly available datasets of scans of young people's retinas but not on images of an infant's retina. As illustrated in Fig. 1, the structure of the retinal blood vessels does not develop appropriately in the fundus picture of a premature infant. Because of this, the blood vessels in the preterm neonatal retina are blurry, and traditional vessel segmentation methods that work well with publicly available retinal image datasets do not work with the images of the infant's retina.

The authors of [10] compared three state-of-the-art DR CNNs using a set of 9 ROP pictures. They concluded that the performance of these networks suffered a considerable setback when applied to ROP images due to the presence of non-uniform illumination and thin and choroidal blood vessels inside the images. They also noted the need for comprehensive datasets and efficient CNNs for vessel segmentation in ROP images. Recently, [32,48] developed a DCNN-based technique for vessel segmentation that accurately separates the retinal vessel map of a preterm infant. In this study, the authors segmented the vessels using the DCNN model U-Net [40], which resulted in the precise vessel map being segmented from the image of the retina of the preterm infants. Additionally, the authors of [1] used three U-Net-based architectures, U-Net, AG-UNet, and SE-UNet, on a large collection of manually labelled retinal images from ROP patients. It employs large-scale ROP picture datasets, for which ophthalmologist professionals manually create retinal vascular maps for use in training, testing, and validation. Recent DL-based retinal vascular segmentation models are summarised in Table 1. The authors used many variants of the U-Net and GAN architectures for vessel segmentation. However, only [1] employed it to segment the retinal vessels in infants. The system's effectiveness is affected by the quality of the dataset used to train the DL model. As a result, the architecture of DL makes use of training datasets that take into consideration demographic characteristics such as those related to race, age, and gender.

To address the issues mentioned earlier, we have proposed a DL-based vessel extraction system capable of operating in an environment where large-scale historical datasets are unavailable and where the accuracy of the results is of the utmost importance. Figure 2 illustrates the proposed system design. It is divided into three sections: image preprocessing, DCNN model training, and testing.

3   Method and System Design

Figure 2 illustrates the proposed system's architecture in detail. It comprises four functional units:

- Fundus imaging (or retinal scanning) unit.
- Image pre-processing.
- Blood vessels segmentation.
- Post-processing.

The Fundus Imaging Unit is responsible for acquiring and maintaining retinal scan images and videos necessary for diagnosing and monitoring retinal disorders. An ophthalmologist uses a fundus camera to see the retina of an infant or young adult. For ROP detection, doctors employ the wide-field imaging fundus camera RitCam-3 shutters (Clarity MSI, Pleasanton, CA, United States). A fundus image is a colour photograph of the retinal membrane of the eye captured by a fundus camera. Ophthalmologists use fundus images in diagnostic and screening processes for various eye disorders. Due to uneven illumination, motion blur, and sudden and rapid changes in the signal, scanned photographs and video data are noisy and prone to several defects. Therefore, it is necessary to improve the quality of these images. The second functional unit, the preprocessing unit, uses image reconstruction and enhancement methods to reduce noise and improve picture quality.

The third functional unit processes the preprocessed image using a DL-based model to segment the vessel's map from the fundus image. In this study, we considered two state-of-the-art pre-trained DL models for the segmentation task: U-NET and GAN. U-Net is widely used for image segmentation applications in the medical field. GAN is a machine learning framework inspired by game theory in which two models, a generator and a discriminator, compete simultaneously, making each other more effective. The DL model is trained with a publicly available fundus image dataset listed in Table 2 and then used for blood vessel segmentation of neonatal fundus images.

The fourth functional unit is the post-processing stage, which utilises image processing and computer vision-based algorithms to extract disease-related characteristics of the retina, such as vascular width, tourist, extent, etc., from the segmented vessel map. The results demonstrating the applicability of the proposed method for Zone-1 ROP and Plus disease screening are illustrated in Sect. 4.6.

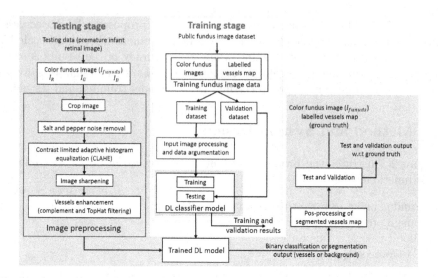

Fig. 2. System flow diagram of Deep Learning based improved vessels segmentation [28].

3.1   Datasets and Material

In this work, we trained and tested both DL models (i.e., GAN and U-net) using a publicly available dataset, including a labelled blood vessel map. The local ROP dataset of infant retinal images was used in the validation phase [27]. The ROP data collection and labelling procedure used in this study is shown in Fig. 3. We gathered 400 posterior and temporal images of ROP patients from the Dr. RP Centre of Ophthalmic Science at AIIMS Delhi, India. During daily screenings, these images are acquired by the RetCam imaging system. RetCam captured images at a resolution of 640 × 480 pixels. The images were taken of infants with gestational ages of between 26 and 30 weeks and birth weights of about 1,250 g. A panel of ROP professionals with training and expertise selected and annotate these images to ROP Zones and Plus disease stage. The acquired images are unprocessed and noisy, and their pre-labelled vessel masks are unavailable. However, a ground truth or gold standard is required for performance verification of blood vessels segmentation approach. Therefore, we manually labelled the blood vessels in the preterm infant's retinal image to create the vessel mask. Therefore, the vascular mask was made by manually labelling the blood vessels in the retinal picture of the premature infant. The labelling procedure is time-consuming and complicated. We have thus just annotated the blood vessels in six photos. But, labelling the OD of these images is less complicated and time-consuming than labelling blood vessel maps. As shown in Fig. 3 of [27], OD is labelled with information on their bounding box's width (a), height (b), and center (C(xc, yc)).

Table 2. Dataset for vessel segmentation [28].

Dataset Name	Number of Images	Resolution (pixels)
ARIA [2]	143	768 × 576 pixels
DRHAGIS [17]	40	4752 × 3168, 3456 × 2304, 3126 × 2136, 2896 × 1944 or 2816 × 1880 pixels
DRIVE [41]	20	584 × 565 pixels
HRF [4]	45	3504 × 2336 pixels
STARE [18]	20	700 × 605 pixels

An output label, i.e., vessel map, is required for the vessel extraction module, but generating these labels manually for the local dataset is impractical. Therefore, a publicly available dataset containing vessel maps was collected for this task, and a DL-based model was trained to generalise the images from the local dataset. Table 2 provides details about the gathered datasets.

Preprocessing and Noise Modeling. The Table 2 dataset is now used to train DL-based vessels segmentation models, such as GAN and U-Net. The collected images for training are from publicly available datasets, which include images with very high contrast for the vessels, making it extremely difficult to generalise the results to the test dataset (ROP image). As shown in Fig. 1, the images' quality and the vessels' nature vary considerably between the two datasets. For these models to work with ROP images, they must be trained to generalise effectively to noisy and low-contrast images.

In order for this model to be functional, it is necessary to recreate the noise and artifacts present in the picture of the local training dataset in the standard training dataset. To make the training dataset (i.e., the compiled dataset) more similar to the test dataset (i.e., the local dataset), we propose a noise modelling

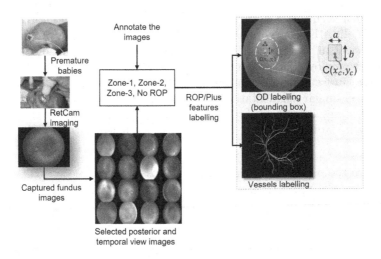

Fig. 3. System flow diagram for dataset preparation.

Table 3. Noise modeling functions [28].

Noise modeling	Description
crop	Image resize to 512 × 512
CLAHE or CLAHE(3.5, (5,5))	CLAHE operation with ClipLimit 3.5 and tileGridSize is (5,5).
medianBlur(3)	Median blur operation with Kernel size is 3
noise or GaussinaNoise((5,5),0)	Gaussian smoothing with Kernek size (5,5) and standard deviation is Zero

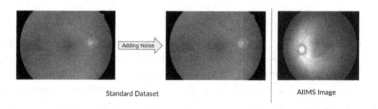

Standard Dataset   AIIMS Image

Fig. 4. Results of Noise modeling and comparison with local dataset [28].

strategy in which noise is added to the input picture and other preprocessing processes are conducted. Table 3 summarises the various noise modelling functions. To reproduce the noises in the training dataset photos, we used image cropping, medianBlur, and Gaussian noise with CLAHE. The results of this noise-modelling-based approach are shown in Fig. 4; the photos from the standard dataset are made to resemble the ROP images in that the blood vessels are blurred and dilated.

Data Augmentation. A further experiment was conducted to increase the size of the training dataset by generating a synthetic dataset using the existing 288 photos from the standard dataset. This experiment was conducted because the vascular segmentation job does not need that much global information, and even if it did, the conventional DCNN layers utilised by the proposed model are inefficient in conveying information over greater spatial distances. However, one might employ dilated convolution layers, requiring a much deeper network. Similarly to vascular segmentation, the model relies primarily on local information; hence, similar augmentation techniques may be used to extend our training sample size, resulting in a more generic model. The approach for the generation of synthetic datasets is shown in Fig. 5. In which it will carry out the following steps:

1. Reduce the resolution of the image (prepossessed and noisy) and the vessel mask to 1024 × 1024 pixels.
2. Create a pool of 18432 smaller partial images by subdividing each image into 128 × 128 grids.
3. After that, 64 random samples are used to make a mosaic picture of 1024 × 1024 pixels, and then 450 of these images are created to form a training dataset.

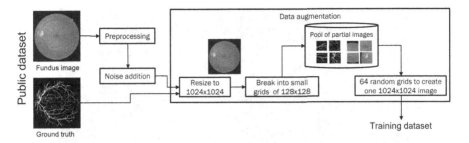

Fig. 5. System flow diagram of data augmentation and training dataset preparation.

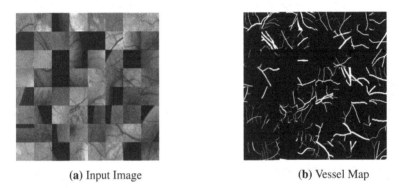

(a) Input Image   (b) Vessel Map

Fig. 6. Sample image from the augmented dataset [28].

Figure 6 shows a sample image and associated vessel map utilised for training purposes using the augmented dataset.

3.2 Image Pre-processing

During the examination of preterm infants' retinas, an ophthalmologist captures images of the retina in raw format. These images suffer from various abnormalities, including motion blur, uneven lighting, abrupt fluctuations in image signals, etc. Images altered by noise may decrease the accuracy of the proposed system's output. Therefore, the quality of the images has to be improved before they can be used for disease diagnosis. Thus, image preprocessing is carried out to enhance the picture quality and reduce the impact of artefacts and noise.

The preprocessing of a picture makes it possible for the retinal blood vessels to be seen more clearly, which is necessary for further segmentation. The preprocessing techniques used by the proposed system to improve the image quality are shown in Fig. 15. The coloured fundus image of a preterm infant is shown in Fig. 1t as a pale yellow colour with a map of blurred blood vessels, which is difficult to distinguish with the naked eye. A colour image frame has three colour channels: red (R), green (G), and blue (B). The R channel is overexposed, while the B channel is underexposed. Consequently, in the R and B channel images,

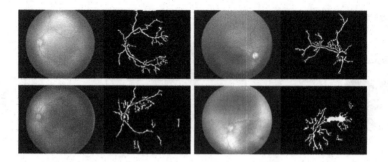

Fig. 7. Blood vessel extraction results.

there is no discernible difference between the brightness of blood vessels and the background. These features are easily distinguishable in the G-channel and are relevant for biological purposes. As a result, we favoured the G-channel (or grey image) and used it for further imaging studies. We also used a mean filter and CLAHE to improve colour image quality and reduce the effects of uneven illumination and motion blur.

3.3   Blood Vessels Segmentation

The third functional unit segmented the vessel's map from the fundus image. For vessel segmentation, first, we used a morphological transformation-based method described in [27]. However, it cannot segment thin and dilated blood vessels in an infant's fundus image as depicted in Fig. 7. Also, statistical evaluation parameters' average accuracy, RSME, PSNR, and SSIM scores are low compared to ground truth, as shown in Table 4. Therefore, we extended our work to include a DL-based technique for blood vessel segmentation and used two advanced pre-trained DL models: U-NET and GAN. U-Net is widely used in medical image segmentation applications. GAN is a machine learning framework inspired by game theory, where two models, a generator and a discriminator, compete simultaneously to improve their effectiveness. Using a publicly available dataset, the DL model segments blood vessels in neonatal fundus images (Table 2). The trained model is validated using the ROP dataset's retinal images from the local hospital.

3.4   Vessels Segmentation and DCNN Architecture

Deep learning (DL) is a method in which a DCNN is trained via historical pathology data relating to different conditions. In this section, we introduce two state-of-the-art DCNNs for vessel segmentation: U-Net and GAN (Pix2Pix), both of which have been included in the system that we have proposed.

U-Net. The architecture of the U-Net model is illustrated in Fig. 8. It consists of a contracting path (left side) to capture context and an expansive path

Table 4. Blood vessels segmentation quality assessment result with premature babies fundus images.

Metrics	Accuracy	RMSE	PSNR	SSIM
Average value	94%	0.23	14.9	0.82

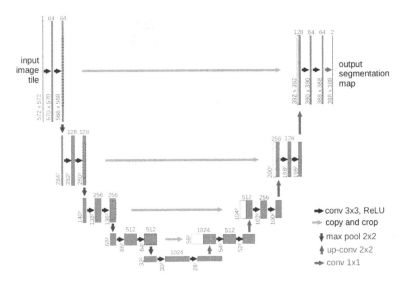

Fig. 8. Architecture of U-Net [40].

(right side) that enables precise localization, similar to an encoder-decoder network. This network performs well with biomedical segmentation because of the model's ability to provide high-quality segmentation results with less training data. Moreover, the network is fast. In total, the network has 23 convolutional layers. In [40], authors have accomplished this by proposing to replace pooling operators with up-sampling layers. As a consequence of this change, the model includes many feature channels, enabling the network to propagate context information to higher resolution layers. This model makes use of a simple pixel-wise soft-max loss, defined as $p_k(x) = exp(a_k(x))/(\Sigma_{k'=1}^{K} exp(a_{k'}(x)))$, in conjunction with cross-entropy loss E. For more detailed architecture, refer to the paper [40].

Pix2Pix GAN Model. The Generative Adversarial Network (GAN) is a machine learning model introduced in 2014 by Ian Goodfellow and colleagues [11]. The architecture of the GAN model is shown in Fig. 9, which comprises two fundamental networks: the generator and the discriminator. This approach has been used for image reconstruction, segmentation, detection, classification, cross-modality synthesis, and many more applications [47]. In recent years, many GAN models, such as deep convolutional GAN (DCGAN), conditional GAN (cGAN), CycleGAN, auxiliary classifier GAN (AC-GAN), Wasserstein-

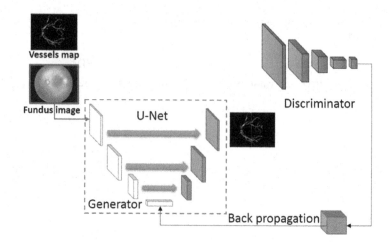

Fig. 9. Pix2Pix GAN architecture in training phase [28].

GAN (WGAN), and least squares GAN (LSGAN), have been created, and this has proved effective in numerous medical image analysis applications [25]. For blood vessel segmentation, we have thus used the cGAN-model Pix2Pix. Pix2Pix was developed in 2016 by [19], which used a U-Net-based model as the generator and another CNN model as the discriminator in the GAN training process (as shown in Fig. 9). These conditional GAN based models work in a way that discriminator D learns to classify between fake (synthesized by the generator) and real input_image, vessel_map tuples and Generator G learns to fool the discriminator. The Objective function to train the GAN is made up of two parts, Conditional GAN loss $\mathcal{L}_{CGAN}$ and traditional L1 loss $\mathcal{L}_{L_1}$ which are mentioned in the equation below.

$$\mathcal{L}_{CGAN}(G, D) = \mathbb{E}_{x,y}[logD(x,y)]+$$
$$\mathbb{E}_{x,z}[log(1 - D(x, D(x,z)))] \quad (1)$$
$$\mathcal{L}_{L_1}(G) = \mathbb{E}_{x,y,z}[\|y - G(x,z)\|_1] \quad (2)$$

And final objective function is combination of both of these.

$$G^* = arg \min_G \max_D \mathcal{L}_{CGAN}(G, D) + \lambda\mathcal{L}_{L_1}(G) \quad (3)$$

4   Experimental Results

The proposed system and its different modules are implemented and tested on a workstation with Intel(R) Xeon(R) 40-Core CPU E5-2630 v4 @ 2.20 GHz with 64 GB RAM and 8 GB NVIDIA GeForce GTX 1070 GPU. The effect of segmentation using U-Net and GAN was studied on local ROP image datasets. Further, we evaluate and compared U-Net and GAN on noisy and augmented fundus datasets with different metrics. We have used following parameter for training the both models: 100 epochs and learning rate of 0.0001.

4.1   Evaluation Metrics

The segmented blood vessel map was evaluated using the following assessment metrics:

1. **Accuracy:** The accuracy of the segmented result is the percentage of pixels correctly classified as True. The given equation calculates accuracy:

$$Accuracy = \frac{(TP + TN)}{(TP + TN + FP + FN)},\tag{4}$$

   where, TP: True Positive, TN: True Negative, FP: False Positive, and FN: False Negative are computed to quantify the impact of the classifier during pixel categorization as foreground or background.

2. **Root Mean Square Error (RMSE):** This metric calculates the root of the mean squared error in these probabilities by using the non-binary pictures that the model created before the binary threshold was applied. This statistic allows us to determine the confidence level of our model. The following expression calculates RMSE:

$$RMSE = \sqrt{\frac{1}{N}\sum_{i=1}^{N}(y_i - \hat{y}_i)^2}\tag{5}$$

   where, $\sum$ = summation ("add up"), y_i = actual image pixel, $\hat{y}_i$ = predicted image pixel and N = total number of image pixels.

3. **Peek Signal to Noise Ratio (PSNR):** This function is primarily used in signal processing and correlates with the RMSE. The following is the formula for PSNR:

$$PSNR = 20log_{10}(MAX_I) - 10log_{10}(MSE)\tag{6}$$

   where, MSE = Mean Squared Error = $(RMSE)^2$ and MAX_I = 255, as image pixel has max value of 255.

4. **Structural Similarity Index (SSIM):** The SSIM index measures the similarity of two images. The SSIM index may be interpreted as a measure of the quality of one of the images being compared, assuming that the other image is of perfect quality. This approach enables us to assess the index's structural similarity quality. This statistic is explained in further depth in [46].

5. **Dice Coefficient:** The segmentation task is evaluated using a similarity metric known as the Dice coefficient. The Dice coefficient is calculated as follows:

$$Dice\ coefficient = \frac{2 * \text{Area of overlap}}{\text{Total pixels combined}}\tag{7}$$

6. **Absolute Mean Brightness Error (AMBE), Contrast (C), and Contrast Improvement Index (CII):** In addition, we evaluated the impact of picture preprocessing on image quality using absolute mean brightness error (AMBE), contrast (C), and contrast improvement index (CII) [16]. The AMBE definition is:

$$AMBE = mean(I_{original}) - mean(I_{enhance}),\tag{8}$$

where $I_{original}$ and $I_{enhance}$ represent the original (or input) and enhanced (or output) images, respectively. CII and C are measured in the following way [6,16]:

$$CII = \frac{C_{processed}}{C_{original}}, \tag{9}$$

$$C = \frac{m_f - m_b}{m_f + m_b}, \tag{10}$$

where, $C_{processed}$ and $C_{original}$ denote the contrast of the processed and original images, respectively, and m_f and m_b denote the average intensity of an image's foreground and background, respectively.

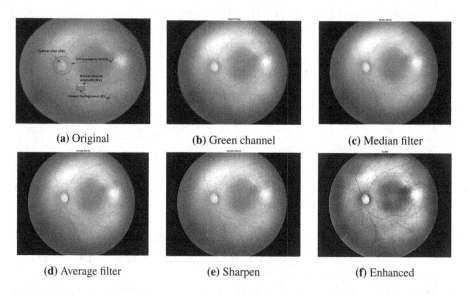

(a) Original   (b) Green channel   (c) Median filter

(d) Average filter   (e) Sharpen   (f) Enhanced

Fig. 10. Output images of different stages of preprocessing of original color (RGB) image [28].

4.2 Preprocessing of Fundus Images

The G channel is chosen for analysis as it provides the highest contrast between blood vessels and the background. Furthermore, a median filter was used in the preprocessing step to eliminate impulsive noise's influence. Sharp and sudden image signal fluctuations may cause impulse noise during acquisition. In the subsequent step, the average filter diminishes the impact of neighbouring pixel intensity changes. Image quality is also improved by applying sharpening and CLAHE, as illustrated in the preprocessing results in Fig. 10. In the sharpening filter, we have used unsharp masking with a standard deviation of 4 for the Gaussian low-pass filter and a sharpening effect intensity of 1.0. CLAHE is used to improve an image's contrast by transforming the intensity image's values.

Here, the number of tiles in a row, column, and contrast enhancement limit has been defined as 8 × 8 and 0.005, respectively. The remaining parameters for the MATLAB R2020b CLAHE[1] function, including the number of histogram bins (= 256), output picture intensity range (= 0 to 255), histogram distribution type (= uniform), and distribution parameters (= 0.4), are set to their default values.

For the evaluation of image preprocessing, we selected two regions of interest (ROIs) in the fundus image: the OD region and the blood vessel segment, as shown in Fig. 10a. It is particularly challenging to isolate blood vessels at the periphery of the fundus image. Therefore, we have selected a blood vessel structure region near the periphery of the image to observe the effect of preprocessing. Additionally, the spatial intensity level is irregularly distributed in fundus photographs of preterm infants. Therefore, we select a background region near the ROI in the preprocessing analysis to minimise the effects of uneven lighting and intensity distributions. Table 5 summarises the results of image preprocessing of neonatal fundus images. Due to image preprocessing, image quality metrics such as contrast, CII, and AMBE are significantly increased. We have illustrated how various preprocessing filters impact the original image (G channel). The CLAHE filter significantly enhances vessels, OD and image contrast compared to many other filters. However, the results in the last row show that image quality metrics are at their highest when all filter algorithms are used sequentially during preprocessing of the neonatal retinal image. This study tested different kernel sizes for the above filters. With a kernel size of 3 × 3, the mean and median filters work better. To do this, we have utilised Matlab 2020b's built-in image enhancement and sharpening functions with its default configuration.

Table 5. Effect of preprocessing on image quality.

Image processing	C_{vessel}	CII_{vessel}	C_{OD}	CII_{OD}	AMBE
Original Image (I_g)	0.0848	–	0.0697	–	–
Average	0.0847	0.9988	0.0696	0.9986	−0.15
Median	0.0851	1.0035	0.0697	1.0014	0.0253
Sharpen	0.0850	1.0024	0.0699	1.0029	0.012
Enhancement (or CLAHE)	0.1821	2.1474	0.1375	1.9727	14.97
Average + Median + sharpen + CLAHE	0.1990	2.3467	0.1394	2.0	24.5602

4.3   DL-Model Training and Testing

DL is a method in which the DCNN model is trained using historical labelled images of pathological information pertaining to various illnesses. In the following section, we have discussed two state-of-the-art DL-based networks for vessel segmentation.

---

[1] https://in.mathworks.com/help/images/ref/adapthisteq.html.

GAN Based Approach. After prepping the data with noise modelling and data augmentation, the pix2pix cGAN model was trained. During training, each model's loss functions for the generator and discriminator are shown in Fig. 11 for each step. In this graph, the loss value is initially quite large owing to the random assignment of weights, but as training goes on, it has decreased and fluctuated. This is due to a property of GAN in general, since both entities operate against and for each other. The pix2pix model's base code may be found in the GitHub repository[2].

In order to find the optimum model, we trained with a large number of different permutations of input picture size, model parameters, data with and without noise modelling, enhanced datasets during training, and models that utilised input images of various types. Table 8 provides more information on each of these permutations.

U-Net Based Approach. The cGAN-based model mentioned in the previous section employs U-Net as a generator. The key difference between GAN and any other encoder-decoder-based networks like U-Net is in the training of the network since the GAN has a conditional-objective GAN function in the training process. Therefore, this might sometimes result in overfitting with a smaller dataset. Experiments were performed using the vanilla version of the U-Net [40] without the GAN loss, which was built for biomedical picture segmentation.

In order to train the U-Net model, the same dataset described in Table 2 was used, together with the noise modelling shown in Sect. 3.1 applied to raw images. Additionally, the U-Net model was trained using the augmented dataset stated in Sect. 3.1 The same combination of models used to train the GAN model was also used to train various U-Net models to identify the best model among all of these combinations.

While training the model, the plot for the best model and nearly all models resembled Fig. 12; from these plots, it can be inferred that the dice co-efficient

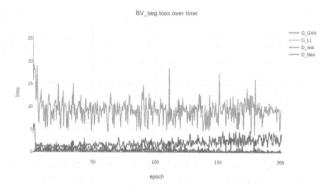

Fig. 11. Training History plot for the GAN model [28].

---

for the validation dataset is increasing, which is a metric for measuring the segmentation model's performance; the loss function on the training dataset is decreasing as training continues. In the testing, the model should have shown good generalizability, as reflected in the findings. The U-Net codebase may be accessed on the GitHub repository[3].

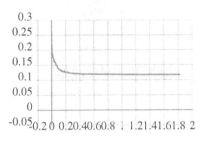
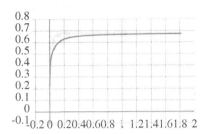

(a) Loss Function v/s time for Train Dataset

(b) Dice coefficient v/s time for Validation Dataset

Fig. 12. Training History for U-Net model [28].

4.4 Blood Vessels Segmentation

This section evaluates how well the proposed system works to separate the vessels in the nascent corpuscle image. We used accuracy, RMSE, PSNR, and SSIM as performance metrics to measure the quality of the segmentation. A high value indicates the best quality.

Segmentation Using U-Net. In the case of U-Net, the model with the augmented dataset did the best out of all the models that were trained. Now, to get a general idea of how well the model works, a qualitative analysis was done on a local dataset, which showed that this model gives good results for our dataset (as shown in Fig. 13). Quantitative analysis was also done on the few labelled examples from the local dataset, just as it was done for the GAN model. Table 6 contains the outcomes of the test. This table shows that this model works well for noisy, overexposed, and underexposed images where the vessels do not stand out well from the background. The performance numbers are also very similar to what the GAN model came up with, but this model is much easier to train and detect than the GAN model.

---

[3] https://github.com/milesial/Pytorch-UNet.

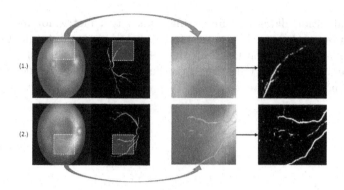

Fig. 13. Retinal vessel segmentation using U-net. In image (1) and (2) patch ROI-1 and ROI-2 are used to analyze the segmented blood vessels map in detail [28].

Table 6. Bench-marking Results from U-Net model [28].

Image	Accuracy	RMSE	PSNR	SSIM
Img_1	97.56	0.15	16.82	0.93
Img_2	97.55	0.16	16.80	0.92
Img_3	92.66	0.27	11.60	0.85
Img_4	97.27	0.16	16.14	0.92
Img_5	97.46	0.15	16.70	0.93
Img_6	97.26	0.17	16.31	0.92
Mean	**96.63**	**0.18**	**15.73**	**0.91**

Segmentation Using GAN. Now for the evaluation of the vessel extraction model, qualitative methods were employed, which required manual inspection of all the results generated by the model for the local dataset. The models trained by noise modelling gave good results, although models trained with augmented dataset displayed some edge like artifacts in the test images due to the nature of mosaic images used in training, this dataset will be used afterwards, and it has shown promising results for other models. The result from the GAN model is shown in the Fig. 14.

Table 7 summarises vessel segmentation results on preterm retinal images from local ROP distastes. We report the results of proposed segmentation techniques when a trainable DL model is used to separate the vessels. From a statistical point of view, the Accuracy, RMSE, PSNR, and SSIM scores are all high and similar for the U-net network. On the other hand, we get an average accuracy of 96.69% for the GAN model, slightly higher than the accuracy of the U-Net model (96.63 %).

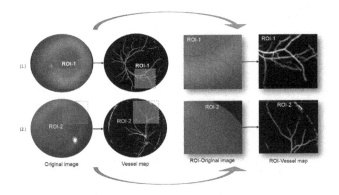

Fig. 14. Retinal vessel segmentation using GAN on local dataset. In image, (1) and (2) patch ROI-1 and ROI-2 are used to analyze the segmented blood vessels map in detail [28].

Table 7. Bench-marking Results from GAN(pix2pix) model [28].

Image	Accuracy	RMSE	PSNR	SSIM
Img_1	97.51	0.16	16.89	0.89
Img_2	97.76	0.15	16.14	0.91
Img_3	92.80	0.27	11.70	0.81
Img_4	97.62	0.15	17.15	0.90
Img_5	97.30	0.16	16.74	0.89
Img_6	97.15	0.17	16.29	0.88
Mean	**96.69**	**0.18**	**16.15**	**0.88**

4.5 Various Combinations for Vessel Extraction Models

While training these models, the validation using any performance metric for segmentation was not carried out due to the absence of ground truth for the local dataset. Multiple experiments were conducted for the vessel extraction model by changing several parameters. While these models were being trained, the validation was not carried out. A large number of experiments were carried out, each involving the modification of different parameters and being followed by a qualitative examination of the data provided by the previous experiment.

- **Noise Modelling.** Proposed noise modelling-based approach in Sect. 3.1 to bridge the gap between training and test datasets as they have very distinct characteristics.

Table 8. Different combinations of models trained for U-net or GAN [28].

Model_name	Pre-processing steps	Color	Resolution	Dice-coeff.
orig	crop	rgb	512 × 512	0.42–0.44
noise	crop + GaussianNoise((9,9),0)	rgb	512 × 512	0.38–0.42
noise + clahe	noise + clahe(3.5,(5,5)) + medianBlur(3)	rgb	512 × 512	0.58–0.6
orig_bw	crop	gray	512 × 512	0.58–0.59
noise_bw	crop + GaussianNoise((5,5),0)	gray	512 × 512	0.52–0.53
noise + clahe_bw	noise + clahe(3.5,(5,5)) + medianBlur(3)	gray	512 × 512	0.59–0.60
noise_bw	crop + GaussianNoise((9,9),0)	gray	512 × 512	0.54–0.55
noise + clahe_bw	noise + clahe(3.5,(5,5))+ medianBlur(3)	gray	512 × 512	0.55–0.56
noise + clahe_bw + bicubic_upscal	noise + clahe(3.5,(5,5)) + medianBlur(3)	gray	512 × 512	0.60–0.64
noise + clahe + bicubic_upscal	noise + clahe(3.5,(5,5)) + medianBlur(3)	rgb	512 × 512	0.57–0.59
noise + clahe_bw + bicubic_upscal	noise + clahe(3.5,(5,5)) + medianBlur(3)	gray	256 × 256	0.60–0.62
noise + clahe + bicubic_upscal	noise + clahe(3.5,(5,5)) + medianBlur(3)	rgb	256 × 256	0.59–0.60
noise + clahe_bw + bicubic_upscal	noise + clahe(3.5,(5,5)) + medianBlur(3)	gray	1024 × 1024	0.61–0.62
noise + clahe + bicubic_upscal	noise + clahe(3.5,(5,5)) + medianBlur(3)	rgb	1024 × 1024	0.48–0.50

Table 9. Different Combinations of models trained for U-Net/GAN with dataset augmented using mosaic generation in input image of size 512 × 512 pixels and its Dice coefficient in the last step [28].

Model_name	rgb/gray	Dice-coeff.	Grid Size
noise+ clahe_bw+ bicubic upscaling	gray	0.678–0.68	32 × 32
noise+ clahe+ bicubic upscaling	rgb	0.685+	32 × 32
noise+ clahe_bw+ bicubic upscaling	gray	0.67–0.68	64 × 64
noise+ clahe+ bicubic upscaling	rgb	0.67+	64 × 64

- **Preprocessing:** This is applied to test and training examples to enhance the contrast using the CLAHE Filter.
- **Color Channels:** During the first part of the experiments, models that used only single-channel (i.e., G-channel) grey-scale images did better at separating blood vessels, so RGB and grey-scale images were used as input for some combinations.
- **Resolution:** Since this parameter could be adjusted, it played a crucial role in the given model and eventually determined how long it would take to train and extract the blood vessels from the image.
- **Grid size for Augmented Dataset:** As described in Sect. 3.1, we experimented with various grid sizes for the enhanced data set.
- **Upscaling Algorithm:** Both models use U-Net either directly or indirectly, and deconvolution is a component of this. Upscaling may be performed in two ways: bilinear and bicubic [40]. U-Net defaults to bilinear upscaling since it has a lower computing cost. However, several investigations have also tested the bicubic upscaling method, which is known to provide superior outcomes at the expense of a greater computational cost.

Table 8 shows the original dataset with all possible permutations that were tested after taking certain preprocessing measures (i.e., without image mosaic-based enhancement). Note that the size of the training dataset was 224 in each of these studies. Table 9 shows the models that were trained with the augmented dataset from Sect. 3.1 using Mosaic. In all of these experiments, the training dataset had 450 samples. In both cases, the model was trained for 100 epochs with a 0.0001 learning rate.

Without noise modelling and preprocessing, the U-Net and GAN models give a dice coefficient of between 0.42 and 0.44 for vessel segmentation with the local dataset. However, using publicly accessible datasets such as DRIVE, STARE or CHASE_DB1, the same network and task [12, 22, 30, 43] showed a dice coefficient higher than 0.70. However, using the proposed system, we significantly improved the Dice Coefficient and the accuracy of vessel segmentation with the ROP dataset. However, since we employed preprocessed (or noise-modelled) images in training datasets, its performance suffered on public datasets.

4.6 Applications of Blood Vessel Segmentation

Zone-1 ROP Screening. Our next set of experiments showed that the GANs based vessel detection had better generalization in terms of quality of vessel maps

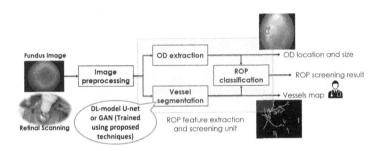

Fig. 15. ROP screening using improved blood vessels segmentation.

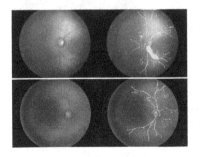 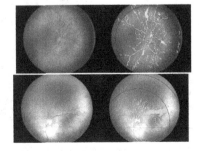

Fig. 16. Visualisation of Zoning algorithm: blue line depict zone boundary (Left side: original image, Right side: ROP zoning based on vessels extent) [28] (Color figure online).

generated and detect thinner vessels on the posterior regions of the fundus image helping in the zoning algorithm (ICROP) [27]. Therefore, we have use the DCNN architecture (Pix2Pix or U-Net) for infant's retinal blood vessels segmentation in [27], which is trained through the proposed method shown in Fig. 15. Zoning algorithm with new ROP screening method gave the accuracy of **88.23%** on the local dataset. However, in [27], zoning algorithm gave the accuracy of **83.33%** on the local dataset is uses the image processing based morphological technique for blood vessels segmentation. The image 16 shows detection of the extent of vessel growth pretty accurately even in case of some tricky images with noise or high exposure or even in case of very dark images, using GANs based vessel detection.

Plus Disease Screening. Only a few DCNN and other image processing imple-mentations [3,8,44] can predict binary labels for Plus illness or generate any quantisation number that may be used to make such predictions when a thresh-old is applied. One of the biggest problems is that there are no image datasets of an infant's fundus for blood vessel segmentation, and there are also no blood vessel map ground truths are available. Labeling blood vessel maps is also an expensive and time-consuming process. In addition, a qualified ophthalmologist or medical professional is required for their labelling. In this case, our proposed method helps to segment the blood vessel map, which is used by the Plus disease screening algorithms to monitor the progression of the disease. Furthermore, it may assist medical professionals in maintaining a more precise disease moni-toring system. Figure 17 shows how the blood vessels are used to measure and monitor the degree of Plus disease. It is also beneficial for ophthalmologists to accurately track the tortuosity index value and the structure of the blood ves-sels as the PLUS disease progresses, especially after treatment (whose tortuosity index exceeds the threshold). In this situation, we have made the assumption that the torture index has a cutoff value of 1.10. In Fig. 17c, all of the vessel segments having a tortuosity index more than 1.10 have been highlighted in red.

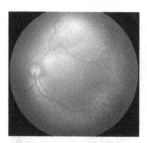 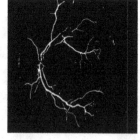 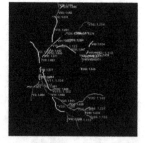

(a) Original image with ROP and Plus

(b) Blood vessel map gener-ation using [29].

(c) Tortuosity index of ves-sel's segment

Fig. 17. Blood vessels analysis (tortuosity index) for plus disease classification and monitoring.

The value of the torture index varies based on a number of variables, including the device used for retinal imaging, the technique of photography used, the lighting conditions, the subject's race, age, and gender, among others.

5 Conclusion

In neonate ophthalmology, accurate segmentation and identification of blood vessels are critical for diagnosing and monitoring ROP and Plus disease effectively. In this study, we propose a novel approach for segmenting retinal vessels using the DCNN architecture in which retinal scans cannot be distinguished from image/video noise, blur, and vessel map background. We have used two existing models of GAN (Pix2Pix) and U-Net for this purpose. The proposed dataset preparation method is used to train and test publicly available datasets and measure how well it works on the ROP dataset. The proposed approach achieves a high Dice coefficient and accuracy rate for the segmentation of retinal blood vessels.

In addition, we tested our approach on retinal scans of premature infants at a nearby hospital. Our approach significantly improves the Zoning based ROP classification as it is based on the extent of blood vessels. However, for the Plus disease requires structural information of the vessel such as tortuosity, branch angle and width. The proposed work provides greater interest in utilising deep learning-based systems in the future to develop similar applications such as disease screening, diagnosis and monitoring using biomedical (retinal) images. The proposed system can be specially used to develop automated applications for fundus imaging-based affordable health care in the future [29,35,37,38]. Therefore, this will require a research study that we expect to significantly improve using the new DL-based vessel segmentation technique in resource-constraint environments.

Acknowledgements. We acknowledge key insights received from Prof. Rohan Chawla and Dr. Abhidnya Surve in discussion that we have done related to this work.

References

1. Agrawal, R., Kulkarni, S., Walambe, R., Deshpande, M., Kotecha, K.: Deep dive in retinal fundus image segmentation using deep learning for retinopathy of prematurity. Multimed. Tools Appl. **81**(8), 11441–11460 (2022). https://doi.org/10.1007/s11042-022-12396-z
2. Bankhead, P., Scholfield, C.N., McGeown, J.G., Curtis, T.M.: Fast retinal vessel detection and measurement using wavelets and edge location refinement. PLoS ONE **7**(3), e32435 (2012)
3. Brown, J.M., et al.: Automated diagnosis of plus disease in retinopathy of prematurity using deep convolutional neural networks. JAMA Ophthalmol. **136**(7), 803–810 (2018)
4. Budai, A., Bock, R., Maier, A., Hornegger, J., Michelson, G.: Robust vessel segmentation in fundus images. Int. J. Biomed. Imaging **2013** (2013)

5. Ding, A., Chen, Q., Cao, Y., Liu, B.: Retinopathy of prematurity stage diagnosis using object segmentation and convolutional neural networks. arXiv preprint arXiv:2004.01582 (2020)

6. Ema, T., Doi, K., Nishikawa, R.M., Jiang, Y., Papaioannou, J.: Image feature analysis and computer-aided diagnosis in mammography: Reduction of false-positive clustered microcalcifications using local edge-gradient analysis. Med. Phys. **22**(2), 161–169 (1995)

7. Fielder, A.R., Wallace, D.K., Stahl, A., Reynolds, J.D., Chiang, M.F., Quinn, G.E.: Describing retinopathy of prematurity: current limitations and new challenges. Ophthalmology **126**(5), 652–654 (2019)

8. Gelman, R., Martinez-Perez, M.E., Vanderveen, D.K., Moskowitz, A., Fulton, A.B.: Diagnosis of plus disease in retinopathy of prematurity using retinal image multiscale analysis. Invest. Ophthalmol. Vis. Sci. **46**(12), 4734–4738 (2005)

9. Gilbert, C., Malik, A.N., Vinekar, A.: Artificial intelligence for ROP screening and to assess quality of care: progress and challenges. Pediatrics **147**(3) (2021)

10. Gojić, G., et al.: Deep learning methods for retinal blood vessel segmentation: evaluation on images with retinopathy of prematurity. In: 2020 IEEE 18th International Symposium on Intelligent Systems and Informatics (SISY), pp. 131–136. IEEE (2020)

11. Goodfellow, I., et al.: Generative adversarial networks. Commun. ACM **63**(11), 139–144 (2020)

12. Guo, C., Szemenyei, M., Yi, Y., Wang, W., Chen, B., Fan, C.: SA-UNet: spatial attention U-Net for retinal vessel segmentation. arXiv preprint arXiv:2004.03696 (2020)

13. Guo, X., et al.: Retinal vessel segmentation combined with generative adversarial networks and dense u-net. IEEE Access **8**, 194551–194560 (2020)

14. Guo, X., Kikuchi, Y., Wang, G., Yi, J., Zou, Q., Zhou, R.: Early detection of retinopathy of prematurity (ROP) in retinal fundus images via convolutional neural networks. arXiv preprint arXiv:2006.06968 (2020)

15. Han, J., Wang, Y., Gong, H.: Fundus retinal vessels image segmentation method based on improved U-Net. IRBM (2022)

16. Henry, A.G.P., Jude, A.: Convolutional neural-network-based classification of retinal images with different combinations of filtering techniques. Open Comput. Sci. **11**(1), 480–490 (2021)

17. Holm, S., Russell, G., Nourrit, V., McLoughlin, N.: DR HAGIS—a fundus image database for the automatic extraction of retinal surface vessels from diabetic patients. J. Med. Imaging **4**(1), 014503 (2017)

18. Hoover, A.D., Kouznetsova, V., Goldbaum, M.: Locating blood vessels in retinal images by piecewise threshold probing of a matched filter response. IEEE Trans. Med. Imaging **19**(3), 203–210 (2000). https://doi.org/10.1109/42.845178

19. Isola, P., Zhu, J.Y., Zhou, T., Efros, A.A.: Image-to-image translation with conditional adversarial networks (2018)

20. Jiang, Y., Liang, J., Cheng, T., Lin, X., Zhang, Y., Dong, J.: Mtpa_UNet: multiscale transformer-position attention retinal vessel segmentation network joint transformer and CNN. Sensors **22**(12), 4592 (2022)

21. Jiang, Y., Liang, J., Cheng, T., Zhang, Y., Lin, X., Dong, J.: MCPANet: multiscale cross-position attention network for retinal vessel image segmentation. Symmetry **14**(7), 1357 (2022)

22. Kamran, S.A., Hossain, K.F., Tavakkoli, A., Zuckerbrod, S.L., Sanders, K.M., Baker, S.A.: RV-GAN: segmenting retinal vascular structure in fundus photographs

using a novel multi-scale generative adversarial network. In: de Bruijne, M., et al. (eds.) MICCAI 2021. LNCS, vol. 12908, pp. 34–44. Springer, Cham (2021). https://doi.org/10.1007/978-3-030-87237-3_4

23. Karaali, A., Dahyot, R., Sexton, D.J.: DR-VNet: retinal vessel segmentation via dense residual UNet. In: El Yacoubi, M., Granger, E., Yuen, P.C., Pal, U., Vincent, N. (eds.) ICPRAI 2022. LNCS, vol. 13363, pp. 198–210. Springer, Cham (2022). https://doi.org/10.1007/978-3-031-09037-0_17

24. Karmakar, R., Nooshabadi, S., Eghrari, A.: Mobile-RetinaNet: a computationally efficient deepnet for retinal fundus image segmentation for use in low-resource settings. Invest. Ophthalmol. Vis. Sci. 63(7), 2064–F0053 (2022)

25. Kazeminia, S., et al.: GANs for medical image analysis. Artif. Intell. Med. 109, 101938 (2020)

26. Kumar, A., Agrawal, R., Joseph, L.: IterMiUnet: a lightweight architecture for automatic blood vessel segmentation. arXiv e-prints, pp. arXiv-2208 (2022)

27. Kumar, V., Patel, H., Paul, K., Surve, A., Azad, S., Chawla, R.: Deep learning assisted retinopathy of prematurity screening technique. In: Proceedings of the 14th International Joint Conference on Biomedical Engineering Systems and Technologies - Volume 5: HEALTHINF, pp. 234–243. INSTICC, SciTePress (2021). https://doi.org/10.5220/0010322102340243

28. Kumar, V., Patel, H., Paul, K., Surve, A., Azad, S., Chawla, R.: Improved blood vessels segmentation of retinal image of infants. In: HEALTHINF, pp. 142–153 (2022)

29. Kumar, V., Paul, K.: mNetra: a fundoscopy based optometer. In: HEALTHINF, pp. 83–92 (2016)

30. Li, L., Verma, M., Nakashima, Y., Nagahara, H., Kawasaki, R.: IterNet: retinal image segmentation utilizing structural redundancy in vessel networks. In: Proceedings of the IEEE/CVF Winter Conference on Applications of Computer Vision, pp. 3656–3665 (2020)

31. Li, M., Zhou, S., Chen, C., Zhang, Y., Liu, D., Xiong, Z.: Retinal vessel segmentation with pixel-wise adaptive filters. In: 2022 IEEE 19th International Symposium on Biomedical Imaging (ISBI), pp. 1–5. IEEE (2022)

32. Luo, Y., Chen, K., Mao, J., Shen, L., Sun, M.: A fusion deep convolutional neural network based on pathological features for diagnosing plus disease in retinopathy of prematurity. Invest. Ophthalmol. Vis. Sci. 61(7), 2017 (2020)

33. Lyu, J., Zhang, Y., Huang, Y., Lin, L., Cheng, P., Tang, X.: AADG: automatic augmentation for domain generalization on retinal image segmentation. IEEE Trans. Med. Imaging 41, 3699–3711 (2022)

34. Megrabov, E., Jamshidi, A., Patange, S.: Retinel vessel segmentation using U-Net and GANs

35. Moshfeghi, D.M., Capone, A.: Economic barriers in retinopathy of prematurity management. Ophthalmol. Retina 2(12), 1177–1178 (2018)

36. World Health Organization, et al.: World report on vision. Technical report. World Health Organization, Geneva (2019)

37. Patel, T.P., et al.: Smartphone-based fundus photography for screening of plus-disease retinopathy of prematurity. Graefes Arch. Clin. Exp. Ophthalmol. 257(11), 2579–2585 (2019). https://doi.org/10.1007/s00417-019-04470-4

38. Paul, K., Kumar, V.: Fundus imaging based affordable eye care. In: HEALTHINF, pp. 634–641 (2015)

39. Qi, X., Wu, Z., Ren, M., Sun, M., Sun, Z.: Robust and efficient segmentation of cross-domain medical images. arXiv preprint arXiv:2207.12995 (2022)

40. Ronneberger, O., Fischer, P., Brox, T.: U-Net: convolutional networks for biomedical image segmentation (2015)
41. Staal, J., Abramoff, M., Niemeijer, M., Viergever, M., van Ginneken, B.: Ridge based vessel segmentation in color images of the retina. IEEE Trans. Med. Imaging **23**(4), 501–509 (2004)
42. Ting, D.S.W., et al.: Artificial intelligence and deep learning in ophthalmology. Br. J. Ophthalmol. **103**(2), 167–175 (2019)
43. Uysal, E.S., Bilici, M.Ş., Zaza, B.S., Özgenç, M.Y., Boyar, O.: Exploring the limits of data augmentation for retinal vessel segmentation. arXiv preprint arXiv:2105.09365 (2021)
44. Wallace, D.K., Jomier, J., Aylward, S.R., Landers, M.B., III.: Computer-automated quantification of plus disease in retinopathy of prematurity. J. Am. Assoc. Pediatr. Ophthalmol. Strabismus **7**(2), 126–130 (2003)
45. Wang, J., Zhao, Y., Qian, L., Yu, X., Gao, Y.: EAR-NET: error attention refining network for retinal vessel segmentation. In: 2021 Digital Image Computing: Techniques and Applications (DICTA), pp. 1–7. IEEE (2021)
46. Wang, Z., Bovik, A.C., Sheikh, H.R., Simoncelli, E.P.: Image quality assessment: from error visibility to structural similarity. IEEE Trans. Image Process. **13**(4), 600–612 (2004). https://doi.org/10.1109/TIP.2003.819861
47. Wang, Z., She, Q., Ward, T.E.: Generative adversarial networks in computer vision: a survey and taxonomy. ACM Comput. Surv. (CSUR) **54**(2), 1–38 (2021)
48. Yildiz, V.M., et al.: Plus disease in retinopathy of prematurity: convolutional neural network performance using a combined neural network and feature extraction approach. Transl. Vis. Sci. Technol. **9**(2), 10 (2020)
49. Zhang, Y., et al.: Development of an automated screening system for retinopathy of prematurity using a deep neural network for wide-angle retinal images. IEEE Access **7**, 10232–10241 (2018)

On the Impact of the Vocabulary for Domain-Adaptive Pretraining of Clinical Language Models

Anastasios Lamproudis[✉] and Aron Henriksson

Department of Computer and Systems Sciences, Stockholm University, Kista, Sweden
{anastasios,aronhen}@dsv.su.se

Abstract. Pretrained language models tailored to the target domain may improve predictive performance on downstream tasks. Such domain-specific language models are typically developed by pretraining on in-domain data, either from scratch or by continuing to pretrain an existing generic language model. Here, we focus on the latter situation and study the impact of the vocabulary for domain-adaptive pretraining of clinical language models. In particular, we investigate the impact of (i) adapting the vocabulary to the target domain, (ii) using different vocabulary sizes, and (iii) creating initial representations for clinical terms not present in the general-domain vocabulary based on subword averaging. The results confirm the benefits of adapting the vocabulary of the language model to the target domain; however, the choice of vocabulary size is not particularly sensitive with respect to downstream performance, while the benefits of subword averaging is reduced after a modest amount of domain-adaptive pretraining.

Keywords: Natural language processing · Clinical language models · Domain-adaptive pretraining · Clinical text

1 Introduction

Large, pretrained language models have come to dominate much of modern natural language processing. In this new paradigm, language models are pretrained using massive unlabeled corpora, which are typically readily available, in a process of self-supervision. Before applying the pretrained language models to specific tasks, they can be fine-tuned using labeled, task-specific data. Pretraining large language models is computationally expensive, while fine-tuning is relatively computationally inexpensive and requires fewer labeled examples compared to using supervised learning to train a new model from scratch. Pretrained language models are sometimes referred to as foundation models and, by utilizing transfer learning techniques, can readily be tailored to carry out a myriad of different tasks in different domains. Fine-tuned language models have obtained state-of-the-art results in many natural language processing tasks.

While language models are generally pretrained on data in the general domain, such as Wikipedia, applying generic language models in specialized domains may lead to sub-optimal performance on many domain-specific tasks. This is likely to be the case

A. C. A. Roque et al. (Eds.): BIOSTEC 2022, CCIS 1814, pp. 315–332, 2023.
https://doi.org/10.1007/978-3-031-38854-5_16

if there are significant differences between the target domain and the general-domain corpora used for pretraining, i.e. differences in terms of, for instance, vocabulary and language use. As a result, sub-optimal representations may be learned during the pretraining process that can not be sufficiently adapted during fine-tuning. This realization has motivated the development of domain-specific language models, such as SciBERT [1] and BioBERT [14].

Several different strategies for developing domain-specific language models have been proposed. While the most obvious approach is to pretrain an entirely new language model from scratch using in-domain data, several strategies are based on the idea of leveraging an existing, generic language model and subsequently adapting it to the target domain. This process typically involves domain-adaptive pretraining, i.e. inheriting the parameters of the generic language model and continuing to pretrain it using in-domain data.

An important consideration when leveraging an existing language model and carrying out further domain-adaptive pretraining is the vocabulary of the language model. The language model has a vocabulary, which is typically constructed from the pretraining data using a particular algorithm, such as WordPiece [26], SentencePiece [10] and Byte-Pair Encoding [18]. The vocabulary and the language model's tokenizer is used for pre-processing the input text; it is also used for creating the mapping of the input data to the representations of the model at its lowest level, namely the embedding table. A possible drawback of continued, domain-adaptive pretraining of an existing, generic language model is that domain-specific words are often tokenized poorly. For example, in Swedish, when tokenizing the common clinical term röntgenundersökning (English: x-ray examination) with a generic language model, it is split into multiple sub-tokens: ['ro','##nt', '##gen', '##under', '##so', '##kning']. This has motivated efforts to adapt the vocabulary to the target domain prior to domain-adaptive pretraining [9,21].

In this study, we investigate how best to adapt an existing, generic language model – pretrained on general-domain corpora – to a specialized domain, in this case the clinical domain, and focus specifically on questions related to the vocabulary of the language model. Specifically, we study the following three research questions:

1. When adapting an existing pretrained language model from the general domain to a specific domain, is it beneficial to adapt or modify the vocabulary of the language model prior to carrying out domain-adaptive pretraining?
2. When adapting the vocabulary of the language model to the target domain, what should the size of the vocabulary be? The size of the domain-specific vocabulary affects the number and ratio of tokens for which it can inherit learned representations from the existing language model. Does the vocabulary size have an impact on the predictive performance of the domain-adapted language model when fine-tuning it on domain-specific tasks?
3. When adapting the vocabulary of the language model to the target domain, should a technique based on subword averaging be used for tokens that are not present in the existing language model prior to carrying out domain-adaptive pretraining? Subword averaging calculates the average of the embeddings for the subwords that

the language model's tokenizer splits a word into, while the alternative is random initialization of the initial embeddings for unknown words.

This paper is an extension of a previous study [13], where preliminary results showed that adapting the vocabulary to the target domain prior to domain-adaptive pretraining is beneficial in the sense that it leads to clinical language models that perform better on downstream tasks in the clinical domain. In this paper, we deepen our study of the impact of the language model's vocabulary when adapting an existing generic language model to the clinical domain through domain-adaptive pretraining. Specifically, we introduce two new experiments:

1. **Vocabulary Sizes.** We develop clinical language models with different vocabulary sizes and study the impact of this design choice on downstream task performance. Initial representations for vocabulary items present in the generic language model are inherited prior to domain-adaptive pretraining, which entails that different vocabulary sizes will inherit representations for different numbers and ratios of tokens.
2. **Subword Averaging.** We evaluate the impact of subword averaging, which is a technique whereby representations for clinical vocabulary items not present in the vocabulary of the generic language model are initialized by averaging the representations of its subtokens. This technique is compared to random initialization of embeddings for words that are not present in the vocabulary of the generic language model. The comparison is, moreover, conducted for all considered vocabulary sizes.

Furthermore, compared to the previous study [13], where the pretrained language models were fine-tuned and evaluated on two downstream tasks, we here extend and strengthen the evaluation to six downstream tasks.

2   Related Work

Several studies have demonstrated the benefits of developing domain-specific language models for specialized domains. In addition to pretraining entirely new domain-specific models with in-domain data, much research has endeavored to exploit the existence of large language models pretrained for the general domain, subsequently adapting them to some target domain.

One research direction to adapt existing, generic language models focuses on developing domain-adaptation techniques without the need for further pretraining with in-domain, which can be useful in domains where access to large amounts of in-domain pretraining data is limited, e.g. the clinical domain. One example of such an effort is KIMERA [25], which is a technique for detecting, retraining and instilling attention heads with complementary domain knowledge in the form of structured ontological data. KIMERA implements a multi-task training scheme, in which attention heads that are least useful for a given downstream task are identified and their representation is then optimized using information from structured data. This technique is shown to lead to improved downstream performance on several datasets in the medical domain. Another example is AVocaDo [8], which treats the vocabulary as an optimizable parameter and allows the vocabulary to be updated during fine-tuning by expanding it with domain-specific vocabulary based on a tokenization statistic. AVocaDo is shown to yield consistent performance improvements in a number of different domains.

Most efforts to adapt an existing language model to a specific domain, however, involve some form of domain-adaptive pretraining, i.e. inheriting the parameters of a generic language model and then continuing to pretrain it with in-domain data. This has shown to lead to rather substantial gains in downstream task performance in the target domain [7]. A notable example of a domain-specific language model in the biomedical domain is BioBERT [14], which inherit its parameters and vocabulary from BERT before carrying out domain-adaptive pretraining with biomedical corpora. Another example from the biomedical domain is BioMegatron [19], which is a larger language model trained with more data, but also uses a domain-specific vocabulary to obtain improved performance on downstream tasks in the target domain. In the clinical domain, Clinical BERT models inherit both its parameters and vocabulary from BERT-Base and BioBERT, respectively, after which domain-adaptive pretraining is carried out using clinical text from MIMIC-III. A similar approach was also taken when developing SweClinBERT [11] – a clinical language model for Swedish – which was shown to outperform a generic language model for Swedish on several downstream tasks in the clinical domain.

The benefits of domain-adaptive pretraining was investigated in a more elaborate study [7], where domain-adaptive pretraining was compared to task-adaptive pretraining, i.e. pretraining on unlabeled task-specific data. Further efforts in adapting existing language models to some target domain have focused on the vocabulary of the language model. With exBERT [21], domain-specific terms were included in the model's vocabulary along with extensions in each self-attention layer. This resulted in a model with slightly more parameters than the original BERT, which was then further pretrained with in-domain data and yielded improved performance on the domain-specific downstream tasks. Similarly, when developing IndoBERTweet [9], the language model's vocabulary was replaced entirely with a domain-specific vocabulary, yielding promising results. In this approach, the language model is initialized using parameters for whole words and subwords and then further pretrained with in-domain data.

As mentioned previously, a different approach to adapting an existing, generic language model to some target domain is to pretrain an entirely new, domain-specific language model from scratch with in-domain data. In one study [6], this approach was shown to outperform domain-adaptive pretraining, albeit requiring substantial computational resources. Similar conclusions were made in two other studies comparing pretraining clinical language models from scratch versus adapting generic language models to the clinical domain [5,24]. Another study [12] compared various pretraining strategies for developing domain-specific language models and found that domain-adaptive pretraining requires less pretraining with in-domain data – in particular when first adapting the vocabulary to the target domain – but that, eventually, a model trained from scratch obtained nearly as good performance as the domain-adapted variants.

3   Data

The clinical corpora[1] used both for domain-adaptive pretraining and for fine-tuning are part of Health Bank[2] – Swedish Health Record Research Bank at DSV/Stockholm University [2]. The Health Bank infrastructure contains health records from Karolinska University Hospital in Stockholm, Sweden. It encompasses health records for over 2 million patients across approximately 500 clinical units from 2007 to 2014.

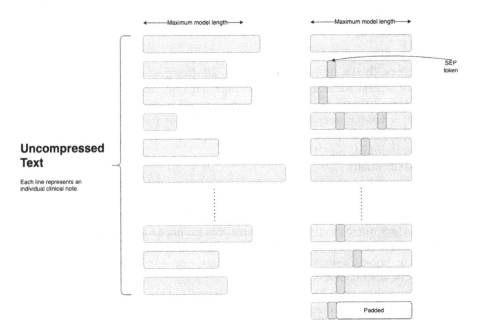

Fig. 1. Illustration of the text preprocessing for the purposes of domain-adaptive pretraining. On the left, the original clinical notes are shown on each line with rotating blue and green colors. On the right, the processed samples are shown with the added separation [SEP] tokens in red. (Color figure online)

3.1   Pretraining Data

From Health Bank and for the purposes of domain-adaptive pretraining, we extract all clinical notes recorded by any healthcare professional. This results in $\sim$ 17.8 GB of uncompressed clinical text written in Swedish. We then process the text by tokenizing it with the BERT tokenizer and create sequences of maximum length for training our BERT models, either by concatenating shorter sequences or by splitting longer ones. To denote the different sentences within a single block, we add separation tokens. This process is illustrated in Fig. 1. This results in $\sim$ 9,000,000 text samples with sequence

---

[1] This research has been approved by the Swedish Ethical Review Authority under permission no. 2019-05679.

[2] http://dsv.su.se/healthbank.

lengths of 512 tokens or $\sim 4,590,000,000$ tokens in total, depending on the vocabulary/tokenizer used.

3.2 Fine-Tuning Data

To evaluate the performance of the domain-adapted language models, six downstream tasks in the clinical domain are used. The downstream tasks include both classification tasks and named entity recognition (NER) tasks and the datasets used for these tasks are described below:

ICD-10 (Classification)

The Stockholm EPR Gastro ICD-10 Corpus consists of 6,062 gastro-related discharge summaries and their assigned ICD-10 diagnosis codes. The data is divided into 10 groups (classes) using a more coarse granularity compared to the full ICD-10 codes; the groups correspond to different body parts and range from K00 to K99. There is, on average, 1.2 labels per sample. This is a multi-class, multi-label classification task. See [17] for more details.

ADE (Classification)

The Stockholm EPR ADE ICD-10 Corpus contains 21,642 clinical documents and a total of 634,000 tokens. The documents are distributed over 12 different ICD-10 codes describing adverse drug events. The task is treated as a binary classification task where positive samples have been assigned a specific ICD-10 code that denotes an adverse drug event. Negative samples in each group have been assigned a code describing a similar condition that was not drug-induced.

Factuality (Classification & NER)

The Stockholm EPR Diagnosis Factuality Corpus encompasses six levels of annotations regarding the factuality of a diagnosis. The corpus consists of 3,710 samples (240,000 tokens) with 7,066 annotated entities: *Certainly Positive, Probably Positive, Possibly Positive, Possibly Negative, Probably Negative*, and *Certainly Negative*. See [22,23] for more details. This corpus is used for creating two downstream tasks: a multi-label document classification task and a NER task.

PHI (NER)

The Stockholm EPR PHI Corpus consists of 4,480 annotated entities and 380,000 tokens. The protected health information (PHI) correspond to nine classes: *First Name, Last Name, Age, Phone Number, Location, Health Care Unit, Organization, Full Date*, and *Date Part*. See [3] for the creation of the gold standard.

Clinical Entity (NER)

The Stockholm EPR Clinical Entity Corpus consists of 70,852 tokens and 7,946 annotated entities corresponding to four clinical entity classes: *Diagnosis, Findings, Body parts* and *Drugs*. See [20] for more details.

4 Methods

In this paper, we investigate ways to adapt an existing, generic language model to the clinical domain, focusing on questions related to the vocabulary of the language model.

We not only compare inheriting the general-domain vocabulary of the existing language model to using a domain-specific, clinical vocabulary; we also (i) investigate the potential impact of different vocabulary sizes when replacing the language model's general-domain vocabulary with a clinical vocabulary prior to domain-adaptive pretraining, and (ii) compare two domain-specific vocabulary initialization techniques prior to domain-adaptive pretraining: subword averaging – i.e. calculating the average of the embeddings for the subwords that the language model's tokenizer splits a non-vocabulary word into – versus random initialization.

The development of the clinical language models includes a (i) vocabulary development and vocabulary swap phase, and (ii) a domain-adaptive pretraining session using in-domain data in the form of clinical text. The domain-adapted language models are evaluated in terms of their predictive performance on six downstream tasks in the clinical domain, with checkpoints saved and evaluated throughout the domain-adaptive pretraining sessions.

4.1   Baseline – Inheriting the General-Domain Vocabulary

As our baseline, we use the clinical language model SweClinBERT [11]. This clinical language model was developed by performing domain-adaptive pretraining on KB-BERT [16] – a general-domain language model for Swedish – using 17.8 GB of uncompressed Swedish clinical text. This model was trained using masked language modeling for one epoch and has been shown to outperform the original generic language model on a number of downstream tasks in the clinical domain.

4.2   Vocabulary Development

To develop the domain-adapted language models by replacing the general-domain vocabulary of the original model with domain-specific, clinical vocabularies, we must first construct the these new vocabularies. Using the WordPiece algorithm [26] and the totality of the domain-adaptive pretraining corpus described in Sect. 3.1, we create five different vocabularies with sizes ranging from 30,000 tokens to 70,000 tokens. In Table 1, we present these vocabularies in terms of their intersection and difference compared to the general-domain vocabulary of the original language model that is adapted through vocabulary replacement and domain-adaptive pretraining.

Table 1. Five clinical vocabularies of different sizes are constructed and used by the domain-adapted language models. We also report the intersection and difference compared to the vocabulary of KB-BERT, the original language model.

Vocabulary Size	Intersection	Difference	Intersecting Ratio
30,000	12,709	17,291	42.3%
40,000	14,747	25,253	36.8%
50,000	16,519	33,801	32.8%
60,000	17,792	42,271	29.5%
70,000	18,984	51,016	27.1%

The vocabulary used by the language model affects the tokenization of the text that is processed during both domain-adaptive pretraining and downstream task fine-tuning, as words not present in the vocabulary are split into multiple tokens. To illustrate this, Fig. 2 shows a comparison of the tokenization of the downstream task data, i.e. in the form of clinical text, when using clinical-domain vocabularies of varying sizes versus using the general-domain vocabulary of the original, generic language model. As can been seen, using the general-domain vocabulary on clinical text leads to a much higher proportion of words being split into two or more WordPieces. Furthermore, as expected, using a larger clinical-domain vocabulary leads to fewer words being split into multiple WordPieces compared to using a smaller clinical vocabulary. However, the difference between using a clinical vocabulary with 30,000 words and 70,000 words is much smaller compared to using a general-domain vocabulary.

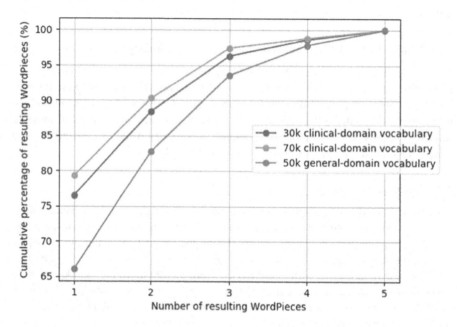

Fig. 2. Comparison of the tokenization of the downstream clinical corpora using three different vocabularies.

After developing the vocabularies we use them to replace the vocabulary of KB-BERT. We do this by replacing the embedding table of the model with a new randomly initialized embedding table. Then, for the intersection – i.e. tokens in the clinical vocabulary that are also present in the general-domain vocabulary – we inherit the parameters from the original embedding table. For the difference – i.e. tokens in the clinical vocabulary that are not present in the general-domain vocabulary – we follow one of the following two approaches:

1. **Subword Averaging.** Using the tokenizer of the original, generic language model to compute sub-tokens, for which there are embeddings in the original embedding table. By calculating the average of these embeddings, we obtain a representation for the clinical term [9].
2. **Random Initialization.** Instead of inheriting any embeddings from the original table, we leave the randomly initialized embeddings in their place.

By experimenting with both of these approaches, we are not only able to evaluate the impact of the size of the clinical vocabulary on the model's predictive performance in downstream tasks, but also whether subword averaging is a beneficial domain-specific vocabulary initialization technique for domain-adaptive pretraining.

4.3 Domain-Adaptive Pretraining

The second step in the development of the domain-adapted language models is the domain-adaptive pretraining session. This is a pretraining session with masked language modeling for approximately one epoch of the pretraining data. For the hyperparameters of the session, we try to follow closely the instructions in [4, 16]. However, following the work in [15], we omit the next sentence prediction task in favor of using only masked language modeling. Furthermore, we omit the shorter sequence length training steps in favor of training only with sequences of the maximum length of 512.

Table 2. Hyperparameters for domain-adaptive pretraining. As described in [11], these are a combination of the hyperparameter values used in [4, 15, 16].

hyperparameters	values
learning rate	10^{-4}
batch size	256
Adam β_1	0.9
Adam β_2	0.999
L2 weight decay	0.01
warm up steps	10,000
learning rate decay	linear
dropout probability	10%
update steps	$\approx 35,000$ or ~ 1 epoch
training sequence length	512
Masked language modeling probability	15%

With the hyperparameter values described in Table 2, we perform the second step in the development of the models described in Sect. 4.2, as well as the baseline:

SweClinBERT [11]. After preprocessing the text with each model's respective tokenizer, we train for a maximum of one epoch of our data; we regularly save checkpoints on each 10th percentile of the domain-adaptive pretraining session. We later use these checkpoints to track the models' performance on each of the evaluation downstream tasks, during different times in their development.

4.4   Downstream Task Fine-Tuning

During the downstream task fine-tuning and evaluation, each downstream dataset is randomly split into training, validation, and test sets, with the training set being 80% of the original dataset and the validation and test sets being 10% each. Each experiment is repeated 10 times with different training, validation, and test splits. The final results reported are the mean values over all ten the experiments, along with standard deviations.

For the **ICD-10** and **PHI** task, we use the same hyperparameters as in [13], while for the remaining downstream tasks a narrow grid search with our baseline is conducted. Note that the hyperpameters used in these downstream task experiments, which are summarized in Table 3, are most likely not the most optimal due to the nature of the narrow grid search that yielded them. However, we aim for a fair comparison between the different models and not for the best possible performance.

Table 3. Hyperparameters for the downstream tasks.

Model	ICD-10	PHI	Clinical Entity	ADE	Factuality Classification	Factuality NER
learning rate	$2 \cdot 10^{-5}$	$3 \cdot 10^{-5}$	$3 \cdot 10^{-5}$	$3 \cdot 10^{-5}$	$2 \cdot 10^{-5}$	$3 \cdot 10^{-5}$
batch size	32	64	64	64	32	64

5   Results

When evaluating the clinical language models, we select the checkpoints during the domain-adaptive pretraining session that produce the best performance over all six downstream tasks. The results are shown in Tables 4 and 5.

From the results in Table 4, we can see that using a domain-specific, clinical vocabulary leads to a slightly better performance on all tasks compared to using the general-domain vocabulary of the original language model. However, there is no obvious pattern with respect to which vocabulary size leads to better performance across tasks: for ICD-10 and ADE classification, using a smaller vocabulary size yields the best results, while for factuality classification, using a somewhat larger vocabulary size instead yields the best results.

Regarding how best to initialize the clinical vocabulary for words that are not present in the vocabulary of the original generic language model – subword averaging or random initialization – there is likewise not one method that invariably outperforms the other. On two out of three classification tasks, using random initialization results in clinical language models with the best performance.

Table 4. The results for the classification downstream tasks. All results are reported in F_1-score and the standard deviations are computed over 10 different runs, each using different validation and test sets. Averaging indicates the vocabulary initialization technique used: 'yes' = subword averaging, 'no' = random initialization.

Model	Epoch progress	Averaging	ICD-10	ADE	Factuality
			Classification	Classification	Classification
SweClinBERT	100%	—	0.830±0.011	0.195±0.023	0.727±0.016
Clinical 30k	90%	yes	0.829±0.015	0.19±0.015	0.728±0.017
	90%	no	0.832±0.01	**0.198±0.018**	0.725±0.02
Clinical 40k	90%	yes	**0.836±0.013**	0.197±0.018	0.735±0.03
	90%	no	0.829±0.012	0.194±0.016	0.733±0.017
Clinical 50k	100%	yes	0.833±0.013	0.196±0.012	0.735±0.028
	90%	no	0.834±0.011	0.188±0.014	0.733±0.019
Clinical 60k	80%	yes	0.832±0.011	0.192±0.019	0.731±0.024
	90%	no	0.831±0.012	0.187±0.013	**0.737±0.02**
Clinical 70k	90%	yes	0.830±0.013	0.185±0.009	0.735±0.018
	90%	no	0.831±0.016	0.189±0.018	0.736±0.02

From the NER results in Table 5, using a domain-specific vocabulary similarly results in clinical language models that outperform SweClinBERT, which uses a general-domain vocabulary, across all three tasks. Similar to the classification results, the choice of vocabulary size does not seem to have a substantial impact on downstream performance of the models, although, in this case, using a larger vocabulary yields better predictive performance on two out of three downstream tasks.

Furthermore, and like in the classification results, there is not clear difference between random initialization and subword averaging of embeddings for words that are not present in the general-domain vocabulary of the original, generic language model before domain-adaptive pretraining. Subword averaging seems to lead to clinical language models that perform best on two out of three downstream tasks, in both cases using a large clinical vocabulary. In fact, when using a larger clinical vocabulary (>50,000), subword averaging leads to equal or better performance than random initialization on all three NER tasks. However, and taking into account the standard deviation, we cannot say conclusively that the improvements are significant.

Finally, we observe that the clinical language models with a clinical vocabulary generally need to carry out domain-adaptive pretraining for the 90% of an epoch to reach the maximum performance. The model that required the least amount of domain-

Table 5. The results of the NER downstream tasks. All results are reported in F_1-score and the standard deviations are computed over 10 different runs, each using different validation and test sets. Averaging indicates the vocabulary initialization technique used: 'yes' = subword averaging, 'no' = random initialization.

Model	Epoch progress	Averaging	PHI	Clinical Entity	Factuality
			NER	NER	NER
SweClinBERT	100%	—	0.926±0.022	0.855±0.009	0.682±0.023
Clinical 30k	90%	yes	0.937±0.011	0.856±0.007	0.693±0.02
	90%	no	**0.938±0.017**	0.857±0.009	0.69±0.021
Clinical 40k	90%	yes	0.932±0.017	0.854±0.011	0.696±0.028
	90%	no	**0.938±0.014**	0.855±0.008	0.687±0.022
Clinical 50k	100%	yes	0.936±0.013	0.857±0.007	0.695±0.026
	90%	no	0.936±0.016	0.853±0.01	0.695±0.017
Clinical 60k	80%	yes	0.937±0.016	0.857±0.008	0.694±0.015
	90%	no	0.930±0.01	0.854±0.008	0.693±0.019
Clinical 70k	90%	yes	0.936±0.017	**0.858±0.008**	**0.706±0.028**
	90%	no	0.936±0.018	0.854±0.019	0.698±0.02

adaptive pretraining was the one with a vocabulary size of 60,000 that needed 80% of an epoch to reach its optimal performance.

In addition to presenting the results of the clinical language models that yielded the overall best results, we also present the average performance across downstream tasks of different checkpoints during the domain-adaptive pretraining session. In Fig. 3, this is illustrated for two domain-adapted clinical language models using a vocabulary size of 30,000 and 70,000, respectively, and in relation to the SweClinBERT baseline, which uses a general-domain vocabulary. As we can see, using a clinical vocabulary – in this case with subword averaging – leads to better performance throughout the domain-adaptive pretraining session, with only a few exceptions. We also observe that, overall, using a larger vocabulary size – 70,000 versus 30,000 – leads to slightly better performance. However, it appears that using a large clinical vocabulary – which means that the intersecting ratio is smaller, see Table 1 – requires more domain-adaptive pretraining before it outperforms models with a smaller clinical vocabulary. When considering the best results of each model, it also seems that the impact of using a (larger) clinical vocabulary is somewhat bigger for NER tasks than classification tasks, albeit even these differences are rather small ($\sim$1 F_1-score point).

We also analyze the impact of the two vocabulary initialization techniques – subword averaging versus random initialization – on downstream performs for various checkpoints throughout the domain-adaptive pretraining session. In Fig. 4, these results are shown for classification and NER, respectively, and with a vocabulary size of 30,000 and 70,000, respectively. One observation is that random initialization requires more domain-adaptive pretraining before reaching a comparable performance to subword

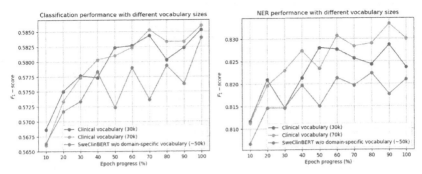

(a) **Classification** performance with different vocabulary sizes

(b) **NER** performance with different vocabulary sizes

Fig. 3. Downstream task performance when using clinical vocabularies of different sizes (30,000 vs. 70,000) with subword averaging embeddings versus using a general-domain vocabulary. We present the two extremes to illustrate the lack of a significant impact of the vocabulary size in the performance of the domain-adapted model.

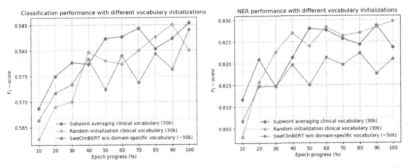

(a) **Classification** performance with two vocabulary initialization methods and a vocabulary size of **30,000**.

(b) **NER** performance with two vocabulary initialization methods and a vocabulary size of **30,000**

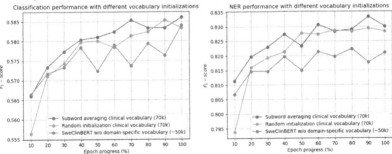

(c) **Classification** performance with two vocabulary initialization methods and a vocabulary size of **70,000**

(d) **NER** performance with two vocabulary initialization methods and a vocabulary size of **70,000**

Fig. 4. Downstream task performance when using two different clinical vocabulary initialization methods and different vocabulary sizes (30,000 vs. 70,000).

averaging. This seems to hold true for both classification and NER tasks, and with both a small (30,000) and large (70,000) clinical vocabulary. In fact, although not surprisingly, random initialization requires 20–40% of an epoch of domain-adaptive pretraining before outperforming using a general-domain vocabulary. Subword averaging, on the other hand, outperforms using a general-domain vocabulary already after 10% of an epoch of domain-adaptive pretraining. It is also worth pointing out that the importance of using a domain-specific, clinical vocabulary is more evident for NER tasks compared to classification tasks.

6   Discussion

The results of this study show that using a domain-specific, clinical vocabulary is beneficial when carrying out domain-adaptive pretraining of a generic language model, i.e. compared to retaining the general-domain vocabulary of the original language model. This further corroborates results from previous studies [9, 12, 13, 21]. One consequence of using a domain-specific vocabulary is that fewer words are split into multiple subtokens, as we showed in Fig. 2. This, in turn, allows better representations for more domain-specific terms to be learned during the domain-adaptive pretraining session, which may be of importance in allowing the model to learn to perform a particular downstream task in the target domain. Of course, in order to allow for good representations to be learned for domain-specific, clinical terminology – in particular when not part of the general-domain vocabulary of the original language model, for which pretrained representations already exist – one needs to have access to sufficient amount of in-domain data for domain-adaptive pretraining. This is especially true when using random initialization for embeddings of words that are not present in the general-domain vocabulary, whereas subword averaging represents an attempt to alleviate this limitation. On the other hand, it is clear (Fig. 3) that using a domain-specific, clinical vocabulary, especially in combination with subword averaging, requires less domain-adaptive pretraining to reach good downstream performance compared to retaining the general-domain vocabulary of the original language model. This can be important in settings where access to large amounts of in-domain data – and possibly also computational resources – for (domain-adaptive) pretraining is limited.

Since using a vocabulary tailored to the target domain leads to the development of better domain-specific language models, one may hypothesize that having a larger vocabulary should lead to even better downstream performance. This hypothesis would be based on the results shown in Fig. 2 and the reasoning above. When averaging the predictive performance results across downstream tasks, as shown in Fig. 3, there is slight advantage of using vocabulary size of 70,000 over 30,000; however, the difference is really very small and most likely not statistically significant. This is further supported by the results in Tables 4 and 5, which fail to reveal a clear pattern: for some tasks, a smaller vocabulary size yields the best predictive performance, while, for other tasks, the opposite is true. In other words, we were not able to verify this hypothesis. In fact, the results rather seem to indicate that choosing an exact size for the domain-specific vocabulary – at least within the range of vocabulary sizes considered in this study – does not have a large impact on the downstream performance of the domain-specific language models, suggesting that this is not an critical design decision. That said, it is possible that using a larger vocabulary requires more domain-adaptive pretraining compared to using a smaller vocabulary, in part because there is a larger portion of words that are not present in the general-domain vocabulary – as shown in Table 1 – and therefore do not have good representations prior to domain-adaptive pretraining, in particular when relying on random initialization. In future studies, this could be investigated further by exposing the models to more epochs of domain-adaptive pretraining.

Concerning the two vocabulary initialization techniques, we wanted to investigate empirically if there is a benefit of subword averaging in conjunction with domain-adaptive pretraining. Again, when looking at the average performance across downstream tasks, subword averaging yielded the best performance for both classification and NER with a vocabulary size of 70,000; with a vocabulary size of 30,000, it yielded the best performance for classification tasks but was outperformed by random initialization for NER tasks (Fig. 4). However, once again, the differences between the two techniques when considering the best checkpoints is very small. Likewise, when considering the best models on specific tasks (Tables 4 and 5), there is no clear pattern and the differences in predictive performance is negligible. That said, subword averaging does indeed seem to outperform random initialization with less domain-adaptive pretraining (Fig. 4). This makes sense since the representations for tokens that cannot be inherited from the original language model – because they do not exist in the general-domain vocabulary – need to learned during the domain-adaptive pretraining session. This is especially apparent when using a larger vocabulary (70,000) – random initialization clearly performs worse after only 10% of an epoch – simply because there are more randomly initialized embeddings as a result of the intersecting ratio between the general-domain and clinical-domain vocabularies being smaller (Table 1). Overall, the benefits of subword averaging over random initialization and other vocabulary initialization techniques, which have been demonstrated in previous work [9], were less evident, albeit not contradicted, in our study.

Finally, it is interesting to note that using a domain-specific, clinical vocabulary leads to bigger improvements in downstream performance for NER tasks compared to classification tasks (Table 5 and Figs. 4b and 4d). On the NER tasks, the SweClinBERT baseline, which relies on a general-domain vocabulary, performs significantly worse than the models with clinical vocabularies. This may indicate that a using a clinical vocabulary is especially important in tasks where the main focus is the entities and their position in the text rather than the complete text as in classification.

7   Conclusions

In this study, we have investigated the impact of the vocabulary for domain-adaptive pretraining of clinical language models. We have focused on the situation where one wishes to leverage an existing generic language model, pretrained on general-domain corpora, and adapt it to some target domain. One option, then, is to replace the vocabulary of the original language model with a domain-specific vocabulary before carrying out domain-adaptive pretraining – the idea being that it would allow for the development of domain-adapted language models that perform better on downstream tasks in the target domain.

The experimental results confirm the benefits of adapting the vocabulary of the language model to the target domain, corroborating previous work. This not only leads to language models with better downstream performance – on classification and named entity recognition tasks alike – but also requires less domain-adaptive pretraining to converge to a good performance. This is an important finding in settings where access to large amounts of in-domain data for pretraining large language models is limited, which is often the case in the clinical domain.

When adapting the vocabulary of a generic language model to the target domain, one needs to decide what the size of the vocabulary should be. In this study, we experimented with five different vocabulary sizes – ranging from 30,000 to 70,000 – and found no clearly significant impact on downstream performance, although using a larger vocabulary yielded the best results overall. It therefore seems that the choice of vocabulary size is not particularly sensitive with respect to downstream performance.

We further investigated two vocabulary initialization techniques – subword averaging and random initialization – for tokens that are not present in the vocabulary of the existing language model. Again, we observed no clearly significant differences in downstream performance after a certain amount of domain-adaptive pretraining, although subword averaging seems to require less domain-adaptive pretraining compared to random initialization and yielded slightly better performance overall.

As future work, it would be interesting to explore the minimum domain-adaptive pretraining steps required to develop competitive domain-adapted models. Furthermore, different parameter inheritance techniques can be tested for the parameters of the new tokens that are not present in the general-domain vocabulary. Finally, when adapting language models to the clinical domain one could investigate the possibility – and potential advantages – of introducing additional domain-adaptive pretraining tasks based on structured data in electronic health records, e.g. diagnosis codes.

References

1. Beltagy, I., Lo, K., Cohan, A.: SciBERT: a pretrained language model for scientific text. In: Proceedings of the 2019 Conference on Empirical Methods in Natural Language Processing and the 9th International Joint Conference on Natural Language Processing (EMNLP-IJCNLP), pp. 3606–3611 (2019)
2. Dalianis, H., Henriksson, A., Kvist, M., Velupillai, S., Weegar, R.: HEALTH BANK- a workbench for data science applications in healthcare. In: CEUR Workshop Proceedings Industry Track Workshop, pp. 1–18 (1 2015). http://ceur-ws.org/Vol-1381/paper1.pdf
3. Dalianis, H., Velupillai, S.: De-identifying Swedish clinical text - refinement of a gold standard and experiments with conditional random fields. J. Biomed. Semant. 1(1), 6 (2010). https://doi.org/10.1186/2041-1480-1-6
4. Devlin, J., Chang, M.W., Lee, K., Toutanova, K.: BERT: pre-training of deep bidirectional transformers for language understanding. In: Proceedings of the 2019 Conference of the North American Chapter of the Association for Computational Linguistics: Human Language Technologies, Volume 1 (Long and Short Papers), pp. 4171–4186. Association for Computational Linguistics, Minneapolis, Minnesota (2019). https://doi.org/10.18653/v1/N19-1423, https://aclanthology.org/N19-1423
5. El Boukkouri, H., Ferret, O., Lavergne, T., Zweigenbaum, P.: Re-train or train from scratch? Comparing pre-training strategies of BERT in the medical domain. In: LREC 2022, pp. 2626–2633 (2022)

6. Gu, Y., et al.: Domain-specific language model pretraining for biomedical natural language processing. ACM Trans. Comput. Healthc. (HEALTH) **3**(1), 1–23 (2021)
7. Gururangan, S., et al.: Don't stop pretraining: adapt language models to domains and tasks. In: Proceedings of the 58th Annual Meeting of the Association for Computational Linguistics, pp. 8342–8360. Association for Computational Linguistics, Online (2020). https://doi.org/10.18653/v1/2020.acl-main.740, https://aclanthology.org/2020.acl-main.740
8. Hong, J., Kim, T., Lim, H., Choo, J.: AVocaDO: strategy for adapting vocabulary to downstream domain. In: Proceedings of the 2021 Conference on Empirical Methods in Natural Language Processing, pp. 4692–4700 (2021)
9. Koto, F., Lau, J.H., Baldwin, T.: IndoBERTweet: a pretrained language model for indonesian twitter with effective domain-specific vocabulary initialization. In: Proceedings of the 2021 Conference on Empirical Methods in Natural Language Processing, pp. 10660–10668 (2021)
10. Kudo, T., Richardson, J.: SentencePiece: a simple and language independent subword tokenizer and detokenizer for neural text processing. In: Proceedings of the 2018 Conference on Empirical Methods in Natural Language Processing: System Demonstrations, pp. 66–71 (2018)
11. Lamproudis, A., Henriksson, A., Dalianis, H.: Developing a clinical language model for Swedish: continued pretraining of generic BERT with In-Domain data. In: Proceedings of RANLP 2021: Recent Advances in Natural Language Processing, 1–3 September 2021, Varna, Bulgaria, pp. 790–797 (2021)
12. Lamproudis, A., Henriksson, A., Dalianis, H.: Evaluating pretraining strategies for clinical BERT models. In: Proceedings of the Language Resources and Evaluation Conference, pp. 410–416. European Language Resources Association, Marseille, France (2022). https://aclanthology.org/2022.lrec-1.43
13. Lamproudis, A., Henriksson, A., Dalianis, H.: Vocabulary modifications for domain-adaptive pretraining of clinical language models. In: HEALTHINF 2022, pp. 180–188. SciTePress (2022)
14. Lee, J., et al.: BioBERT: a pre-trained biomedical language representation model for biomedical text mining. Bioinformatics **36**(4), 1234–1240 (2020)
15. Liu, Y., et al.: RoBERTa: a robustly optimized BERT pretraining approach. arXiv preprint arXiv:1907.11692 (2019)
16. Malmsten, M., Börjeson, L., Haffenden, C.: Playing with words at the national library of Sweden-making a Swedish BERT. arXiv preprint arXiv:2007.01658 (2020)
17. Remmer, S., Lamproudis, A., Dalianis, H.: Multi-label diagnosis classification of Swedish discharge summaries - ICD-10 code assignment using KB-BERT. In: Proceedings of RANLP 2021: Recent Advances in Natural Language Processing, RANLP 2021, 1–3 September 2021, Varna, Bulgaria, pp. 1158–1166 (2021)
18. Sennrich, R., Haddow, B., Birch, A.: Neural machine translation of rare words with subword units. In: Proceedings of the 54th Annual Meeting of the Association for Computational Linguistics (Volume 1: Long Papers), pp. 1715–1725. Association for Computational Linguistics, Berlin, Germany (2016). https://doi.org/10.18653/v1/P16-1162, https://aclanthology.org/P16-1162
19. Shin, H.C., et al.: BioMegatron: larger biomedical domain language model. In: Proceedings of the 2020 Conference on Empirical Methods in Natural Language Processing (EMNLP), pp. 4700–4706 (2020)
20. Skeppstedt, M., Kvist, M., Nilsson, G.H., Dalianis, H.: Automatic recognition of disorders, findings, pharmaceuticals and body structures from clinical text: an annotation and machine learning study. J. Biomed. Inform. **49**, 148–158 (2014)

21. Tai, W., Kung, H., Dong, X.L., Comiter, M., Kuo, C.F.: exBERT: extending pre-trained models with domain-specific vocabulary under constrained training resources. In: Proceedings of the 2020 Conference on Empirical Methods in Natural Language Processing: Findings, pp. 1433–1439 (2020)
22. Velupillai, S.: Automatic classification of factuality levels: a case study on Swedish diagnoses and the impact of local context. In: Fourth International Symposium on Languages in Biology and Medicine, LBM 2011 (2011)
23. Velupillai, S., Dalianis, H., Kvist, M.: Factuality levels of diagnoses in Swedish clinical text. In: User Centred Networked Health Care, pp. 559–563. IOS Press (2011)
24. Verkijk, S., Vossen, P.: MedRoBERTa.nl: a language model for Dutch electronic health records. Comput. Linguist. Neth. J. **11**, 141–159 (2021)
25. Winter, B., Figueroa, A., Löser, A., Gers, F.A., Siu, A.: KIMERA: injecting domain knowledge into vacant transformer heads, pp. 363–373 (2022)
26. Wu, Y., et al.: Google's neural machine translation system: bridging the gap between human and machine translation. arXiv preprint arXiv:1609.08144 (2016)

A Systematic Literature Review of Extended Reality Exercise Games for the Elderly

Yu Fu[1]([⊠])[iD], Yan Hu[1][iD], Veronica Sundstedt[1][iD], and Yvonne Forsell[2][iD]

[1] Blekinge Institute of Technology, 371 79 Karlskrona, Sweden
{yu.fu,yan.hu,veronica.sundstedt}@bth.se
[2] Karolinska Institutet, 171 77 Stockholm, Sweden
yvonne.forsell@ki.se

Abstract. In recent years, with the rise of the ageing population worldwide, the health of the elderly has attracted increasing attention. This study explored existing extended reality (XR) game applications aiming at physical exercise for the elderly. Through the review of 1847 papers from the Scopus database, 17 articles were included. Based on these papers, we explored the existing contributions of exercise XR games for the elderly, the development opportunities and challenges of such games, and their special considerations in adapting to the characteristics and requirements of the target user. The results were organized into several perspectives: publication information and keywords, immersive technologies and game concepts, teamwork and social games, evaluation, opportunities and challenges, and adapting designs. We found the elderly interested in and accepted using XR games. The reported research results proved positive effects on such games' physical and mental health. XR exercise games for the elderly should considerably adapt to the elder's cognition, behaviour, and demand. Although problems existed, such as simulator sickness, safety risks, device problems, and cost, there were opportunities and space for research and future developments. Researchers and developers could refer to this paper for XR exercise games for the elderly and create or enhance future XR applications by learning from existing work.

Keywords: Virtual reality · Augmented reality · Mixed reality · Extended reality · Game · Physical training · Exercise · Elderly · Old people · Health

1 Introduction

There is an increasingly serious ageing problem all over the world. The ageing and health report from the WHO pointed out that as people live longer, more and more ageing populations are burdened by all countries [64]. They predicted people aged over 60 years populations will be one out of every six people in the world range by 2030. By 2050, the number was expected to be 2.1 billion. With the ageing problem, there are many challenges for society and families, especially in terms of the health challenges faced by the elderly, such as the presence of musculoskeletal pain, diabetes, depression, and dementia. This challenge is not only in individual diseases but also in multimorbidity. In order to take up the challenges, the WHO recommend changing lifestyle factors,

A. C. A. Roque et al. (Eds.): BIOSTEC 2022, CCIS 1814, pp. 333–352, 2023.
https://doi.org/10.1007/978-3-031-38854-5_17

such as increased regular physical exercise and training, which could directly or indirectly improve physical and mental health [64].

According to the "Active Ageing A Policy Framework" by WHO, active ageing not only means expectancy extending a healthy life but also the quality of life for all people. One of the key goals of active ageing is maintaining independence. To achieve the aim, the activities of daily living (ADL) function need to be sufficient [63]. Compelling evidence from longitudinal observational studies proves that the risk of declining ADL could be decreased by sufficient levels of physical activity [13,16,43]. Another term often used is frailty [17]. It has many definitions; however, they all include a decrease in physical function or independence [13,19]. Evidence was also sufficient that physical exercise has a positive effect for the frail elderly [8], such as supporting cognitive functions [61] and reducing effects on the ageing brain [13]. Evidence was limited on what kind of physical exercise would be the most effective. The observational studies included various activities for the elderly health, such as cycling, dancing, and walking. The various types of exercise programs were also used in intervention studies [45]. However, most physiotherapists recommended the combination of strength and aerobic exercises.

	Mixed Reality (MR)			
Real world	Augmented Reality (AR)	Augmented Virtuality (AV)	Virtual Reality (VR)	Extended Reality (XR)

Fig. 1. The relationship of AR/VR/AV/MR technique [47].

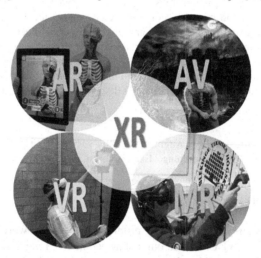

Fig. 2. Examples of AR/VR/AV/MR/XR techniques.

'Game' is one of the keywords of this paper, which is defined by Juul as a rule-based formal system with a variable and quantifiable outcome, where different outcomes assigned different values. Players exert effort in order to influence the outcome and feel attached to the outcome [35].

The in-home exercise was often done by a treadmill or bicycle. However, poor health conditions, lack of company [49] and varied stimuli in the surrounding could previously decline the rate of exercise [39]. The digital game was proven beneficial for engagement and motivation through providing a fun and plentiful user experience [18]. Digital games could also support the aims and tasks with a serious propose, such as training and exercise [18,57]. Such games are also referred to as serious games, not only for entertainment, but also for meaningful activities, for example, training, education, and treatment [20]. Serious games have game attributes; and are more easily accepted as well as used more continuously than non-game concepts, to achieve serious aims [65]. Moreover, Deterding et al. summarised relevant studies and developments, and they pointed out the other commonly used concept: "gamification", which refers to the design of elements characteristic for games in non-game contexts [18].

Except for "elderly", "health", "exercise", and "game", immersive techniques are included in the keywords of this study. According to Milgram and Kishino's study of the real to the virtual [47], we adopted their description as shown in Fig. 1. Extended reality (XR) is a collection of immersive technologies (including augmented reality/virtual reality/mixed reality), referring to all virtual technologies generated by computers [15], as shown in Fig. 2. The mixed reality (MR, or hybrid reality) merges the natural world and immersive techniques. In a sense, the relationship from left to right in Fig. 1 is the transition from reality to virtual reality (VR), diminishing the real objects' composition, and increasing virtual objects progressively. There are no digital objects in the real environment; augmented reality (AR) adds digital objects to the real environment; augmented virtuality (AV) is the opposite, adding real objects to a virtual world, which could be seen as the complement set of AR to a certain extent. VR has the highest proportion of digital objects, which simulates a virtual world completely; in other words, all objects are computer-generated [59]. Especially in head-mounted displays (HMDs), VR cuts off the perception of the real environment. Audible, visual and interactive objects are all computer-presented [59].

Some previous work showed that XR games could benefit mental and physical health [66]. XR games were thought popular due to their unique immersive experience [53]. While XR games were widely concerned, expectations and opportunities of XR technology were not only on digital games. Except for games and entertainment, the industry practitioners believed healthcare had once again become the top application field of the most easily subverted by XR techniques (34% in 2020, 38% in 2021), pointed out by the XR industry insider survey by Perkin Coie LLP and XR Association (2021) [53]. The report claimed that due to the COVID-19 pandemic's effect, people stayed at home for several months; it strengthened the prospects of XR techniques, especially in the healthcare and education fields [53]. Moreover, consumers' experience online and virtually was more comfortable, which means the potential trend and more feasibility of XR games providing solutions for elders' physical health.

Thus, this study aims to explore XR games for elderly physical exercise and training. Through the literature review of such existing games in academic research, we could summarise the games' characteristics and attributes, opportunities and challenges, user attitudes, and the functions, features or other designs adapted to elderly users. This study included papers paying attention to physical exercise and training and excluded articles with the background motivation on physical training for a particular disease. In other words, this paper excluded the XR game applications that aim at rehabilitation/treatment/prevention of certain diseases (such as stroke, Alzheimer's disease, and cognition training). To address the research aim, this study was conducted with the following three research questions:

- RQ1: What existing research contributions on XR game applications target elderly physical health training?
- RQ2: What are the opportunities and challenges on XR game applications for elderly physical health training?
- RQ3: What are the design principles and adapted considerations for XR exercise games for elderly users?

This paper is an extended version of our previous study, "A Review of Extended Reality Exercise Games for Elderly" [24], published at the 15th International Joint Conference on Biomedical Engineering Systems and Technologies (BIOSTEC-2022). Both papers have the same overall research topic, but with an additional research question (RQ3), an extended time range in the retrieval, and a different analysis view (Sect. 4.6 Adapting design) presented in this work. The previous results were also restructured and revised.

The rest of this paper is structured as follows. Relevant research were summarised in Sect. 2. Section 3 illustrates the retrieval process of the systematic literature review. Section 4 describes the review result in six parts: publication information and keywords, immersive technologies and game concepts, teamwork and social games, evaluation, advantages and disadvantages, as well as the special design guidelines and considerations adapted to the elderly. Section 5 discusses the results with relevant works, and Sect. 6 presents the conclusions and future work.

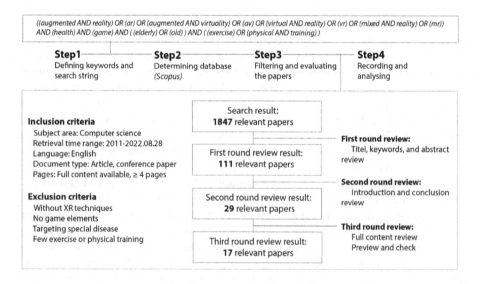

Fig. 3. Publication retrieval process.

2   Related Work

In our previous literature review of the XR game applications in healthcare, we reviewed 3793 papers from six databases [22]. Of the 88 included papers, 16 mentioned that the elderly were the target user. XR games aiming for mental and psychological treatment or prevention (9) were more frequent than those for physical health (7). Fall prevention training (3) and cognitive training (5) were the top topics. Ten included papers did not define the end-user age group, but the elderly are a high-risk group for the diseases they target, such as Type 2 diabetes, Parkinson's and Post-stroke rehabilitation. In total, the XR games that were relevant to elderly users were 24 (27%). However, the difference between the proportion of mental health (11) and physical health (13) was insignificant.

Miller et al. conducted a systematic review (2000.01.01 to 2012.07.10), aimed at older adults (over 45 years), to explore the effectiveness of VR/gaming systems for in-home physical activity, as well as evidence supporting its feasibility. Their review result of 17 included articles found there was weak evidence and a high risk of bias to support the effectiveness and feasibility of how VR/gaming could address impairments, as well as limitations of activity and participation [48]. Moreover, they pointed out the issues affecting feasibility, such as the high dependence on training and assistance, acceptability problems, safety problems, high cost, etc. In addition, they claimed the higher function required for safely using VR game activities at home; and users had higher dependence on training and assistance at the beginning of use. They concluded that VR games encourage motivation and social engagement. Furthermore, they discussed technique costs for developers and end-users and believed the development trend of devices would be towards more sophisticated motion-sensing equipment [48].

Campo-Prieto et al. also conducted a literature review of VR games for the elderly, focusing on immersive VR (IVR) applied in physical therapy and rehabilitation. Their 11 included papers were filtered from the 765 publications before 2019.06 in four medical science databases. They indicated few VR games for elderly health. Among them, most research paid attention to the acceptability and usage analysis of immersive techniques, such as VR headsets and their simulator sickness [10]. Moreover, they used the Simulator Sickness Questionnaire (SSQ), Self-Assessment of Communication (SAC), or System Usability Scale (SUS) to evaluate, and the blood pressure and heart rate monitor for increasing accuracy in the applications' protocols, in the included papers [10]. They believed the differences between VR and IVR in the literature were not significant, but more IVR was used in physical therapy [10]. HMDs of the Oculus Rift, HTC Vive, Meta Quest, and Samsung Gear VR headset were the most common [10]. The exergame device combinations with VR were applied more often, such as a bike or treadmill [10]. Campo-Prieto et al. believed therapists and developers should work together to achieve the requirements of the target users and enhance the attractiveness of user experiences [10]. They highlighted the challenges of VR games for the elderly as well, including device problems and content improvements [10]. Despite these challenges, they believed IVR could help with traditional treatment and rehabilitation through encouragement and fun [10].

3   Systematic Literature Review

To address the research questions, we explored existing contributions of academic studies in XR exercise and training games targeting elderly physical health (RQ1), the opportunities and challenges of features or attributes of such XR exercise games (RQ2), as well as the special designs to adapt the characteristics and requirements of the elderly (RQ3). This study followed the four steps of the retrieval process in the guidelines of Keele et al. [37]: 1) defining keywords and search string, 2) determining the database, 3) filtering and evaluating the papers, and 4) recording and analysing. We conducted this systematic literature review using the Scopus database. According to the keywords of this paper (virtual reality, augmented reality, mixed reality, extended reality, game, physical training, elderly, old people, health) and their abbreviations (AR/VR/MR) and related words like (old), we generated the search string: "((augmented AND reality) OR (ar) OR (augmented AND virtuality) OR (av) OR (virtual AND reality) OR (vr) OR (mixed AND reality) OR (mr)) AND (health) AND (game) AND ((elderly) OR (old)) AND ((exercise) OR (physical AND training))" for the paper retrieval process.

As shown in Fig. 3, the search results were limited to the publication years (2011-01-01 to 2022-08-28), using language (English), and document type (journal article and conference paper). We excluded the papers which equal to or less than four pages, or without being available as full text online (based on databases access right in the library of the Blekinge Institute of Technology). Moreover, according to the UN convention, referring to the elderly was an age over 60-year-old [38]. In some other research in countries and territories with shorter life expectancy, the age could be narrowed to 55-year-old [21]. To cover more research, we used 55-year-old as the criteria baseline for the elderly and excluded studies targeting younger people.

The review of the title, keywords and abstract was the first round review. It narrowed down the search results from 1847 to 111. The following second round review was mainly focused on the introduction and conclusions sections and excluded 82 of 111 based on the exclusion criteria. Finally, the remaining 29 papers were previewed, reviewed, and checked in the third round review in full content. Seventeen of them matched all inclusion criteria, as the included papers for this review study were analysed further. As previously mentioned above, this study only focuses on the research targeting "pure" exercise and physical training for the elderly. Papers relevant to treatment/prevention/rehabilitation of specific diseases and health issues were excluded (such as stroke, fall, dementia, Parkinson's disease, cognitive training, memory training, and Alzheimer's disease). Moreover, some paper search results were also excluded in the second or third round review due to not mentioning XR techniques (7), being without game elements (1), had less than four pages (1), or the full content was not available (6).

4   Results

Based on the 17 included papers, we analysed the reviewed research and answered the research questions. There were four included papers [1,52], [5,28] which came from two projects, respectively, with different research content. Thus, we treated them as four individual studies in the analysis. To address the research questions about contributions of the academic studies of XR game applications for elderly exercise and physical training (RQ1), opportunities and challenges of such game applications (RQ2), and adapting designs for the elderly (RQ3), we analysed the included papers in six areas as previously mentioned. These were: 1) publication information and keywords, 2) immersive technologies and game concepts, 3) teamwork and social games, 4) opportunities and challenges, 5) evaluation, and 6) adapting designs for elderly users.

4.1 Publication Information and Keywords

All included papers came from 2016 to 2022. The included studies in 2021 were the highest and reached four papers; the following were three in 2020 and 2022; two each in 2016, 2019, and 2018; and only one published in 2017. The authors of these 17 papers involved 14 countries and regions. More than 65% (11/17) of the included papers are research institutions from Europe and the USA (Spain, Norway, Sweden, Denmark, US., Italy, Germany, Netherlands), followed by Asian countries and regions (South Korea, Brazil, Japan, China, Hong Kong China, Australia). Moreover, South Korea, Norway, Denmark, Italy, and Brazil have more than one paper included in this study.

Almost all 17 included papers were conducted by academic researchers; they usually came from different departments, such as medical subjects (neurology, health sciences, psychology, geriatrics, etc.), computer and engineering subjects (electronic information, ICT and natural sciences, industrial technology and automation, etc.), and media and communication subjects. Only two studies involved authors from a hospital or nursing home, and one study mentioned software developers.

The included papers mentioned 73 keywords which could be grouped into four classes: computer science (including AR/VR/MR and simulation/immersive, hardware, user, evaluation), medical science (including task and activity), game, and others. The top three were elderly and related words (8), virtual reality (8), exergame (4), and exercise (4). In addition, we could see virtual reality (exposure) therapy, augmented reality, and user experience in the computer science groups with more than a one-time frequency. In the medical science group, it was ageing, rehabilitation, and physical activity. Even if the included paper was purely targeting elderly exercise and physical training, there were still keywords relevant to diseases, such as fall prevention, physical balance, COVID-19, and rehabilitation. It is worth noting that social and multi-user relevant words were mentioned in the included papers, such as collaboration, competition, and social media.

4.2 Immersive Technologies and Game Concepts

As shown in Table 1 and 1, more than 59% (10/17) of the included studies used VR techniques. Three of them created a non-immersive VR environment by applying the large screen and other equipment. Only one involved using a CAVE (cave automatic virtual environment), while the other six studies achieved the IVR experience by HMDs. About the AR technique, three articles mentioned the Kinect, while a VR paper also used the Kinect. The MR-based study only included one with the HoloLens. In the same project, the authors transformed and updated their display device from a CAVE [52] to a large screen [1].

Table 1. The analysis of the included papers based on technology, game, and evaluation viewpoints.

		1 [12]	2 [44]	3 [56]	4 [31]	5 [28]	6 [52]	7 [40]	8 [1]	9 [5]
Technology	Technique	VR	VR	VR	VR	VR	VR	VR	VR	VR
	Display	HMD				HMD/TV	CAVE	TV (curved screen)	Big screen	TV
	Controlling/interaction device	null	Hand controller, Ankle controller	null	null	WiFi microcontroller (on pedal)	Hardware interface	Hardware interface	Hardware interface	null
	Tracker/Sensor	Limb motion trackers	null	null	Speed sensor	null	Cycle-ergometer/Arduino/motion tracking system,	Arduino/hall effect sensor (on chassis)/inertial sensor (on headset)	Arduino, cycle-ergometer	Arduino
Game	Use posture	Sitting	Stand	Sitting						
	Use type	Single							Single/multiple	Single
	Game genre	Simulation	Action game	Simulation						
	Activity/Task	Handball/football/gate-keeping	Change action by different shape and color/feed animals	Cycling						
Evaluation	Participants number	135	20	20	null		5	5	null	24
	Age group	62.7	≥65	63.6			≥59	≥65		null
	Method	Experiment/questionnaire	Experiment/questionnaire				Experiment/questionnaire	Experiment/questionnaire		Experiment/questionnaire
	Quality index	Usefulness/user experience	Usefulness/user experience				Usability	Usability/acceptability		User experience
	Standard scale	null	Player Experience (PX)	Stress arousal checklist(SAC)/Simulator sickness questionnaire (SSQ)/ITC sense of presence inventory (ITC-SOPI)/Borg rate of perceived exertion scale(RPE)			System usability scale (SUS)	SUS/SSQ		Intrinsic Motivation Inventory (IMI)

(continued)

Table 1. (*continued*)

		10 [34]	11 [50]	12 [33]	13 [51]	14 [6]	15 [25]	16 [36]	17 [58]
Technology	Technique	VR	AR	AR	AR	MR	VR	VR	VR
	Display	null	null	Screen		HoloLens	HMD	null	
	Controlling/interaction device	Kinect					Hand controller		
	Tracker/Sensor					null	Motion sensor		
Game	Use posture	Stand					Sitting/stand	Sitting	Stand
	Use type	Single/multiple	Single	Single/multiple	Single	Multiple	Single/multiple	Single/multiple	Single/multiple
	Game genre	Simulation		Action game	Adventure	Shooting	Simulation		
	Activity/Task	Bowling	Put bird into cage	Imitate actions	Island adventure	Shooting rabbit	Rowing/shooting/water surfing/fishing/recalling objects	Collecting/avoiding bubbles	Grabing/moving objects
Evaluation	Participants number	19	57	27	3	null	null	38	10
	Age group	68	≥65	≥65	43–62			41.5–84.33	64–82
	Method	Experiment/questionnaire	Experiment/questionnaire		Experiment and interview	Experiment and interview		Experiment/observation and field notes/interviews	Experiment/questionnaire/interview/field observation
	Quality index	Usafulness/user experience	Usability/usability/acceptability	Usafulness/user experience	Usafulness/user experience	User experience		User experience	Acceptability/user experience
	Standard scale	Physical Exercise Adherence Questionnaire/Game Experience Questionnaire (GEQ)	SUS/Usefulness/Satisfaction/Ease of Use/Happiness/Importance	Exercise Self-Efficacy Scale (ESE)	null	Game experience questionnaire (GEQ)		null	null

[1] In the "Age" column, the unit is the year; numbers without signs and intervals represent the average.
[2] In the Table, "null" means did not mention such information in the papers.

The indoor bike was the most common sport, which used a hardware user interface on a stationary bike to interact with users [40,52]. Sensors were also used on the stationary bike, such as speed sensor [31], Hall effect sensor, and inertial sensors [40]. It is worth noting that two indoor cycling games mentioned heart rate detection. Sakhare et al. used the Borg rate of perceived exertion (RPE) scale and heart rate to calculate the exercise intensity [56], while Arlati et al. used the heart rate to adjust the bicycle ergometer, thereby maintaining a constant level of effort [1].

The Kinect was mainly used in AR games to capture motion, interact, and control systems as the motion sensor and way to interact. One paper [44] used two hands and two wearable ankle controllers to detect hand and ankle movements, while Yu et al. only proposed to use hand controllers [25]. Moreover, the WiFi microcontroller was mentioned in one of the indoor cycling games on the pedal of the stationary bike [28]. The HoloLens was both the display device and the interaction device by capturing and recognizing the gesture for the MR study [8]. In addition, the 12 XR games which mentioned developing software were all created using Unity.

From the viewpoint of game genres and tasks, the 17 included papers had overlap to some extent. Seven studies used an indoor bike as their game content. The simulation game was the most common game genre, not only for cycling games but also for other game content, such as bowling [34] and rowing game [25]. Although this study's scope is the "pure" XR exercise games for the elderly, some included papers combined physical training with mental training tasks named "double tasks". For example, Arlati et al. asked users to find animals along the way whose names started with a particular letter [1] and guess the city name based on the landmarks. The study by Munoz et al. also used animals as the game objects [50]. Their XR game could train the shoulders by asking players to raise their arms and put birds into a cage [50]. Chau et al. created a set of VR games facing a different group of users [12]. They covered physical training with ball games (such as handball for upper limbs and football for lower limbs) [12].

Game genres of the included papers also covered action, adventure, and shooter games. The VR game developed by Li et al. aimed to impact the cognitive and physical health of the elderly [44]. Users were asked to change posture and location by following different shapes/colours of objects. Jeon and Kim's game was an action game for elderly exercise, which asked users to follow the non-player character's actions and achieve the aim of physical training [33]. Nishchyk et al. created an adventure AR game according to a story on an island with a pirate, parrot, and treasure chests [51]. The physical exercise revolved around treasure hunting (including climbing stairs and "flying" by controlling the parrot). Moreover, Buckers et al. used shooting rabbits as the game task to exercise the whole body [6].

In the included papers, using posture in sitting or standing had equal amounts, which was dependent on the game tasks. For example, the cycling games used a sitting position, while the bowling game or the action following game used a standing position. However, there was a game aiming at the upper limbs exercise but used a standing posture [50]. Chau et al. pointed out that the training intensity of the sitting playing position was not sufficient to improve functional mobility [12]. Moreover, rewards, avatars, and points were game elements used in the included papers. Among them, the points element was the most commonly used.

4.3 Teamwork and Social Games

The work by Júnior et al. presented an XR exercise game for the elderly, and explored the team member user or a single user difference in fitness tests, physical exercise adherence, and game experience before, between, and after use [34]. They pointed out that the results of the physical fitness test increased significantly in the team-playing scenario [34]. The score for sensory and imaginative immersion was higher in the team. Teammates could also provide support when players felt sad/pain/difficulties to help them continue training. Moreover, Arlati et al. provided a social VR bike game [1], which allowed users to train with other players. In multiplayer mode, users had voice contact, training collaboratively, or competitively with others [1,25,36]. It could help with physical health and reduce the risk of social isolation as well [1]. Furthermore, Buckers et al. presented a virtual dodgeball game in which two users could play together and shoot balls at the rabbit target [6]. They thought this multi-user game was more attractive and engaging [6]. It is worth noting that the multiple-user game usually operates online, while the single-user game typically uses offline mode. However, there were exceptions: a single-user game could connect with the web client [50], while a multiple-user game could identify two users in offline mode [33].

4.4 Evaluation

From the viewpoint of evaluation, except for the four included papers, which did not mention assessment, the main evaluation method was combining an experiment and questionnaires. The effectiveness and usefulness were studied by comparing the before and after use health situation or obtaining satisfaction in subjective user feedback at the end of the experiment. As shown in Table 1 and 1, the standardized scales were the most common questionnaire tool. Usability, simulator sickness, and game/player experience obtained the most attention from the included papers. Moreover, the number of participants ranged from 3 to 135. They were usually classified as experiment and control groups randomly. However, studies aimed to compare the differences between age groups and divided the respondents by age (elderly vs. younger) [56]. Unlike other research, Karaosmanoglu et al. conducted eight session tests with different themes and interviewees, which included the ordinary elderly, the older adults with dementia, physiotherapists, healthcare professional, and trainer, and the topic covered the game task, user study, social value, etc. [36].

4.5 Opportunities and Challenges

The evaluation results of the included papers showed that an overall attitude toward XR games for the elderly physical health and exercise training was positive. However, there were still some problems reported to be addressed in the future. Some studies claimed the elderly may have a negative tendency toward new technologies [29,41]. However, the evaluation results from the included papers were on the opposite positive. Sakhare et al. pointed out that age did not significantly influence the feasibility of using VR for the elderly [56]. Even during the experiment, the most receptive were the oldest (75–80) [50]. Positive comments also included the high levels of learnability and ease and confidence in use [40] of the elderly when they use VR techniques. There were interesting and engaging [51], innovative, fun, exciting, and interactive [12], and benefiting physical and mental health as well [33,34,44,50].

Challenges could be grouped into three categories: simulator sickness, device problems, and content improvement. Three included articles that used SSQ achieved similar results: symptoms such as dizziness, nausea, and disorientation during use, but all mild and acceptable [12,40,56]. Sakhare et al. thought use time was the significant effect factor of simulator sickness, not age [56]. Chau et al. also supported this view. They indicated that over 50% of the simulator sickness reports come from the first four times of use [12]. The research by Lee et al. listed both the simulator sickness problems and some solutions, such as limiting and reducing the viewing range and content amount, using active instead of passive VR experiences and more realistic VR photography technology, stabilizing the viewpoints, as well as displaying on curved TVs instead of a HMD [40].

The problems of devices were mainly focused on HMD and controller/sensor's low user experience. Chau et al. reported the HMD would be more portable, and the sensor would be unnecessary for upright operation [12]. The studies from Lee et al. and Li et al. obtained negative user feedback on VR headsets [40,44]. These feedback were a bit heavy weight from the HMDs for users [36,44], disorientation due to the head pressure [40], and improper wearing easily leading to mistakes [44].

The comments on improved content were not as much as the above two problems and were usually specific to the different applications. Chau et al. advised improving the scoring system to improve the sense of accomplishment and enrich the personalized scoring [12]. The study by Arlati et al. also pointed out similar enhancement requirements in rewards for the application design; increasing the value rewards to add motivation and enjoyment [1]. Moreover, their study found that game content linked with full of users' memories (such as familiar scenes to the users) was more popular [12]. Júnior et al. believed avatars in games as stimulus could increase participation [34]. In addition, Nishchyk et al. pointed out that feedback was necessary when the player made mistakes, as well as a skip feature for jumping the background video story [51]. Improving the sense of reality was raised repeatedly by the respondents [5]. Similar comments were also from Pedroli et al., such as increasing objects' identification, reducing interference, enhancing realism, and improving proactive interaction [52]. The content enhancements were not common comments and were usually specific to the application. Karaosmanoglu et al. conducted eight prototyping sessions and interviews in different version iterations to optimize the game. The results of these sessions and interviews indicated that game object properties need to be improved in size, speed, height, difficulty, etc. [36]. Their content also improved by removing the cumbersome game flow, slowing the tutorial, and avoiding providing too much information. Last but not least, they commented on a safety issue, the movements based on game content probably had too wide crossing activity which inclinations to fall [36].

4.6   Adapting Design

Colder et al. pointed out that a considerable part of the existing sports games is aimed at general users of commercial games. They are usually not especially designed or adapted for the elderly [14]. Such games are not the best solution for elderly to do exercise [30]. Pisan et al. agreed with it; they claimed most of the exercise games were commercial and not designed for the elderly physical training [54]. They had limitations, such as a lack of usability and accessibility for users with low technology tolerance and low safety levels [54]. To summarise, there is a lack of exercise games designed and developed for the elderly in particular [51]; sports training games should match the performance level and aims of their target users [30].

Based on the included reviewed papers, the XR exercise games aimed at the elderly users, they have mentioned several considerations in the design process and product to adapt to the characteristics and requirements of the target user group.

From the viewpoint of design, Yu et al. presented a conceptual design of a VR rowing game for the elderly [25], which used Hunicke et al.' MDA framework (standing for Mechanics, Dynamics, and Aesthetics) and is based on the design principles of exercise games [9] and human-computer interaction for seniors [42]. To match the elderly target users, they proposed several adapting design: 1) simplify the equipment and operations to reduce the use complexity, 2) set up different activities and tasks to fit different health conditions and target exercise body parts, 3) provided roles and modes variously to motivate the elderly users, and 4) presented the UI design that matched the elderly' preferences (such as simple layout, simple terminology, and clear and straightforward navigation paths and type-specific help) [25].

Jorge et al. invited the elderly to design and develop together [34]. In this way, they could understand the motivation of the elderly using exercise games, adjust the game mechanics to optimize persistence and enjoyment of the game and test functional abilities/motivation/persistence to the exercise game, based on first-hand data from the end users. The elderly also contributed to selecting and confirming game types and sports. At the same time, by taking part in the development process, end users could see their suggestions adopted before the game goes live and feel valued in the development process [3,4]. Nishchyk et al. also mentioned the importance of including the end users in the development process [51]. They used the user-centered method in the design to obtain the needs of potential users, a deeper understanding of their faced problems, and help articulate how to generate a product where they could benefit the most [11]. Moreover, after each iteration of the design and development, they conducted user evaluations to identify problems and confirm the quality [51].

From the viewpoint of game content, several included papers mentioned it should be based on the physical and psychological characteristics of the elderly [40], for example, the interface [51] and navigation [12]. Munoz et al. believed graphical user interface elements and workflows were designed with the sensory, physical, and technical lack of the elderly in mind [50]. They also thought graphical elements, such as avatars, could help make the system easier to understand and enjoy for the elderly users [50]. Furthermore, the exercise program content adapted to older people was considered by Nishchyk et al. They chose the low-intensity resistance training program with slow movement (LST method) proposed by Ishii [62] (recommended by The National Health Service, the publicly funded healthcare system of the United Kingdom). It was claimed that the LST method increases muscle mass and strength, could help reduce some possible injuries, and be safe and effective for the elderly [62]. The indisputable fact is mental and physical health could affect each other [26]. Based on this interplay, "Double tasks (DT)" and "Social" were considered in some XR games in the included papers. In the physical exercise, they added mental training or communication with other users at the same time. Cadore et al. and Inokuchi et al. pointed out DT had been suggested as a more effective method to improve cognitive and motor performance [7,32]. Moreover, due to the more positive statements related to playing with the peer group, social interaction was one of the main motivations leading the elderly to use exercise games [27,46,60]. Thus, some included papers designed the communication function in their XR games to increase engagement in exercise and benefit mental health [1,34,52].

From the viewpoint of hardware, the adapting for elderly were mainly on two points: ease of use and safety. Lee et al. thought the immersive devices on the market were not easy to use for the elderly; the functionality of the hardware interface should be minimized and designed to be easy for the user to operate [40]. On the other hand, Lee et al. [40], and Sakhare et al. [56] paid attention to simulation sickness. They believed that compared with younger adults, the elderly were more likely to experience severe side effects during immersive experiences using HMDs, due to age-related sensory processing degradation [2,55]. They solved the problem using a similar strategy: replacing HMDs with curved TVs, desktop monitors, and projector screens.

Finally, the interaction method was considered in several included papers to adapt elderly characteristics and requirements. Interaction design with new technologies based on older adults' experiences of interacting in the real world makes it easier to apply their existing skills and skills to new areas, as pointed out by Zhang et al. [67]. The XR exercise game by Junior et al. followed three design principles from Zhang et al.: 1) the representation should be as similar as possible to the real world to help the elderly understand the games, 2) the manipulation should show how the elderly manipulate objects in motor games, 3) the design should be meaningful, including memory and emotion [67]. According to the principles, Junior et al. proposed a bowling XR game familiar to the elderly, which was specially designed in a controlling way for the elderly based on body movement [34]. A similar design idea was shown in the work by Munoz et al.. They preferred more natural and intuitive interaction techniques, such as recognition of gesture [50]. It was designed to simplify the use of the system by the elderly with poor technical skills [50]. In their future design, biometric identification via facial or voice recognition was mentioned to reduce the burden of the user logging in [50].

Moreover, in the XR exercise game by Chau et al., they noticed reaction time and motion sensitivity issues. They thought the elderly commonly have longer response times and cannot use buttons to operate controls due to their weaker fine motor skills [12]. Thus, the game by Pui et al. used a loose tolerance range tailored to the elderly motion detection sensitivity for evaluating motion correction during exercise performance to compensate for limited motor skills in older adults [12,50]. Buttonless limb movement trackers allowed users to engage in the game with simple limb movements without relying on fine motor controls [12]. In addition, Pui et al. used the seated position in their XR exercise game to ensure the safety of the elderly [12]. Without moving or bending forward, and reducing agile body and head movements, thereby this game decreased simulation sickness, such as vertigo and nausea for the elderly. At the same time, their game allowed the standing use posture and playing with one or more limbs to suit different users [12].

5   Discussion

This study's results were similar to the consequences of related studies [23,66]: there was increased attention to XR game applications for the physical health of the elderly. Even though all included papers in this review were published after 2015, the rise in the academic study was obvious in the following years. Significantly, the included papers in 2021 doubled compared to 2018 and 2019; in the first three quarters of 2022 had exceeded every single full year in 2016–2019 and equal to 2020. In addition, judging from the data from the researchers and organisations, the number of studies on such applications in Europe and the United States had apparent more. Especially, South Korea, Norway, and Denmark had two included papers. Furthermore, since such applications are interdisciplinary, the researchers' academic background was mainly computer and engineering, but it tended to involve other subjects, such as media and communication and medical science.

Different immersive techniques did not have equal attention. Only one paper aimed at the augmented virtuality exercise game for the elderly in the search result but was excluded due to that it targeted the health problem belonging to mental health. In addition, the VR technique had more focus than AR/MR. Particularly, the HMD VR contributed to the most existing solutions for elderly physical exercise games. Although, IVR had the most attention and HMD was the most used display device. There were still three included papers using the screen as the display in non-immersive VR, based on the consideration of safety, experience, and cost. As mentioned in the results, the replacement of the CAVE to the screen was also for this consideration.

From the viewpoint of the attributes and characteristics of the elderly, some existing studies presented the considerations in the design and development, game content, hardware, and interaction methods. Regardless of which adapting designs, the design core of those included papers tries to match the physiological or psychological changes brought about by ageing. However, some viewpoints were clear, such as the exercise intensity, reaction time, and exercise sensitivity of the elderly are commonly lower than in other age groups; they prefer natural, direct, simplified interaction; and higher requirement of hardware safety and easy to use. However, the preference for the sitting and standing posture was not. In the included papers, they were equal in amounts. Both had positive and negative outcomes; more safety with the sitting posture for users and more exercise effectiveness with the standing posture.

From the viewpoint of gamification, we obtained similar conclusions to the related work [10,48], that applying gamification techniques and game elements aimed to increase the fun and interest, motivate the use of the applications, and achieve the exercise goals. According to the review results, the interaction and control of XR exercise games for the elderly should be simple and directed to the target users. Thus, a development trend could be less equipment, an easier interface, and a better experience.

Even if this paper targeted specifically the elderly physical health, it is undeniable that physical and mental health affect each other. The research by Sauvé et al. suggested the effect of digital games on the elderly to cover three dimensions of quality of life: 1) psychological, 2) physical, and 3) social [57]. So, the other development trend could be "double tasks"; in other words, matching the requirements of both physical and mental health issues in an XR game. Some authors design their exercise XR games with mental training activities and tasks [1,52] or with benefits for memory, cognition and attention [44]. The existing studies also mentioned another term, which was social games. Some other researchers added the multi-user mode in their games to approve teamwork and social interaction [1,34], which was beneficial for mental health.

For the opportunities of XR game exercise for the elderly, there was evidence of acceptance of those techniques by the elderly. They have positive attitudes towards such techniques applied for their physical health improvements. The evidence of the effectiveness of VR exercise games was also proven acceptable. However, due to the limitations of this review paper on the database, published year, and search string, we could not say the review result represents all elderly attitudes. A more universal result could be obtained by extending the study in the future. According to our earlier survey [23], the three largest obstacles to mass adoption were user experience, content offering, and cost to the consumers. What needed attention in the research and development of such games was a more straightforward operation in the design, fixing the challenges of simulator sickness and content, clear training of use for users, and device improvements.

Some included papers conducted an user evaluation, focusing on the simulator sickness after using their games and obtaining acceptable test results [12]. Many of them stood on prevention standpoints in the design and implementation stages, and a few studies also focused on how to avoid being uncomfortable, such as Lee et al. propose to stabilize the viewpoints, decrease the viewing range, etc., to reduce VR dizziness [40]. Moreover, the fact that with the increase in use time, it was proven that the uncomfortable symptoms were reduced [56]. Thus, simulator sickness might not be avoided but could be under control. The comments for content improvement were the most detailed and specific. Except for the advice about in-time feedback, rewards, avatars, and shared memory, user participation in the design and evaluation should be noted. The VR experience was more dependent on the device than the AR experience. Thus, the comments of HMDs were mentioned most in device-relevant comments, which outcome is similar to our previous surveys: the uncomfortable weight and cables and low experience of HMDs [23,66].

6 Conclusions and Future Work

Aiming to review the contributions from existing research about XR exercise game applications targeting the elderly, its opportunities and challenges in academic study and development, as well as the adapting design for the elderly, this study conducted a systematic literature review in the Scopus database. From the 1847 search results, 17 papers were filtered and included for deeper analysis, by three rounds of review.

Analysing the included papers from six different perspectives, we found the development of XR exercise games for the elderly in the recent 12 years. It includes segmenting the elderly as an independent target user group, designing games that match their characteristics and needs, researching their adaptability and acceptance of immersive technologies, improving hardware and software to reduce safety risks and discomfort, and innovating in functionality and technology.

The elderly, as a vulnerable group, need to be more considered their characteristics and vision in the future of XR exercise games for them. Future work could fully use the advantages of gamification and immersion technology, and integrate them with the content, thereby improving the motivation and interest of use to help the elderly maintain a healthy mind and body. At the same time, the continuous development of new technologies requires future research and development to focus on the new challenges and risks that come with them.

Acknowledgement. This research was funded partly by the Knowledge Foundation, Sweden, through the Human-Centered Intelligent Realities (HINTS) Profile Project (contract 20220068).

References

1. Arlati, S., et al.: A social virtual reality-based application for the physical and cognitive training of the elderly at home. Sensors **19**(2), 261 (2019)
2. Arns, L.L., Cerney, M.M.: The relationship between age and incidence of cybersickness among immersive environment users. In: 2005 IEEE Proceedings of Virtual Reality, VR 2005, pp. 267–268. IEEE (2005)
3. Bellei, E.A., Biduski, D., Lisboa, H.R.K., De Marchi, A.C.B.: Development and assessment of a mobile health application for monitoring the linkage among treatment factors of type 1 diabetes mellitus. Telemed. e-Health **26**(2), 205–217 (2020)
4. Biduski, D., Bellei, E.A., Rodriguez, J.P.M., Zaina, L.A.M., De Marchi, A.C.B.: Assessing long-term user experience on a mobile health application through an in-app embedded conversation-based questionnaire. Comput. Hum. Behav. **104**, 106169 (2020)
5. Bruun-Pedersen, J.R., Serafin, S., Kofoed, L.B.: Motivating elderly to exercise-recreational virtual environment for indoor biking. In: 2016 IEEE International Conference on Serious Games and Applications for Health (SeGAH), pp. 1–9. IEEE (2016)
6. Buckers, T., Gong, B., Eisemann, E., Lukosch, S.: VRabl: stimulating physical activities through a multiplayer augmented reality sports game. In: Proceedings of the First Superhuman Sports Design Challenge: First International Symposium on Amplifying Capabilities and Competing in Mixed Realities, pp. 1–5 (2018)
7. Cadore, E.L., et al.: Multicomponent exercises including muscle power training enhance muscle mass, power output, and functional outcomes in institutionalized frail nonagenarians. Age **36**(2), 773–785 (2014)
8. Campbell, E., et al.: The effect of exercise on quality of life and activities of daily life in frail older adults: a systematic review of randomised control trials. Exp. Gerontol. 111287 (2021)
9. Campbell, T., Ngo, B., Fogarty, J.: Game design principles in everyday fitness applications. In: Proceedings of the 2008 ACM Conference on Computer Supported Cooperative Work, CSCW 2008, pp. 249–252. Association for Computing Machinery, New York (2008). https://doi.org/10.1145/1460563.1460603
10. Campo-Prieto, P., Cancela, J.M., Rodríguez-Fuentes, G.: Immersive virtual reality as physical therapy in older adults: present or future (systematic review). Virtual Reality 1–17 (2021)
11. Ceccacci, S., Germani, M., Mengoni, M.: User centred approach for home environment designing. In: Proceedings of the 5th International Conference on PErvasive Technologies Related to Assistive Environments, pp. 1–8 (2012)
12. Chau, P.H., et al.: Feasibility, acceptability, and efficacy of virtual reality training for older adults and people with disabilities: single-arm pre-post study. J. Med. Internet Res. **23**(5), e27640 (2021)
13. Colcombe, S.J., et al.: Aerobic fitness reduces brain tissue loss in aging humans. J. Gerontol. A Biol. Sci. Med. Sci. **58**(2), M176–M180 (2003)

14. Colder Carras, M., et al.: Commercial video games as therapy: a new research agenda to unlock the potential of a global pastime. Front. Psych. **8**, 300 (2018)
15. Çöltekin, A., et al.: Extended reality in spatial sciences: a review of research challenges and future directions. ISPRS Int. J. Geo Inf. **9**(7), 439 (2020)
16. Daskalopoulou, C., Stubbs, B., Kralj, C., Koukounari, A., Prince, M., Prina, A.M.: Physical activity and healthy ageing: a systematic review and meta-analysis of longitudinal cohort studies. Ageing Res. Rev. **38**, 6–17 (2017)
17. Dent, E., Kowal, P., Hoogendijk, E.O.: Frailty measurement in research and clinical practice: a review. Eur. J. Intern. Med. **31**, 3–10 (2016)
18. Deterding, S., Dixon, D., Khaled, R., Nacke, L.: From game design elements to gameful-ness: defining "gamification". In: Proceedings of the 15th International Academic MindTrek Conference: Envisioning Future Media Environments, pp. 9–15 (2011)
19. Devereux, N., Ellis, G., Dobie, L., Baughan, P., Monaghan, T.: Testing a proactive approach to frailty identification: the electronic frailty index. BMJ Open Qual. **8**(3), e000682 (2019)
20. Djaouti, D., Alvarez, J., Jessel, J.P.: Classifying serious games: the G/P/S model (PDF) (2015). http://www.ludoscience.com/files/ressources/classifying_serious_games.pdf. Accessed 05 Jan 2019
21. Ferreira, M., Kowal, P.: A minimum data set on ageing and older persons in sub-Saharan Africa: process and outcome. Afr. Popul. Stud. **21**(1) (2006)
22. Fu, Y., Hu, Y., Sundstedt, V.: A systematic literature review of virtual, augmented, and mixed reality game applications in healthcare. ACM Trans. Comput. Healthc. (HEALTH) **3**(2), 1–27 (2022)
23. Fu, Y., Hu, Y., Sundstedt, V., Fagerstrom, C.: A survey of possibilities and challenges with AR/VR/MR and gamification usage in healthcare. In: 14th International Joint Conference on Biomedical Engineering Systems and Technologies (BIOSTEC)/14th International Conference on Bio-inspired Systems and Signal Processing (BIOSIGNALS)/14th International Conference on Biomedical Electronics and Devices (BIODEVICES), pp. 733–740. SciTePress (2021)
24. Fu, Y., Hu, Y., Sundstedt, V., Forsell, Y.: A review of extended reality exercise games for elderly. In: 15th International Conference on Health Informatics (HEALTHINF) held as part of 15th International Joint Conference on Biomedical Engineering Systems and Technolo-gies (BIOSTEC), Virtual, Online, 09–11 February 2022, pp. 201–210. No. 15th International Conference on Health Informatics (HEALTHINF) held as part of 15th International Joint Conference on Biomedical Engineering Systems and Technologies (BIOSTEC), SciTePress (2021)
25. Fu, Y., Hu, Y., Sundstedt, V., Forsell, Y.: Conceptual design of an extended reality exercise game for the elderly. Appl. Sci. **12**(13), 6436 (2022)
26. Fu, Y., Hu, Y., Sundstedt, V., Forsell, Y.: A review of extended reality exercise games for elderly. In: Proceedings of the 15th International Joint Conference on Biomedical Engineer-ing Systems and Technologies - HEALTHINF, pp. 201–210. INSTICC, SciTePress (2022). https://doi.org/10.5220/0010907800003123
27. Goršič, M., Cikajlo, I., Novak, D.: Competitive and cooperative arm rehabilitation games played by a patient and unimpaired person: effects on motivation and exercise intensity. J. Neuroeng. Rehabil. **14**(1), 1–18 (2017)
28. Grani, F., Bruun-Pedersen, J.R.: Giro: better biking in virtual reality. In: 2017 IEEE 3rd Workshop on Everyday Virtual Reality (WEVR), pp. 1–5. IEEE (2017)
29. Hauk, N., Hüffmeier, J., Krumm, S.: Ready to be a silver surfer? A meta-analysis on the relationship between chronological age and technology acceptance. Comput. Hum. Behav. **84**, 304–319 (2018)

30. Henrique, P.P., Colussi, E.L., De Marchi, A.C.: Effects of exergame on patients' balance and upper limb motor function after stroke: a randomized controlled trial. J. Stroke Cerebrovasc. Dis. **28**(8), 2351–2357 (2019)
31. Ijaz, K., Wang, Y., Milne, D., Calvo, R.A.: VR-rides: interactive VR games for health. In: Marsh, T., Ma, M., Oliveira, M.F., Baalsrud Hauge, J., Göbel, S. (eds.) JCSG 2016. LNCS, vol. 9894, pp. 289–292. Springer, Cham (2016). https://doi.org/10.1007/978-3-319-45841-0_33
32. Inokuchi, S., Matsusaka, N., Hayashi, T., Shindo, H.: Feasibility and effectiveness of a nurse-led community exercise programme for prevention of falls among frail elderly people: a multi-centre controlled trial. J. Rehabil. Med. **39**(6), 479–485 (2007)
33. Jeon, S., Kim, J.: Effects of augmented-reality-based exercise on muscle parameters, physical performance, and exercise self-efficacy for older adults. Int. J. Environ. Res. Public Health **17**(9), 3260 (2020)
34. Júnior, J.L.A.D.S., et al.: A bowling exergame to improve functional capacity in older adults: co-design, development, and testing to compare the progress of playing alone versus playing with peers. JMIR Ser. Games **9**(1), e23423 (2021)
35. Juul, J.: Half-Real: Video Games Between Real Rules and Fictional Worlds. MIT Press, Cambridge (2011)
36. Karaosmanoglu, S., Kruse, L., Rings, S., Steinicke, F.: Canoe VR: an immersive exergame to support cognitive and physical exercises of older adults. In: CHI Conference on Human Factors in Computing Systems Extended Abstracts, pp. 1–7 (2022)
37. Keele, S., et al.: Guidelines for performing systematic literature reviews in software engineering. Technical report, Ver. 2.3 EBSE Technical Report. EBSE (2007)
38. Kowal, P., Dowd, J.E.: Definition of an older person. proposed working definition of an older person in Africa for the MDS project. World Health Organization, Geneva (2001). https://doi.org/10.13140/2.1.5188.9286
39. Lee, N., Choi, W., Lee, S.: Development of an 360-degree virtual reality video-based immersive cycle training system for physical enhancement in older adults: a feasibility study. BMC Geriatr. **21**(1) (2021). https://doi.org/10.1186/s12877-021-02263-1
40. Lee, N., Choi, W., Lee, S.: Development of an 360-degree virtual reality video-based immersive cycle training system for physical enhancement in older adults: a feasibility study. BMC Geriatr. **21**(1), 1–10 (2021)
41. Lee, Y., Kozar, K.A., Larsen, K.R.: The technology acceptance model: past, present, and future. Commun. Assoc. Inf. Syst. **12**(1), 50 (2003)
42. Leonardi, C., Mennecozzi, C., Not, E., Pianesi, F., Zancanaro, M.: Designing a familiar technology for elderly people. Gerontechnology **7**(2), 151 (2008)
43. Li, T., et al.: Cognitive training can reduce the rate of cognitive aging: a neuroimaging cohort study. BMC Geriatr. **16**(1), 1–12 (2016)
44. Li, X., Niksirat, K.S., Chen, S., Weng, D., Sarcar, S., Ren, X.: The impact of a multitasking-based virtual reality motion video game on the cognitive and physical abilities of older adults. Sustainability **12**(21), 9106 (2020)
45. Lindsay-Smith, G., Eime, R., O'Sullivan, G., Harvey, J., van Uffelen, J.G.: A mixed-methods case study exploring the impact of participation in community activity groups for older adults on physical activity, health and wellbeing. BMC Geriatr. **19**(1), 1–15 (2019)
46. Mehra, S., et al.: Attitudes of older adults in a group-based exercise program toward a blended intervention; a focus-group study. Front. Psychol. **7**, 1827 (2016)
47. Milgram, P., Kishino, F.: A taxonomy of mixed reality visual displays. IEICE Trans. Inf. Syst. **77**(12), 1321–1329 (1994)

48. Miller, K.J., Adair, B.S., Pearce, A.J., Said, C.M., Ozanne, E., Morris, M.M.: Effectiveness and feasibility of virtual reality and gaming system use at home by older adults for enabling physical activity to improve health-related domains: a systematic review. Age Ageing **43**(2), 188–195 (2014)

49. Moschny, A., Platen, P., Klaaßen-Mielke, R., Trampisch, U., Hinrichs, T.: Barriers to physical activity in older adults in Germany: a cross-sectional study. Int. J. Behav. Nutr. Phys. Act. **8**(1), 1–10 (2011)

50. Muñoz, G.F., Cardenas, R.A.M., Pla, F.: A kinect-based interactive system for home-assisted active aging. Sensors **21**(2), 417 (2021)

51. Nishchyk, A., Geentjens, W., Medina, A., Klein, M., Chen, W.: An augmented reality game for helping elderly to perform physical exercises at home. In: Miesenberger, K., Manduchi, R., Covarrubias Rodriguez, M., Peňáz, P. (eds.) ICCHP 2020. LNCS, vol. 12376, pp. 233–241. Springer, Cham (2020). https://doi.org/10.1007/978-3-030-58796-3_28

52. Pedroli, E., et al.: Characteristics, usability, and users experience of a system combining cognitive and physical therapy in a virtual environment: positive bike. Sensors **18**(7), 2343 (2018)

53. PERKINSCOIE, Association, X.: 2021 augmented and virtual reality survey report (2021)

54. Pisan, Y., Marin, J.G., Navarro, K.F.: Improving lives: using Microsoft kinect to predict the loss of balance for elderly users under cognitive load. In: Proceedings of The 9th Australasian Conference on Interactive Entertainment: Matters of Life and Death, pp. 1–4 (2013)

55. Rebenitsch, L., Owen, C.: Review on cybersickness in applications and visual displays. Virtual Reality **20**(2), 101–125 (2016). https://doi.org/10.1007/s10055-016-0285-9

56. Sakhare, A.R., Yang, V., Stradford, J., Tsang, I., Ravichandran, R., Pa, J.: Cycling and spatial navigation in an enriched, immersive 3D virtual park environment: a feasibility study in younger and older adults. Front. Aging Neurosci. **11**, 218 (2019)

57. Sauvé, L., Renaud, L., Kaufman, D., Dupláa, E.: Can digital games help seniors improve their quality of life? pp. 179–192 (2017). https://doi.org/10.1007/978-3-319-63184-4_10

58. Shah, S.H.H., Hameed, I.A., Karlsen, A.S.T., Solberg, M.: Towards a social VR-based exergame for elderly users: an exploratory study of acceptance, experiences and design principles. In: Chen, J.Y.C., Fragomeni, G. (eds.) HCII 2022. LNCS, vol. 13317, pp. 495–504. Springer, Cham (2022). https://doi.org/10.1007/978-3-031-05939-1_34

59. Slater, M., Sanchez-Vives, M.V.: Enhancing our lives with immersive virtual reality. Front. Robot. AI **3**, 74 (2016)

60. Taylor, L., Kerse, N., Klenk, J., Borotkanics, R., Maddison, R.: Exergames to improve the mobility of long-term care residents: a cluster randomized controlled trial. Games Health J. **7**(1), 37–42 (2018)

61. Valenzuela, M., Sachdev, P.: Can cognitive exercise prevent the onset of dementia? Systematic review of randomized clinical trials with longitudinal follow-up. Am. J. Geriatr. Psychiatry **17**(3), 179–187 (2009)

62. Watanabe, Y., Tanimoto, M., Ohgane, A., Sanada, K., Miyachi, M., Ishii, N.: Increased muscle size and strength from slow-movement, low-intensity resistance exercise and tonic force generation. J. Aging Phys. Act. **21**(1), 71–84 (2013)

63. WHO: Active ageing a policy framework (2002)

64. WHO: Ageing and health (2019)

65. Wilkinson, P.: A brief history of serious games. Entertainment computing and serious games, pp. 17–41 (2016)

66. Yu Fu, Yan Hu, V.S.: A survey on AR/VR games for mental and physical public health. In: eTELEMED 2021, The Thirteenth International Conference on eHealth, Telemedicine, and Social Medicine. ThinkMind (2021)

67. Zhang, H., Shen, Z., Lin, J., Chen, Y., Miao, Y.: Familiarity design in exercise games for elderly. Int. J. Inf. Technol. **22**, 1–19 (2016)

Simulating the Vital Signs of a Digital Patient Undergoing Surgery, for the Purpose of Training Anaesthetists

Hugo Boisaubert[1], Lucas Vincent[2], Corinne Lejus-Bourdeau[3,4],
and Christine Sinoquet[1(✉)]

[1] Nantes University, Ecole Centrale Nantes, CNRS, LS2N, UMR 6004, 44000 Nantes, France
`{hugo.boisaubert,christine.sinoquet}@univ-nantes.fr`
[2] INRAE, 78352 Jouy-en-Josas, France
`lucas.vincent@inrae.fr`
[3] Experimental Universitary Laboratory for Simulation in Intensive Care (LESiMU) of Nantes University, 44035 Nantes, France
`corinne.lejus@chu-nantes.fr`
[4] Nantes University Hospital, 1 place Alexis Ricordeau, 44093 Nantes, France

Abstract. More than half a million surgeries with anaesthesia are performed every day worldwide, making the safety and quality of intraoperative care a major health issue.

We present SVP-OR (Simulation of Virtual Patient at the Operating Room), a novel approach designed for computer-assisted anaesthesia training. For this purpose, we simulate the evolution of the physiological state of a virtual patient, depending on the actions of the simulator user (anaesthetist in training) and the other medical agents.

We present the problem as a case-based reasoning approach. When a new medical action is initiated, we first identify real patients whose anaesthetic profiles show a region most similar to the recent history of the virtual patient; then we predict the near future of the virtual patient (a multivariate time series) from the time series of these real patients.

Our contribution is fourfold. First, we have designed a contextualized multidimensional pattern recognition approach focused on temporal data. Second, using the concept of contextualized multidimensional pattern, we have developed a generic framework for predicting the evolution of a virtual patient's state in the operating room. Thirdly, the choice of a relevant dissimilarity measure for real-time comparison of many short time series is crucial for our simulation problem. We have designed an experimental protocol to achieve the comparative analysis of 8 candidates. Fourthly, we have evaluated the realism of the SVP-OR simulations. We have examined how the prediction ability varies along the phases of the surgery studied.

Keywords: Training in simulation-assisted anaesthesia · Digital patient ·
Case-based reasoning · Data mining · Pattern recognition · Temporal data ·
e-Health record · Event log · Multivariate time series

A. C. A. Roque et al. (Eds.): BIOSTEC 2022, CCIS 1814, pp. 353–376, 2023.
https://doi.org/10.1007/978-3-031-38854-5_18

1   Introduction

Simulation is a modern educational tool for learning and maintaining skills in the health sciences. Around the world, intensive care simulation platforms are hosted by university hospitals, to train medical interns and nurses, together with more experienced practitioners. Especially, the Experimental Universitary Laboratory for Simulation in Intensive Care (LESiMU) in Nantes offers training in seven medical specialities, including anaesthesia. To this end, LESiMU uses high-fidelity mannequins, with the trainee immersed in an interdisciplinary medical team. With the exception of the trainee, the members of the factice team play roles. At the present time, the training scenarios are written in advance. There is therefore little variability in the scenarios. Besides, during a scenario, the trainer is compelled to manually modify the vital signs of the mannequin, in response to the medical actions (including those of the trainee).

The justification for our work is based on a real need expressed by LESiMU. The latter wishes to vary the scenarios to be offered to anaesthesia interns and nurse anaesthetists, in initial training, as well as to more experienced practitioners, in continuing education. We proposed to develop a digital simulation modality, which leverages the database of anaesthetic profiles recorded by Nantes University Hospital since 2000.

To implement this modality, we need an automatic generator of reactive scenarios. The software program to be run by the trainee is set up with the surgery of interest, age, sex, weight and medical history (*e.g.*, hypertensive subject) of the digital patient to be simulated. The rest of the medical team is simulated very simply by means of icons that act on the patient and transmit information on the computer screen in front of which the trainee is seated. The medicine of the future will be personalized and predictive, thanks to digital technology. In particular, serving our training objective also meets the need for prediction, to anticipate risks in the operating room.

To generate reactive scenarios, one must be able to predict the evolution of the physiological parameters of the digital patient, in response to an action of the medical team (including the trainee). Since 2000, Nantes University Hospital has collected more than 500,000 anaesthetic profiles. An anaesthetic profile is composed of a multivariate time series recorded *via* monitoring, and of the log of all actions taken on the patient during the surgery. In the time series, the observed values are measured with a constant frequency, for physiological parameters such as heart rate, blood pressure, oxygen saturation. In the action log, the actions are time-stamped on a continuous time scale. In the following, we will also use the term "variables" to refer to the physiological parameters.

Given a cohort of patients who have undergone the same surgery and belong to the same "class" as the digital patient to be simulated (age, sex, weight and medical history), the time series and action logs of the cohort contain knowledge that makes it possible to predict the evolution of the digital patient after the initiation of a given action. We can exploit this cohort data by considering either a modelling approach or a data mining approach.

Our proposal relies on a case-based reasoning (CBR) technique adapted for temporal data. Our approach avoids the need to learn and evaluate a machine learning model. We consider a cohort of real patients with same surgery, age, sex, weight and medical history as the digital patient to be simulated. After a medical action A has been taken, such as the administration of an anaesthetic product, we want to evolve the digital patient until the next (unknown) action is initiated. We refer to a **reactive simulation scenario** as the dynamic process whereby the actions of a user (the trainee) cause a virtual patient to evolve, complementing the actions of the rest of the medical team, which is virtual. At the end of the reactive scenario, we obtain a multivariate time series and a log of the actions performed by the trainee and the medical team during the whole surgery.

In order to predict the short-term evolution of digital patient after it has just undergone action A, we rely on the observed evolution of real patients who have already undergone action A. We must also take into account the actions preceding action A. Indeed, some of them are likely to interfere in the evolution of the digital patient because their effect has not yet dissipated. Moreover, interfering actions do not necessarily exert the same combined impact, depending on the time-stamps at which these actions were triggered.

Therefore, in our case-based reasoning framework, we need to identify real patients whose temporal data include a region similar to the recent past of the digital patient. A patient's temporal data encompass a multivariate time series and an action log. We thus have to deal with two pattern recognition problems, one where the query is a sequence of time-stamped actions, the other where the query is a multivariate time series.

The remainder of the paper is organized as follows. Section 2 briefly presents some related work. Section 3 describes the general CBR-based algorithm SVP-OR (Simulation of Virtual Patient at the Operating Room). Then the section details the two main components of the approach, that is (i) a contextualized pattern recognition method and (ii) a strategy for predicting the short-term evolution of the digital patient. Section 4 presents the evaluation of the SVP-OR simulator for the case of laparoscopic inguinal hernia surgery. Section 5 concludes and opens up future directions of research.

From now on, we denote nbv the number of variables described in any anaesthetic profile of the patient cohort of interest.

This paper is an extended version of [1]. In our work, we did not intend to design from the outset a dissimilarity measure able to compare two multivariate time series. Instead, if we handle nbv variables, we rely on a common univariate dissimilarity measure D, to compute the multivariate dissimilarity as the average of nbv dissimilarities. The choice of D is crucial for the real-time comparison of many time series, as is the case in our simulation problem. In addition, the targeted application compares short time series, a situation never studied before. In this extended version, we provide more insights on the study we have conducted to compare 8 candidates for D. As another major difference, in Sect. 4, we have incorporated an analysis of local variability in the realism of the simulation over the course of the surgery.

2   Related Work

The literature reports a number of works dedicated to the prediction of multivariate time series. They all rely on models from the machine learning domain. Our approach is unprecedented as it uses case-based reasoning, focusing on short-term prediction on the fly for multivariate time series. Indeed, the application goal (the management of reactive scenarios simulating a surgical operation) implies a real-time response.

In the last decade, **digital simulation** has made its way into hospitals, particularly for **training purposes**. The range of aids on offer extends from replaying scenarios on the computer from a selection of real-life scenarios, or from artificial but pre-formatted scenarios, to immersion in a virtual operating room [22,23].

Artificial intelligence has an important role to play in extracting knowledge from operating room (OR) data.

Machine learning techniques allow the automatic detection and prediction of surgical tasks, for example by using hidden Markov models [18] or random forests [28]. In particular, deep learning has produced considerable advances in the recognition of surgical procedures from video sequences [12,14].

Work in the area of **data mining** has produced advances in predicting the possible surgeons' subsequent tasks by exploiting low-level surgical tasks [7] and predicting the remaining intervention time [8]. The literature reports works on the three main types of process mining tasks applied in a healthcare context. Besides discovery and conformance checking, enhancement aims to enrich and extend an existing process model using process data [6,21].

Time series forecasting has become a very intensive area of research, specifically with regard to multivariate time series. The reader is directed to the recent review in [17] which surveys multiple methods and models from the fields of statistics, classical machine learning and deep learning. In our application, the dynamic process we wish to simulate presents a specific difficulty: medical actions are likely to exert a combined effect on some of the digital patient's parameters, and the resulting effect also depends on the times at which the actions were taken. Under these conditions, the design and training of a prediction model in the field of machine learning domain, capable of jointly modelling time series and event traces, is a real challenge.

Case-based Reasoning (CBR) is fundamentally different from other major approaches in the field of artificial intelligence. The latter methods rely on general knowledge of a problem domain, or establish associations between the problem descriptors and the conclusion. In contrast, CBR solves a new problem by finding a similar previously experienced case, and leveraging its specific knowledge in the new situation. CBR has been widely used for diagnosis, classification, recommendation and therapeutic planning in medicine (see for example [3] for illustrations). CBR is a promising data-driven self-adaptive approach well suited for problems whose solutions require knowledge that is difficult to specify but for which there are enough data. However, whereas it is easy to perform a majority vote from classes, or to calculate the average from the target continuous outputs of the k nearest neighbours of a given query, it is not straightforward to construct a novel time series from those of the k nearest neighbours. Besides, defining or choosing a similarity measure suitable for time series is not an easy task either. Therefore, to date, relatively little work has been done to exploit temporal data in the CBR framework, and even less to take advantage of knowledge of patients' temporal data.

In the work reported in [27], a temporal similarity measure is designed to cope with irregularly measured laboratory test data, with the aim of measuring similarity between care trajectories. In [9], the authors feed a time-graph structure with the temporal data of patients, to quantify similarity between patients in terms of disease progression. The temporal data considered in these two works are medical events. In their recent work, Mulayim and co-authors advance CBR in the presence of massive data, such as applied to millions of patients' longitudinal records. Their solution is to integrate an anytime lazy k-nearest neighbor (kNN) algorithm to the CBR framework, to avoid unnecessary neighbor assessments [19]. For the situations where this speed-up is not sufficient, the CBR approach can be interrupted before completion, to return the best $kNNs$ obtained so far, together with a confidence value attached to each of them.

Our approach is innovative in the field of CBR: on the one hand, it allows the prediction of non-scalar features instead of more standard outcomes (classes or real values), in an informed context (a subtrace of events), which avoids the artificial use of windows of size to be determined by the user; on the other hand, the prediction task is repeated throughout a simulation scenario, in response to external sollicitations (medical acts in our case).

3   Case-Based Reasoning Framework

To make the digital patient evolve during a surgical operation, we simulate its multivariate time series between the triggers of two consecutive actions, and we iterate this process until the end of the operation.

In this section, we depict our CBR framework, which relies on a Contextualized Multidimensional Pattern Retrieval approach. We first define the concept of Contextualized Multidimensional Pattern, the cornerstone of our proposal. The general principle of our proposal is then described in Sect. 3.2. Two main tasks are involved. Section 3.3 explains how we identify real patients most similar to the digital patient, from the cohort of patients belonging to the same class as the digital patient. Section 3.4 details how we predict the near future of the digital patient from the real patients who are most similar to it. Finally, Sect. 3.4 provides additional comments to Sect. 3.2.

3.1   Contextualized Multidimensional Pattern

The data provided to our CBR approach are composed of multivariate time series, each annotated with a time-stamped event trace. Each event corresponds to the initiation of a given action (a medical action in our case).

An action may impact several variables in parallel. Second, we consider only variables that are influenced by at least one action. Thirdly, a variable impacted by several actions is subject to the combined effect of these actions, initiated or not at different time-stamps.

Our main goal is to predict the evolution of the digital patient after an action, say action A, has been initiated. Contextual information is needed for the most accurate prediction: the recent history of the digital patient provides the context in which action A has been initiated. Such context is composed of the *action-signature*, that is the most recently initiated actions, as well as the recent evolution of the virtual patient's variables until the initiation of action A. In Fig. 1, the action-signature is (C, B, A), and a *contextual time window* is defined, that extends from the initiation of action C to that of action A. A **Contextualized Multidimensional Pattern** (CMP) can therefore be defined for

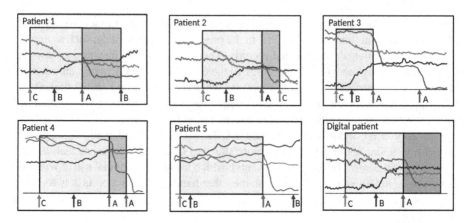

Fig. 1. Simulation of the evolution of a digital patient by using the concept of Contextualized Multidimensional Pattern. In this toy example, the mutivariate time series of a real or digital patient describes three variables respectively represented in red, violet and orange. Actions A, B and C respectively influence the variables represented in red, violet and orange. Action A induces a sharp decline. Action B entails a slow growth. Action C generates a slow decrease. The influence of each of these three actions is no longer observable after a certain duration of action, after which the stabilisation of the affected variable is observed. In this example, the past actions beyond the three last actions are assumed to have no more effect on the variables: the size of the action-signature is set to 3. Real patients 1 to 5 each have an action signature (C, B, A) similar to that of the digital patient in their histories. In this illustration, the corresponding region in the mutivariate time series of patients 1, 2 and 4 (in the yellow boxes) is supposed to be sufficiently similar to the recent time series of the digital patient. Therefore, in the case-based reasoning framework, we can use the multivariate time series of patients 1, 2 and 4 (green boxes bounded on the right at the initiation of the action subsequent to action A) to predict the short-term evolution of the digital patient (blue box). (Color figure online)

the digital patient. The CMP is composed of the action-signature annotated with the durations between two successive action initiations, and of the restriction of the digital patient's multivariate time series to the contextual time window. The number of actions in the action-signature, further referred to as nba, is specified through the expertise of anaesthesiologists. For instance, if nba is set to 4, (D, 28, C, 80, B, 10, A) represents an action-signature in which the time intervals between two successive action initiations are respectively 28, 80 and 10 numbers of time-steps.

3.2   Outline of Algorithm

Algorithm 1 presents the outline of our proposal.

In line 1, we select the appropriate cohort of real patients. It is composed of the patients who belonged to the same class $Class$ as the virtual patient VP (in terms of age, sex, weight, and medical history) when they underwent the surgical operation $Surg$. In line 2, we initialize the first values of VP's multivariate time series, with the initial values of a patient drawn at random in $Cohort$ and we maintain a steady state around these values. Then, the reactive scenario is constructed iteratively (lines 3 to 11) until the surgery is over. At the initiation of action act (line 4), we first build VP's CMP, which is composed of action-signature $\mathcal{T}_{CMP}$ and of the time subseries m_{CMP} defined over the time window encompassed by $\mathcal{T}_{CMP}$ (line 6). The action-signature $\mathcal{T}_{CMP}$ encompasses the $nba - 1$ latest actions in $\mathcal{T}$ annotated with the corresponding time intervals, together with last action act annotated with Δ_t, the time interval between the initiations of the penultimate action and the current action act.

Section 3.3 will detail how the action subtrace $\mathcal{T}_{CMP}$ annotated with time intervals, together with the subseries m_{CMP}, drive the CMP retrieval step. This step outputs the k real patients most similar to VP, also referred to as the VP's k nearest neighbours. Section 3.4 will explain the short-term prediction step, where we build m^+ from the k nearest neighbours. The VP is then updated: in line 9, the short-term prediction m^+ is used to grow the multivariate time series m; in line 10, the action trace $\mathcal{T}$ is extended by adding action act together with its time-stamp.

The simulation continues until no further action is initiated.

Algorithm 1. SVP-OR (Simulation of Virtual Patient in the Operating Room).

FUNCTION simulate_reactive_scenario($Surg$, $Class$, nba, k)
INPUT:
  ▷ $Surg$, surgical operation of interest
  ▷ $Class$, class of virtual patient (VP)
  ▷ nba, number of actions in Contextualized Multidimensional Pattern (CMP)
  ▷ k, required number of nearest neighbours for the VP

OUTPUT:
  ▷ $\mathcal{T}$, action trace of VP
  ▷ m, multivariate time series of VP

VARIABLES:
  ▷ $Cohort$, cohort of real patients having undergone surgical operation $Surg$ and belonging to the same class $Class$ as VP
  ▷ t, time-stamp of current action act initiated by the user
  ▷ Δ_t, time ellapsed between the penultimate action's initiation and t
  ▷ $CMP = (\mathcal{T}_{CMP}, m_{CMP})$, Contextualized Multidimensional Pattern of VP, with
    - $\mathcal{T}_{CMP}$, action-signature of VP, of size nba, including current action act
    - m_{CMP}, time subseries of m corresponding to the CMP' s time window defined by $\mathcal{T}_{CMP}$

1: $Cohort \leftarrow$ **select_cohort** ($Surg$, $Class$)
2: $(\mathcal{T}, m) \leftarrow$ **initialize_virtual_patient**()

3: **while** (scenario is not over)
4:     $(act, t, \Delta_t) \leftarrow$ **wait_for_action**()
5:     **if** no action is initiated **then exit end if**

6:     $(\mathcal{T}_{CMP}, m_{CMP}) \leftarrow$ **build_current_cmp**($\mathcal{T}, m, nba, act, \Delta_t$)
7:     $neighb \leftarrow$ **identify_patients_most_similar_to_VP**($k, \mathcal{T}_{CMP}, m_{CMP}$)
8:     $m^+ \leftarrow$ **build_short_term_prediction**($neighb$)
9:     $m \leftarrow$ **update_multivariate_time_series**(m, m^+)
10:    $\mathcal{T} \leftarrow$ **update_action_trace**($\mathcal{T}, t, act$)
11: **end while**

3.3   Identifying the k Nearest Neighbours of the Digital Patient

The current CMP of the digital patient will be further referred to as the query. We recall that nba, the number of actions in a CMP, is a constant set by the trainers, in our case, anaesthesia experts. This number nba includes the last action (act) initiated by the user (the trainee). Our aim is to design a score Sim, to rank real patients according to their similarity to the digital patient.

Matching Between Action Subtraces. The first subtask in the CMP retrieval step is to recognize real patients'subtraces containing regions similar to the action-signature of the digital patient. We allow strict pairwise matches between the actions of real and digital patients. Nonetheless, thanks to experts, we are able to categorize actions: for instance, it is possible to replace an anaesthetic by another. Therefore, we accept matches between actions belonging to the same category. The score Sim_a contributes to the computation of the final score Sim; it rewards the pairwise matching of actions in the action-signatures $\mathcal{T}_{CMP}^{VP}$ and $\mathcal{T}_{CMP}^{RP}$ of virtual and real patients:

$$Sim_a = \frac{1}{nba} \sum_{i=1}^{nba} \delta(\mathcal{T}_{CMP}^{VP}[i], \mathcal{T}_{CMP}^{RP}[i]), \tag{1}$$

where $\mathcal{T}_{CMP}^{x}[i]$ denotes i^{th} action in the action-signature of patient x, and $\delta(a, a') = 1$ if $a = a'$ and 0 otherwise.

As regards the time intervals between any two successive action initiations, we allow some flexibility in the pairwise matches. We gradually penalize deviations according to the more recent nature of the action. In other words, the older the actions are in the action-signature, the more tolerant we are of possible discrepancies when matching time intervals. Given a relaxation percentage P, the allowed deviation gradually decreases as follows:

$$\mathcal{D}ev(r) = P \left(1 - \frac{r-1}{nba-1} \right), \tag{2}$$

where r stands for the rank of the pair of successive actions under examination in the action-signature. In practice, specifying parameter P (not shown in Algorithm 1) will automatically dismiss any real patient deviating from the digital patient, at rank r, beyond threshold $\mathcal{D}ev(r)$. For example, in the action-signature (D, 28, C, 80, B, 10, A), the rank of the pair (C,B) is 2. Considering this action-signature of size nba equal to 4, and percentage $P = 20\%$, Eq. 2 yields the three following relaxation percentages: $\mathcal{D}ev(1) = 20\%$, $\mathcal{D}ev(2) = 13,3\%$, and $\mathcal{D}ev(3) = 6.7\%$. This means that for a real patient, we accept that the time interval between C and B's initiations varies in range $80 \pm 13.3\%$.

The score Sim_i rewards the pairwise matching of time intervals in the two action-signatures $\mathcal{T}_{CMP}^{VP}$ and $\mathcal{T}_{CMP}^{RP}$:

$$Sim_i = \frac{\epsilon_{max} - \epsilon}{\epsilon_{max} - \epsilon_{min}}, \tag{3}$$

$$\epsilon = \sum_{i=1}^{nba-1} \left| \mathcal{T}_{CMP}^{VP}[[i]] - \mathcal{T}_{CMP}^{RP}[[i]] \right|, \tag{4}$$

where $\mathcal{T}^x_{CMP}[[i]]$ denotes the time interval between i^{th} and $i+1^{th}$ actions in the action-signature of patient x, and ϵ_{min} and ϵ_{max} stand for the smallest and largest values of ϵ observed over all real patients in $Cohort$ that harbour an action-signature compatible with the virtual patient.

Similarity Between Time Subseries. The second subtask in the CMP retrieval step consists in identifying formerly preselected candidates whose multivariate time series are locally similar to m_{CMP}. The computation of a multivariate dissimilarity measure, for example the Dynamic Time Warping (DTW) multivariate distance, is costly from dimension 3 [2,24]. It is beyond the scope of this work to explore this issue further. As an alternative, we compute the multivariate dissimilarity D_m between two nbv-dimensional time series by averaging the nbv dissimilarities calculated with some univariate dissimilarity measure D over all dimensions:

$$D_m = \frac{1}{nbv} \sum_{i=1}^{nbv} D_i, \tag{5}$$

with D_i the dissimilarity obtained using D for i^{th} variable.

From D_m, we compute the similarity score Sim_s

$$Sim_s = \frac{D_{mmax} - D_m}{D_{mmax} - D_{mmin}}, \tag{6}$$

where D_{mmin} and D_{mmax} stand for the smallest and largest values of D_m observed over all real patients in $Cohort$ that harbour an action-signature compatible with the virtual patient.

Ranking the Candidates. On the basis of scores Sim_a, Sim_i and Sim_s, we compute the final similarity score Sim as the weighted sum:

$$Sim = \alpha_a Sim_a + \alpha_i Sim_i + \alpha_s Sim_s. \tag{7}$$

This score is used in line 7 (Algorithm 1), to select the k nearest neighbours of the digital patient.

3.4   Predicting the Short-Term Evolution of the Digital Patient

Once the k nearest neighbours of the digital patient have been identified, a novel time series fragment can be generated for the digital patient. Each of the k sub-series used falls within a time window delimited as follows: the lower boundary coincides with the discretized initiation time of the current action act (line 4 in Algorithm 1); the upper boundary b_i ($1 \leq i \leq k$) is defined by the discretized initiation time of the action that followed act. In Fig. 1, these time windows are highlighted in green.

Figure 2 shows the chunk-wise construction of the whole time series of the digital patient.

Our objective is that the new fragment predicted is as long as possible: we wish to limit the risk that the end of this fragment is reached before a new action can allow us to generate a novel fragment (*i.e.*, a novel prediction). To simulate the time series over the largest possible time interval, our choice is to average iteratively over a decreasing number of fragments defined as follows, in each dimension (*i.e.*, each variable). We consider h iterations, where h is the number of distinct upper boundaries b_i ($1 \leq i \leq k$) mentioned in the above paragraph. At first iteration, we average over those of the k fragments defined over the window time lower bounded by act initiation time and upper bounded by b_1. At iteration j ($2 \leq j \leq h$), we average over those of the k fragments defined over the time window $[b_{j-1}, b_j]$. When repeated over the nbv variables, this process allows to make evolve the nbv physiological parameters of the virtual patient for some time after an action has been initiated. Figure 3 illustrates the case where all b_i's ($1 \leq i \leq k$) are distinct.

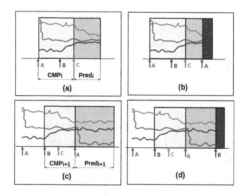

Fig. 2. Chunk-wise generation of the digital patient's multivariate time series, for a whole simulation scenario, following a k-nearest neighbour strategy. In this example, $nbv = 3$ (number of variables) and $nba = 3$ (number of actions in the Contextualized Multidimensional Pattern). Actions A, B and C each influence the variables represented in red, violet and orange. Action A entails a steep decrease. Action B generates a slow increase. Action C induces a slow decline. The Contextualized Multidimensional Pattern CMP_i drives Prediction $Pred_i$. (a) Based on CPM_i, the k nearest neighbours of the digital patient are identified. Their evolution under the influence of the sequence of actions A, B, C allows to build $Pred_i$. (b) When a new occurrence of action A is initiated, $Pred_i$ becomes obsolete from the initiation of A. (c) A novel prediction $Pred_{i+1}$ is produced based on the updated Contextualized Multidimensional Pattern CMP_{i+1} with sequence of actions B, C, A. (d) Again, when a novel occurrence of action B is initiated, $Pred_{i+1}$ becomes obsolete from the initiation of B. (Color figure online)

Discussing the Approach Proposed. In order not to impede the flow of the presentation with details, Algorithm 1 described our CBR approach in a nutshell. We now provide more details.

At the beginning of the scenario, when r^{th} action is performed ($r < nba$), we cannot use a CMP of size nba to identify the k nearest neighbours. Instead, in line 6, we simply proceed with a CMP of size r.

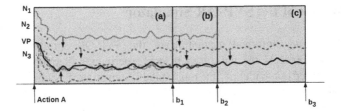

Fig. 3. Generation of the virtual patient's time series, at action A initiation, through an averaging strategy. Principle shown for one dimension (*i.e.,* one variable) of the multivariate time series. $k = 3$ neigbours. VP: virtual patient. In this example, the time series obtained for the neighbours N_1, N_2 and N_3 after action A's initiation all have different lengths and are respectively upper bounded by b_1, b_2 and b_3. (a) The 3 fragments from N_1, N_2 and N_3 defined until b_1 are shifted along y-axis such that their values at A's initiation coincide with the value of VP; these fragments (in red) are annotated with arrows indicating the direction of the shift. The average of the shifted fragments (in green) defines the VP's time series (in black), over the considered time interval. (b) N_1 and N_2 contribute to the generation of VP's time series over time interval $[b_1, b_2]$. (c) The remaining neighbour N2 defined over $[b_2, b_3]$ is shifted to ensure the continuity of the time series under construction. (Color figure online)

Second, to eliminate the risk of obtaining no nearest neighbour, we run several searches in parallel, parameterized by various percentages P (see Eq. 2). In this way, we can ensure real-time responsiveness, at the cost of relaxing the similarity between virtual patient and nearest neighbours. In a training simulation framework, this relaxation is not a problem.

On the other hand, the reader must be aware that whenever a short-term prediction has been generated, for a number of time-steps (never known in advance), this prediction must be consumed time-step by time-step using a timer. Importantly, in the scenario that is being played out, there is always a risk that no action is initiated before one reaches the end of the latest prediction generated. In this case, we switch to a degraded operating mode: we generate stable univariate time series to wait until an action is initiated or a timeout is reached. The management of the timer and that of the switch to the degraded operating mode are low-level processes that are not presented in Algorithm 1.

The averaging-based prediction strategy operates over less and less neighbours. In our case-based reasoning frame, we put forward that the same causes (same sequence of actions in the CMP) entail the same dynamic behaviours. Thus, not only are the current k-nearest neighbours similar to the VP, but any two of them are also expected to show the same general trends (*e.g.*, a moderate increase, a sharp rise). Moreover, in the case of anaesthesia, it is expected that the influence of the actions encompassed in the CMP fade the further away from the moment of latest action's initiation. Thirdly, in a training framework, our aim is a realistic, not an exact, simulation. The three previous remarks strengthen our conviction that the decrease in the number of neighbours contributing to the average is not an issue.

4   Evaluation of the SVP-OR Simulator

We carried out an empirical evaluation of the SVP-OR simulation framework. Section 4.1 first presents the data used in our experiments. Section 4.2 outlines the experiments carried out to identify the most suitable univariate dissimilarity measure for our application, and provides the conclusions obtained. Section 4.3 details the implementation and parameterization used for the SVP-OR simulator. Section 4.4 explains the experimental set up employed to assess the realism of the simulations obtained with the SVP-OR approach. The results are presented and discussed in Sect. 4.5.

4.1   Data Set

SVP-OR is fed with anaesthetic profiles. Due to legal limitations on access to sensitive health data, we were compelled at this stage of our research project to generate our own realistic data. We used our own generator, the BDLBS tool (from the name of the four authors). It was designed based on the expertise of anaesthesiologists. It should be noted that this contribution, the generation of realistic data from scratch in the medical field, based on expertise, represents an unprecedented effort. The BDLBS tool will be thoroughly described in detail in a separate paper, along with the protocol used to validate its ability to reproduce time series distributions similar to those of the real data.

   The data set will be further referred to as the BDLBS data set. It consists of 1000 univariate time series of length around 200 time steps, with measure points spaced every 30 s. These time series describe the evolution of heart rate and diastolic, systolic and so-called average blood pressures, for 1000 male patients aged 30 years, weighing 80 kg, with no medical history. The surgery of interest is inguinal hernia operation under laparoscopy and with prosthetics setting. Figure 4 shows an illustration of how this surgical procedure can be performed. The data set is publicly available at https://github.com/alpharty/BDLBS_dataset.

4.2   Selection of the Univariate Dissimilarity Measure

We define the dissimilarity measure D_m used in Eq. 6 as the average of the nbv dissimilarities obtained for the nbv variables, using a univariate dissimilarity measure D (Eq. 5).

   We recall the reader that our CBR-based approach involves comparisons of time subseries defined over CMPs. As will be mentioned in Sect. 4.3, medical experts recommended that we set nba, the number of actions in a CMP, to 4. This results in time subseries that vary in length from about 10 to 30 measure points, with very few exceptions. The literature reports several studies focused on the comparison of dissimilarity measures dedicated to time series [11,15,16,29]. However, these studies focus on time series of greater length than ours. Furthermore, some of these studies target applications such as classification, clustering or detection of changes. The others evaluate the insensitivity - or robustness - of dissimilarity measures to perturbations of various natures and amplitudes.

Phases	Subphases	Steps
Enter	Setting up	Patient enter
		Patient setting
	Monitoring	Heart rate monitoring
		Arterial pressure monitoring
		Oxygen saturation monitoring
		BIS monitoring
		TOF check
		Bair hugger
	Premedication	Venous route installation
		Prophylactic antibiotic
		Vascular filling
Induction	Preoxygenation	Facial mask
		Preoxygenation administration
	Medication	Morphinic
		Analgesia
		Hypnotic
		Curare
	Intubation	Controled mechanical ventilation
		Eyelid closing
		Intubation
	Control and end of induction	Controled ventilation
		Maintenance of anesthesia
		Oxygen 30%
		Pulmonar auscultation
		Intubation balloon presure check
		Lung volume recruitment
		Temperature monitoring

Phases	Subphases	Steps
Procedure	Procedure preparation	Surgery setting
		Pulmonar auscultation
		Support point check
		Ready for surgery
	Procedure	Incision
		Ubumbilical trocar
		Pneumoperitoneum inflation
		Pulmonar auscultation
		Lung volume recruitment
		Preperitoneal space dissection
		Spermatic cord dissection
		Hernia space dissection
		Prosthetics setting
		Pneumoperitoneum deflation
		Closing
		Bandage
Exit	Decurarization	Decurarization check
		Decurarization
	Ending	Patient setting before exit
		Patient exit

Fig. 4. Surgery for the laparoscopic inguinal hernia operation with prosthetics setting.

Our aim is quite different. We want to select a candidate that exhibits contrast and can be computed quickly to satisfy the real-time responsiveness constraint of the SVP-OR system. We define by contrast the behavior whereby an increase in the degree of perturbation of a (univariate) time series leads to an increase in dissimilarity between the initial time series and the perturbed version.

We carried out an extensive comparative analysis of eight pre-selected univariate dissimilarity measures, to identify a relevant candidate for D. Table 1 briefly describes the 8 pre-selected univariate dissimilarities.

We compared the 8 dissimilarity measures using the BDLBS data set and 26 other data sets from the UCR repository made available to study time series [5].

In a nutshell, the experimental protocol used to evaluate the contrast for the dissimilarity measures starts by drawing at random three subseries of size 10, 20 and 30 (measurement points) respectively for each time series of the 27 reference data sets. We thus obtained $3 \times 27 = 81$ data sets. Each sequence of these sets will be further referred to as a reference.

Then, we applied 6 types of perturbation on each reference. For each perturbation type, we considered 5 degrees of perturbation. Thus, for a given type of perturbation, we obtained 5 perturbed time series per reference. Table 2 details these perturbations.

The degree of perturbation is denoted by d. The possible values for d depend on the perturbation type. With a slight abuse of language, in this paper we only refer to degrees $d \in \{1, 2, \ldots, 5\}$. For instance, if d takes its values in $\{5, 10, 15, 20, 25\}$, instead of $d = 10$, we will refer to $d = 2$ (relatively slight perturbation).

For each of the 81 reference data sets S, each of the 5 perturbation types P, and each of the 8 dissimilarity measures analyzed D, we assessed the dissimilarity between any reference and each of its 5 perturbed versions. Such computation is referred to as

Table 1. The 8 univariate dissimilarity measures compared. DTW: Dynamic Time Warping.

DTWc: classical DTW (pyts library; https://github.com/johannfaouzi/pyts)   Global alignement of the two time series compared [24]
DTWdtai: fast exact DTW (dtaidistance library; https://github.com/wannesm/dtaidistance)   Exact implementation of DTW in Cython language
DTWf: fast DTW (heuristic) (pyts library)   Global alignment of the two time series using a hierarchical approach recursively refining the alignment from coarse to fine resolution [26]
DTWsc: Sakoe-Chiba DTW (heuristic) (pyts library)   Global alignment between the two time series by constraining the warping region to a band of user-specified width along the diagonal of the alignment matrix, the Sakoe-Chiba band [25]
DTWi: Itakura DTW (heuristic) (pyts library)   Global alignment between the two time series by constraining the warping region in the alignment matrix, to the Ikatura parallelogram, a region whose largest width and slope of the steeper side are specified by the user [13]
DTWm: multiscale DTW (heuristic) (pyts library)   Global alignment between the two time series by constraining the warping region thanks to the optimal path obtained by aligning the two downsampled initial time series and projecting this path on the original scale [20]
MPDist (MatrixProfile library, https://matrixprofile.docs.matrixprofile.org/install.html)   Feature-based dissimilarity measure [10]
tsfresh-based measure tsfresh (https://tsfresh.readthedocs.io/en/latest/)   Euclidian distance computed for the numerical representations of the two time series, obtained through the tsfresh feature extraction package [4]

"Reference *versus* Perturbed" (**RvP**). Thus, for each triplet (S, P, D), we obtained 5 distributions of dissimilarity values $\mathcal{D}_1 \cdots \mathcal{D}_5$ corresponding to the 5 degrees of perturbation.

We repeated the experiment in another setting. This time, we conducted the RvPO ("Reference *versus* Perturbed versions of Others") experiment, in which distributions $\mathcal{D}_1 \cdots \mathcal{D}_5$ are collections of dissimilarities between references and perturbed versions of *other* references drawn at random.

The trends observed for computational costs on short series are the same for lengths 10, 20 and 30. Figure 5(a) underlines that on short series, using heuristics to compute DTW is still beneficial, except for multiscale DTW (DTWm). Regarding speed performance, the four DTW heuristics are ranked as follows, in the range [1.4s-1.9s]: DTWf, DTWsc-DTWi, DTWm. The tsfresh-based measure performs similarly as the fastest DTW heuristic (DTWf). Cython implementation (DTWdtai) reduces computing time to about one twentieth. MPDist and DTWdtai have roughly the same computational cost.

Figure 5(b) to (d) provides an excerpt of the results obtained for the RvP and RvPO experiments. In a nutshell, MPDist and the tsfresh-based measure were discarded from the candidates, because of lack of contrast, partial lack (*i.e.*, for some degrees only), or even inverted contrast (contrast decreasing as degree increases) for some perturbations. The RvPO experiment had also the merit of disqualifying the tsfresh-based measure which shows a contrast in this experiment. Moreover, we checked that DTW variants are relevant in presence of very short to short time series, as is the case in the SVP-OR framework. This result is not trivial. The above conclusions are broadly valid for all 27 benchmark data sets.

Amongst the DTW variants, DTWdtai was chosen for its greatest speed.

Table 2. Description of the 6 types of perturbation considered, and parameter values corresponding to the increasing degrees of perturbation. To note, in our experiments, the 7th perturbation elast is never used alone. [1]std: standard deviation of the distribution of amplitudes in the reference; [2]avg: average of amplitudes over the reference. [3] polynomial of degree 4 obtained by linear regression of the reference. a_{ref}: amplitude for the time series to be perturbed (*i.e.*, the reference), at some time-stamp. a_{pert}: amplitude for the perturbed version of the reference.

Perturbation	Description
ampl_gauss	modifies the amplitude at each time-stamp $a_{pert} \sim Norm\left(a_{ref}, (std \times d/100)^2\right)$ [1] 5 degrees: $d \in \{5, 10, 15, 20, 25\}$
ampl_noise	modifies the amplitude at $p\%$ time-stamps $a_{pert} = a_{ref} \times (1 + sign_{aleat} \times d/100), sign_{aleat} \in \{+, -\}$ 5×3 degrees: $d \in \{5, 10, 15, 20, 25\}$, $\qquad\qquad p \in \{50, 75, 100\}$
ampl_unif	moves the time series upwards, along the y-axis $a_{pert} = a_{ref} + (avg \times d/100)$ [2] 5 degrees: $d \in \{5, 10, 15, 20, 25\}$
dilat_unif	increases amplitude at each time-stamp, depending on initial amplitude $a_{pert} = a_{ref} \times (1 + d/100)$ 5 degrees: $d \in \{5, 10, 15, 20, 25\}$
dilat_biunif	increases all amplitudes that were above the polynomial fitted to the initial time series [3], depending on initial amplitude; symmetrically, decreases all amplitudes that were below the polynomial $a_{ref} > a_{pol} : a_{pert} = a_{ref} + ((a_{ref} - a_{pol}) \times d/100)$ $a_{ref} \leq a_{pol} : a_{pert} = a_{ref} + ((a_{pol} - a_{ref} \times d/100)$ 5 degrees: $d \in \{20, 40, 60, 80, 100\}$
elast	inserts $d\%$ novel values at time-stamps drawn at random, the inserted value being the average between preceding and next values 5 degrees: $d \in \{10, 20, 30, 40, 50\}$
dilat_biunif$_e$	applies dilat_biunif and then elast perturbations 5×5 degrees: $d_{elast} \in \{10, 20, 30, 40, 50\}$, $\qquad\qquad d_{dilat\_biunif} \in \{20, 40, 60, 80, 100\}$

4.3 Implementation and Parameterization

The SVP-OR framework has been implemented in Python 3.10.0. Following the advice of anaesthesia experts, we set nba at 4 (see Subsect. 3.1).

We ran five similarity searches in parallel, each driven by the relaxation percentages $P_1 = 1\%, P_2 = 5\%, P_3 = 10\%, P_4 = 20\%, P_5 = 50\%$ (see Eq. 2).

We recall that the similarity score $\mathcal{S}im$ used in these searches is the weighted combination of similarity scores on event traces and time series (Eq. 7). We fixed the weights as follows: $\alpha_a = \alpha_i = 1$ (event traces), $\alpha_s = 2$ (time series).

4.4   Experimental Set Up to Assess the Realism of the SVP-OR Simulations

Our aim is to evaluate how the simulated trajectories (*i.e.*, simulated multivariate time series) depart from observed trajectories.

To achieve this evaluation, n_s digital patients have been subjected to the same sequences of medical actions as n_s patients of the BDLBS data set.

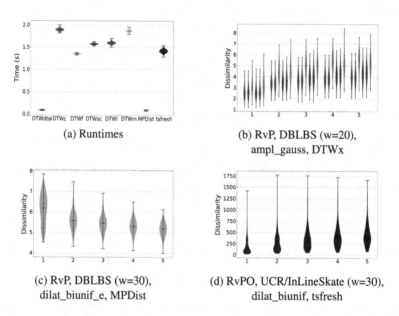

(a) Runtimes

(b) RvP, DBLBS (w=20), ampl_gauss, DTWx

(c) RvP, DBLBS (w=30), dilat_biunif_e, MPDist

(d) RvPO, UCR/InLineSkate (w=30), dilat_biunif, tsfresh

Fig. 5. Comparison of the 8 dissimilarities. (a) Running times. (b) to (d) Partial overview of the trends observed. x-axis: increasing degree of perturbation. w: length of the time series in the reference data set considered. See Table 1 for abbreviations. DTWx: DTWdtai: pink; DTWc: red; DTWf: orange; DTWsc: brown; DTWi: light green; DTWm: dark green; MPDist: light blue; tsfresh: navy blue. (Color figure online)

To start the simulation for i^{th} digital patient, we inititialized its nbv variables to those of ith real patient, observed at the beginning of the surgical operation.

Under the normal conditions of use of the SVP-OR simulator, the trainee is a human being. However, in our experiment, the trainee is virtual: we therefore modified the interface of SVP-OR (line 4 of Algorithm 1), to notify SVP-OR of all medical actions in the real scenario observed. It is important to note that this particular context of using the SVP-OR system eliminates the issue of having to initiate the actions that are not performed by the trainee.

We considered two parameter settings for our SVP-OR approach. On the one hand, we focused on the strategy where a single nearest neighbour is used at each short-term prediction ($k = 1$). On the other hand, setting k to 10 offered a compromise between calculation time and willingness to consider a number of nearest neighbours that is not too small.

Figure 6 offers a visual comparison between real and predicted time subseries for the strategy relying on a single nearest neighbour, for one complete simulation.

When we simulated i^{th} digital patient, we temporarily excluded i^{th} real patient from the set $Cohort$, so as never to accept i^{th} real patient as a k nearest neighbour. For each of the n_s simulations, we computed the dissimilarity between the real and predicted subseries, using Eq. 5. A normalized similarity Sim_n was then defined, considering the two experiments driven by $k = 1$ and $k = 10$:

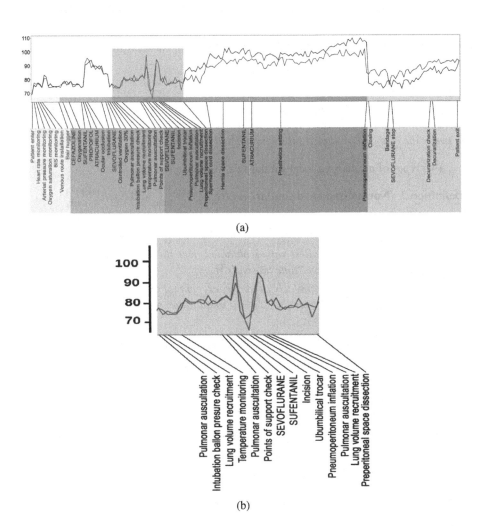

(a)

(b)

Fig. 6. Comparison of real and simulated time series obtained with the SVP-OR simulator parameterized with $k = 1$. The illustration shows the evolution of heart rate. Medical actions relevant to anaesthesia are indicated in capital letters. Black line: real time series. Blue line: simulation. (b) Magnified partial view of (a) encompassing the end of the induction phase and the beginning of the procedure phase. (Color figure online)

Definition 1 (Normalized Global Similarity Sim_n).
$Sim_n = \frac{D_{m\,max} - D_m}{D_{m\,max} - D_{m\,min}}$, where $D_{m\,max}$ and $D_{m\,min}$ are respectively the largest and smallest values obtained over all $2 \times n_s$ simulations obtained with parameter settings $k = 1$ and $k = 10$.

We considered a first category of distributions of normalized similarities:

Notation 1 (Distribution $\mathcal{D}_{Sim_n}$).
The distribution of normalized global similarities obtained over the $2 \times n_s$ simulations is denoted $\mathcal{D}_{Sim_n}$.

In addition to computing the global similarity Sim_n for each simulation, we computed local similarities:

Definition 2 (Local dissimilarity $D_m{}_{\tau_p}^{\tau_q}$).
Given two successive actions p and q in the jth simulation scenario, and their discretized initiation times τ_p and τ_q, following Eq. 5, we define $D_m{}_{\tau_p}^{\tau_q}$ as the dissimilarity between the real and predicted subseries defined over $[\tau_p, \tau_q]$.

Two types of normalized local similarities were then defined:

Definition 3 (Normalized local similarities $Sim_n^{(int,k)\tau_q}{}_{\tau_p}$ and $Sim_n^{(int)\tau_q}{}_{\tau_p}$).

- $Sim_n^{(int,k)\tau_q}{}_{\tau_p} = \frac{D_m{}_{\tau_p\,max}^{\tau_q} - D_m{}_{\tau_p}^{\tau_q}}{D_m{}_{\tau_p\,max}^{\tau_q} - D_m{}_{\tau_p\,min}^{\tau_q}}$ where $D_m{}_{\tau_p\,max}^{\tau_q}$ and $D_m{}_{\tau_p\,min}^{\tau_q}$ are respectively the largest and smallest values obtained over the n_s simulations performed with parameterization k, in "time intervals $[\tau_p, \tau_q]$".
- $Sim_n^{(int)\tau_q}{}_{\tau_p}$ is calculated similarly as above, except that the maximum and minimum considered are obtained over the $2 \times n_s$ simulations performed with $k = 1$ and $k = 10$, in "time intervals $[\tau_p, \tau_q]$".

Note that we abusively use "time intervals $[\tau_p, \tau_q]$" for simplicity, but the reader should bear in mind that the simulations differ from each another by τ_p and τ_q, the discretized initiation times of the two successive actions p and q present in all the simulated scenarios.

We considered the following distributions:

Notation 2 (Distributions $\mathcal{D}_{Sim_n^{(int,k)\tau_q}{}_{\tau_p}}$ and $\mathcal{D}_{Sim_n^{(int)\tau_q}{}_{\tau_p}}$).
The distributions of normalized local similarities defined over "time intervals $[\tau_p, \tau_q]$" across the n_s, and $2 \times n_s$ simulations respectively are denoted $\mathcal{D}_{Sim_n^{(int,k)\tau_q}{}_{\tau_p}}$ and $\mathcal{D}_{Sim_n^{(int)\tau_q}{}_{\tau_p}}$.

4.5 Results and Discussion

We set the number of simulations n_s to 1000.

Figure 7 allows to compare the abilities to simulate a digital patient in a realistic way, according to the two parameter settings of SVP-OR.

We conclude that for the surgery of interest, the distributions obtained using a unique nearest neighbour and 10 nearest neighbours are characterized by the same median global normalized similarity (0.84). Thus, we show that both simulation strategies are equally capable of producing realistic results. However, the simulation using 10 nearest neighbours entails more variability than the other simulation, with 25%- and 75% interquartiles at 0.75 and 0.96, with respect to 0.81 and 0.88. An additional conclusion is that, even in the context of the chunk-wise construction of the final time series of ith digital patient (see Sect. 3.4), the potentially continuous change of the single nearest neighbour nevertheless keeps the **whole** simulated time series close to that of ith real patient.

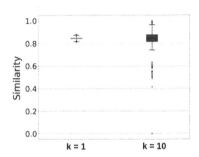

Fig. 7. Comparison between the multivariate time series of real patient and digital patient simulated through the SVP-OR approach. k is the number of nearest neighbours considered in our case-based reasoning approach. The scenario of interest studied is the inguinal hernia operation under laparoscopy and with prosthetics setting, for a male patient aged 30 years, weighing 80 kg, with no medical history. Each box plot represents $\mathcal{D}_{Sim_n}$ (see Notation 1), the distribution of normalized global similarities (see Definition 1). These distributions were obtained for 1000 real patients and 1000 digital patients simulated by using the same 1000 medical action sequences as for the real patients.

Figure 8 highlights that for the surgery of interest and a patient without complications, the simulation is carried out with a relatively high degree of realism throughout the operation, for every strategy (*i.e.*, parameter setting).

Using the normalized similarity $Sim_n^{(int,k)}{}^{\tau_q}_{\tau_p}$, we observe the same general trend for both parameterizations: (i) the similarity is rather stable for 5 out of 7 intervals in ENTER phase and 5 out of 6 intervals in EXIT phase for the two parameterizations; (ii) in contrast, the similarity varies continuously, from one interval to another in the INDUCTION and PROCEDURE phases. The variation is a little more pronounced in the induction phase, in the case of a single nearest neighbour. These results are explained by the fact that more variability is expected in longer phases, in contrast to short routine phases. We learn that INDUCTION, which is however not specific to the inguinal hernia operation, shows variations all through the phase, as for the PROCEDURE phase. In constrast, we are less surprised by the variations observed locally within the procedure phase, which is specific to each type of surgery.

Figures 9(a) and (b) focus on the local similarities normalized within each interval, but with the two strategies $k = 1$ and $k = 10$ taken together ($Sim_n^{(int)}{}^{\tau_q}_{\tau_p}$).

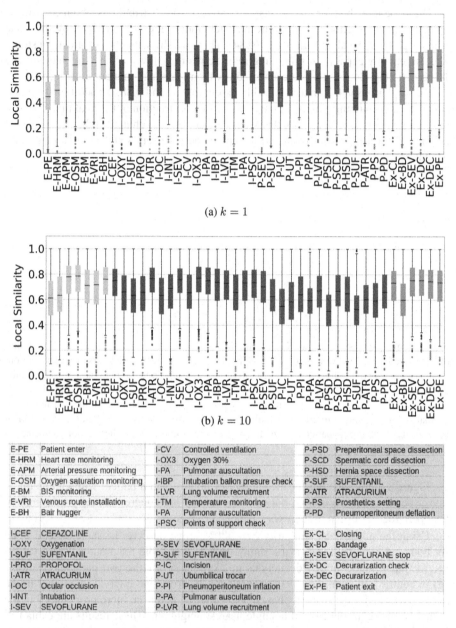

(a) $k = 1$

(b) $k = 10$

E-PE	Patient enter	I-CV	Controlled ventilation	P-PSD	Preperitoneal space dissection
E-HRM	Heart rate monitoring	I-OX3	Oxygen 30%	P-SCD	Spermatic cord dissection
E-APM	Arterial pressure monitoring	I-PA	Pulmonar auscultation	P-HSD	Hernia space dissection
E-OSM	Oxygen saturation monitoring	I-IBP	Intubation ballon presure check	P-SUF	SUFENTANIL
E-BM	BIS monitoring	I-LVR	Lung volume recruitment	P-ATR	ATRACURIUM
E-VRI	Venous route installation	I-TM	Temperature monitoring	P-PS	Prosthetics setting
E-BH	Bair hugger	I-PA	Pulmonar auscultation	P-PD	Pneumoperitoneum deflation
		I-PSC	Points of support check		
I-CEF	CEFAZOLINE			Ex-CL	Closing
I-OXY	Oxygenation	P-SEV	SEVOFLURANE	Ex-BD	Bandage
I-SUF	SUFENTANIL	P-SUF	SUFENTANIL	Ex-SEV	SEVOFLURANE stop
I-PRO	PROPOFOL	P-IC	Incision	Ex-DC	Decurarization check
I-ATR	ATRACURIUM	P-UT	Ubumbilical trocar	Ex-DEC	Decurarization
I-OC	Ocular occlusion	P-PI	Pneumoperitoneum inflation	Ex-PE	Patient exit
I-INT	Intubation	P-PA	Pulmonar auscultation		
I-SEV	SEVOFLURANE	P-LVR	Lung volume recruitment		

Fig. 8. Comparison of real and digital patients within each strategy, in the intervals between the initiations of two successive medical actions. k is the number of nearest neighbours. The four main phases of the surgical procedure are highlighted in light blue (ENTER), green (INDUCTION), red (PROCEDURE) and orange (EXIT). Each box plot represents $\mathcal{D}_{Sim_n^{(int,k)}}{}_{\tau_p}^{\tau_q}$ (see Notation 2), the distribution of local similarities normalized within each interval and each strategy (see Definition 3). (Color figure online)

In the 7 subphases of the ENTER phase, the mean local similarity $Sim_n^{(int)^{\tau_q}}_{\tau_p}$, varies in range [0.39, 0.74] for $k = 1$ and in range [0.72, 0.83] for $k = 10$. In the 16 intervals of the INDUCTION phase, the respective ranges are [0.47, 0.74] and [0.72, 0.82]. In the PROCEDURE phase, the means in the 14 intervals range in [0.43, 0.69] and [0.63, 0.78], respectively. The 6 intervals of the phase EXIT are characterized by variations in [0.44, 0.69] and [0.71, 0.79]. Thus, using several nearest neighbours makes the digital patient **locally** more similar to the real patient than when using the nearest neighbour. In particular, for $k = 1$, we find 19 intervals out of 43 with local similarity means below 0.6 for $k = 1$, and none for $k = 10$. Nine intervals out of 43 show a local similarity above 0.7, for $k = 1$; 37 intervals out of 43 are in this case, for $k = 10$.

This type of normalized similarity, $Sim_n^{(int)^{\tau_q}}_{\tau_p}$, clearly highlights the fact that the use of several nearest neighbours constitutes the most favourable situation to obtain a

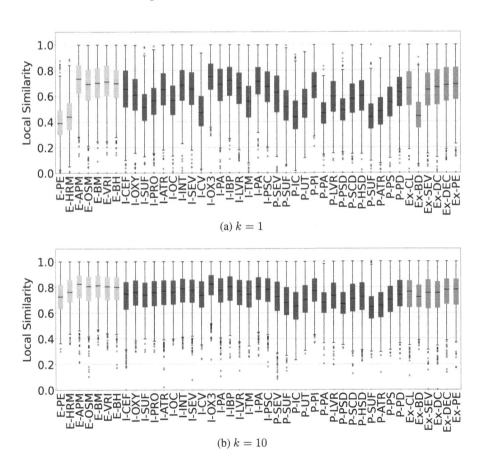

(a) $k = 1$

(b) $k = 10$

Fig. 9. Comparison of real and digital patients across the two strategies, in the intervals between the initiations of two successive medical actions. Each box plot represents $\mathcal{D}_{Sim_n^{(int)^{\tau_q}}_{\tau_p}}$, the distribution of local similarities normalized within each interval and taking strategies $k = 1$ and $k = 2$ together. See Notation 2 and Definition 3.

realistic simulation. Second, using more nearest neighbours homogenizes the ability to predict realistically throughout the surgery. In this respect, a contrast in the variabilities between the two parameterizations for the INDUCTION and PROCEDURE phases is clearly visible. Finally, the $Sim_n^{(int)^{\tau_q}}{}_{\tau_p}$ normalized similarity allows to point out nine steps of the surgery for which the evolution is more difficult to simulate than the others: E-PE, E-HRM; I-CV; P-IC*, P-PA*, P-PSD*, P-SUF*, P-ATR*; EX-BD, where * indicates a trend common to both strategies, and no annotation indicates that only the parameterization with $k = 1$ suffers from this lower ability.

The main conclusion to draw is that under any parameterization, the SVP-OR approach produces trajectories sufficiently similar to real trajectories, when constrained by real scenarios. Anyway, it is more the realism (reproducing the main trends for responses to medical actions) than the accuracy of the prediction that is important for our training application.

5   Conclusion and Future Work

We have proposed the framework SVP-OR (Simulation of Virtual Patient at the Operating Room), which relies on a case-based reasoning approach to make evolve the vital signs of a digital patient in response to the actions of a user and a virtual medical team. The aim is to provide a digital training aid to the user (trainee). Three main functions have been developed: contextualized multidimensional pattern retrieval, short-term prediction from the histories of real patients, and global chunk-wise prediction for the dynamic behaviour of the digital patient.

In order to be used for training purposes, our simulation software will need to trigger the medical actions performed by the virtual agents. One of our future works will be to design a model to subsume the observed event logs for a cohort of patients undergoing a surgery of interest. This synthetic representation will allow SVP-OR to automatically program the actions of the virtual agents. In addition, it will provide a means of identifying inappropriate actions by the trainee.

We also plan to integrate in the SVP-OR framework human factors that may cause the user to make a mistake. These factors include, for example, novel situations, stressful situations, and instances of interactions within the medical team that are likely to perturb the trainee.

One of our next works will also be to deploy SVP-OR on other surgeries, especially surgeries with a more variable course from one patient to another, than inguinal hernia surgery.

The ability to simulate the dynamic behaviour of a digital patient in response to external stimuli offers opportunities beyond the training objective considered here.

First, we can use SVP-OR to generate complex realistic data consisting of interdependent time series and event traces. Whereas the medical data input to SVP-OR is protected, the realistic data output by SVP-OR can be shared with the outside world. This potentiality offers an alternative to data anonymization, a task impossible to achieve in the case of complex dependencies existing within temporal data. By helping to make data available, SVP-OR can thus contribute to the development of research collaboration between university hospitals and the outside world.

Second, by circumventing the need to define and train a complex model in machine learning, SVP-OR allows us to develop a digital twin for a patient undergoing a surgery. In this way, in the context of personalized medicine, we can for example predict the risks associated with given phases of a surgical process, for patients with a medical history.

Acknowledgements. The authors are grateful for the financial support of the thesis of H. Boisaubert, by the Pays de la Loire regional research project RFI OIC EXAN. Funding for the internship work of L. Vincent was provided by the FAME research cluster (Human Factors for Medical Technologies, NExT/ANR-16-IDEX-0007). The authors wish to thank F. Dama, PhD student, for her key contribution to the development of the BDLBS generator. The experiments were carried out at the CCIPL (Centre de Calcul Intensif des Pays de la Loire, Nantes, France).

References

1. Boisaubert, H., Vincent, L., Lejus-Bourdeau, C., Sinoquet, C.: Simulation of the evolution of a virtual patient's physiological status in the operating room: application to computer-assisted anaesthesia training. In: 15th International Joint Conference on Biomedical Engineering Systems and Technologies, BIOSTEC2022, vol. 5: HEALTHINF, pp. 228–239 (2022)
2. Cao, D., Liu, J.: Research on dynamic time warping multivariate time series similarity matching based on shape feature and inclination angle. J. Cloud Comput. **5**(1), 1–9 (2016). https://doi.org/10.1186/s13677-016-0062-z
3. Choudhury, N., Begum, S.: A survey on case-based reasoning in medicine. Int. J. Adv. Comput. Sci. Appl. **7**(8), 132–136 (2016)
4. Christ, M., Braun, N., Neuffer, J., Kempa-Liehr, A.: Time Series FeatuRe Extraction on basis of Scalable Hypothesis tests (tsfresh - a Python package). Neurocomputing **307**, 72–77 (2018)
5. Dau, H., et al.: Hexagon-ML: the UCR time series classification archive (2018). https://www.cs.ucr.edu/~eamonn/time_series_data_2018
6. Erdogan, T., Tarhan, A.: A goal-driven evaluation method based on process mining for healthcare processes. Appl. Sci. **8**(6), 894 (2018)
7. Forestier, G., Petitjean, F., Riffaud, L., Jannin, P.: Automatic matching of surgeries to predict surgeons' next actions. Artif. Intell. Med. **81**, 3–11 (2017)
8. Franke, S., Meixensberger, J., Neumuth, T.: Intervention time prediction from surgical low-level tasks. J. Biomed. Inform. **46**(1), 152–09 (2013)
9. Ganzinger, M., Schrodt, J., Knaup-Gregori, P.: A concept for graph-based temporal similarity of patient data. Stud. Health Technol. Inform. **264**, 138–142 (2019)
10. Gharghabi, S., Imani, S., Bagnall, A., Darvishzadeh, A., Keogh, E.: Matrix profile XII: MPdist: a novel time series distance measure to allow data mining in more challenging scenarios. In: IEEE International Conference on Data Mining (ICDM), pp. 965–970 (2018)
11. Giusti, R., Batista, G.E.A.P.A.: An empirical comparison of dissimilarity measures for time series classification. In: Brazilian Conference on Intelligent Systems (BRACIS), pp. 82–88 (2013)
12. Guédon, A., Meij, S., Osman, K., et al.: Deep learning for surgical phase recognition using endoscopic videos. Surg. Endosc. **35**(11), 6150–6157 (2021)
13. Itakura, F.: Minimum prediction residual principle applied to speech recognition. IEEE Trans. Acoust. Speech Signal Process. **23**(1), 67–72 (1975)
14. Khalid, S., Goldenberg, M., Grantcharov, T., Taati, B., Rudzicz, F.: Evaluation of deep learning models for identifying surgical actions and measuring performance. JAMA Netw. Open **3**(3), e201664 (2020)

15. Kianimajd, A., et al.: Comparison of different methods of measuring similarity in physiologic time series. IFAC-PapersOnLine **50**(1), 11005–11010 (2017)
16. Lhermitte, S., Verbesselt, J., Verstraeten, W.W., Coppin, P.: A comparison of time series similarity measures for classification and change detection of ecosystem dynamics. Remote Sens. Environ. **115**(12), 3129–3152 (2011)
17. Liu, Z., Zhu, Z., Gao, J., Xu, C.: Forecast methods for time series data: a survey. IEEE Access **606–617**, 3091162 (2021)
18. Meißner, C., Meixensberger, J., Pretschner, A., Neumuth, T.: Sensor-based surgical activity recognition in unconstrained environments. Minim. Invasive Ther. Allied Technol. **23**, 198–205 (2014)
19. Mülâyim, M., Arcos, J.: Fast anytime retrieval with confidence in large-scale temporal case bases. Knowl.-Based Syst. **206**, 106374 (2020)
20. Müller, M., Mattes, H., Kurth, F.: An efficient multiscale approach to audio synchronization. In: International Conference on Music Information Retrieval (ISMIR), pp. 192–197 (2006)
21. Munoz-Gama, J., Martin, N., Fernandez-Llatas, C., et al.: Process mining for healthcare: characteristics and challenges. J. Biomed. Inform. **127**, 103994 (2022)
22. Nagendran, M., Gurusamy, K., Aggarwal, R., Loizidou, M., Davidson, B.: Virtual reality training for surgical trainees in laparoscopic surgery. Cochrane Database Syst. Rev. **8**, CD00657 (2013)
23. Qi, D., Ryason, A., Milef, N., et al.: Virtual reality operating room with AI guidance: design and validation of a fire scenario. Surg. Endosc. **35**(2), 779–786 (2021)
24. Sakoe, H., Chiba, S.: A dynamic programming approach to continuous speech recognition. In: ICA, Paper 20 CI3 (1971)
25. Sakoe, H., Chiba, S.: Dynamic programming algorithm optimization for spoken word recognition. IEEE Trans. Acoust. Speech Signal Process. **26**(1), 43–49 (1978)
26. Salvador, S., Chan, P.: Toward accurate dynamic time warping in linear time and space. Intell. Data Anal. **11**(5), 561–580 (2007)
27. Sha, Y., Venugopalan, J., Wang, M.: A novel temporal similarity measure for patients based on irregularly measured data in electronic health records. In: Seventh ACM International Conference on Bioinformatics, Computational Biology, and Health Informatics (BCB), pp. 337–344 (2016)
28. Stauder, R., Okur, A., Peter, L., et al.: Random forests for phase detection in surgical workflow analysis. In: International Conference on Information Processing in Computer-Assisted Interventions, pp. 148–157 (2014)
29. Wang, X., Mueen, A., Ding, H., Trajcevski, G., Scheuermann, P., Keogh, E.: Experimental comparison of representation methods and distance measures for time series data. Data Min. Knowl. Disc. **26**(2), 275–309 (2013)

A Multi-Modal Dataset (MMSD) for Acute Stress Bio-Markers

Mouna Benchekroun[1,2(✉)] , Dan Istrate[1] , Vincent Zalc[1] ,
and Dominique Lenne[2]

[1] Biomechanics and Bioengineering Lab, University of Technology of Compiègne (UMR CNRS 7338), Compiègne, France
mouna.benchekroun02@gmail.com, dan.istrate@utc.fr
[2] Heudiasyc Lab (Heuristics and Diagnosis of Complex Systems), University of Technology of Compiégne (UMR CNRS 7338), Compiègne, France

Abstract. The experiment presented in this study aimed at eliciting two affective states at pre-determined periods including relaxation and stress using various stressors. We advance the hypothesis that it is possible to observe patterns and variations in physiological signals caused by mental stress. In this chapter, an exhaustive description of the experimental protocol for signal acquisition is provided to ensure both reproducibility and repeatability. Details are presented on the whole process from the choice of sensors and stressors to the experimental design and the collected data so that the potential user of our database can have a global view and a deep understanding of the data.

Four physiological signals are recorded throughout the experiment in order to study their correlation with mental stress: electrocardiogram (ECG), photoplethysmogram (PPG), electrodermal activity (EDA) and electromyogram (EMG).

A statistical analysis is carried out for preliminary results and for protocol validation before a deeper analysis using artificial intelligence algorithms in future work.

Keywords: Stress · Multi-modal dataset · Emotion recognition · Stress bio-markers · Physiological data · Affective computing · Stroop test

1 Introduction

Stress has been a topic of growing interest to many different fields including medical professionals, researchers, psychologists as well as social scientists. It is proven to be very harmful to both physical and mental well being and the number of stress victims is growing at an alarming rate with millions of people on stress relief medication today [19]. According to The National Institute for Occupational Safety & Health, stress is responsible for 70% to 90% of employees hospital visits each year and causes huge financial losses to individuals as well as companies due to stress-related ailments [19]. Despite these alarming facts, there are still very few, if any, reliable stress assessment

Supported by INSEAD-Sorbonne University Behavioural Lab.

A. C. A. Roque et al. (Eds.): BIOSTEC 2022, CCIS 1814, pp. 377–392, 2023.
https://doi.org/10.1007/978-3-031-38854-5_19

systems available today. Given the multidimensional nature of stress, three different methods can be used to assess stress including psychological, behavioural and physiological approaches. Psychological methods include questionnaires based on subjective feedback, which is not always accurate. Besides, they are by definition influenced by various systematic measurement errors and bias [15]. Behavioural approaches on the other hand rely on body gestures and facial expressions. While they are part of the stress response, they can also be conscious and intentional. Furthermore, they can be influenced by environmental factors such as room lightening and temperature. Finally, the gold standard physiological stress measurement modality is through cortisol levels in the saliva, blood or urine. This approach is however punctual and delayed.

These limitations together with the development of wearable bio-sensors enhance the need for more reliable, continuous stress detection systems. One way of achieving this goal is using bio-signals involved in the stress response [31] related to heart, skin, muscle activity or other physiological modalities. The main advantage of such physiological signals is that they offer a continuous, real-time stress detection alternative.

2 Physiology of Stress

Selye was the first to introduce and popularize stress as a medical and scientific concept in 1936. He defined stress as the non-specific body response to any demand [35], being an internal or external factor threatening the homeostasis balance.

When a person perceives an upcoming event as a threat, a cascade of physiological processes occurs which are subsumed under the term "stress response" [15]. This response is mainly regulated by the Autonomic nervous system (ANS) and hypothalamic-pituitary-adrenocorticol (HPA) [13, 26] which releases corticotropin-releasing hormone (CRH). This hormone stimulates the secretion of adrenocorticotropic hormone (ACTH), which in turn, is released into the blood stream and eventually reaches the adrenal cortex and stimulates the secretion of cortisol, known as the stress hormone [24]. Energy is then diverted to the organs that need it most such as the skeletal muscles, brain and heart by contracting certain blood vessels while dilating others for less critical body functions such as digestion and reproduction systems [38].

Stress can be either acute or chronic. The acute stress response is generally adaptive and punctual. It can become maladaptive if it is repeatedly or continuously activated [35, 38].

Physiological changes due to increased sympathetic activity during the stress response include higher heart rate and skin temperature faster breathing [17, 20, 25], pupil dilatation [28], muscle contraction, higher skin conductance [14, 27, 29] ....

These physiological changes have been studied by many scientists for mental stress detection. Previous studies involve the monitoring of ECG, BVP, EDA (or Galvanic Skin Response GSR), HRV [30, 32], EMG, skin temperature and various other modalities.

Although many studies have been carried out on the subject, access to data remains very complicated since only few datasets are made public. One of the first stress datasets was published by Healey et al. [18]. It includes trapezius EMG, ECG, EDA and respiration signals from 24 subjects during real-world driving tasks. Koelstra et al. also published a stress dataset (DEAP) including Electroencephalograms (EEG) combined with other modalities [21]. 32 subjects were recorded while watching videos inducing different affective states. Another publicly available dataset is the $SWELL - KW$ collected in an experiment on 25 subjects in their work spaces while they performed typical knowledge work under stressful conditions such as time pressure and email interruptions [22]. More recently, *Schmidt et al.* published a multi-modal dataset (WESAD) of physiological and motion data from 15 subjects during a lab study where three affective states were induced : neutral, stress and amusement [33].

One of the main limitations common to the studies cited above is the small sample size which is under 30 participants for most. Besides, subjects are generally of the same age group and have similar occupational fields (usually students). Moreover, the use of self-assessment through hand-crafted or validated questionnaires as ground truth may be biases in some cases. Finally, stress is highly personalized phenomenon impacted by individual vulnerability and resilience... [12]. These parameters should be somehow considered in the experimental design.

The present study was designed to avoid some of these limitations. Firstly, thanks to the higher sample size as well as the diversity of the participants in terms of age, gender, occupation . . . , it is possible to draw more reliable conclusions and statistical generalisations. Secondly, protocol validation is achieved using both psychological self-reports and cortisol levels considered as gold standard for stress detection today. Finally, physiological differences and constraints such as cortisol fluctuation and subjects' profiles were taken into consideration in the study design.

The protocol was approved by The INSEAD Institutional Review Board (IRB : 202077) on August 2020 and the study was carried out in collaboration with INSEAD Behavioural Lab team which took charge of subject's recruitment and management.

3 Experimental Setup

3.1 Hardware

A market study was carried out to select the appropriate sensors in accordance with our needs. Four main criteria were taken into consideration in our choice :

- Access to raw data: Data had to be stored locally in the raw format for further signal processing of our choice.
- Wireless and real-time data collection: Raw data had to be collected via Bluetooth, displayed and stored in real-time.
- Research Validation: Sensors had to be validated for use in biomedical-oriented research applications.
- Ergonomic value: Sensors had to be designed to be wearable, free from wired constraints and light weighted.

Given these four constrains, sensors from the company Shimmer Sensing were selected. The advantage is that the company offers a specific sensor for each physiological signal of interest. All the sensors can be synchronised very easily using a dock board from the same company.

Some tests were performed to determine the optimal position for each sensor based on signals quality. Below is the final configuration in Fig. 1.

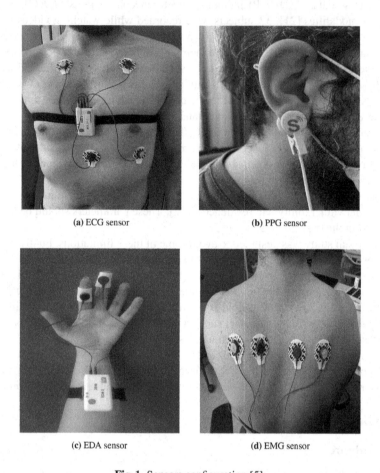

(a) ECG sensor   (b) PPG sensor

(c) EDA sensor   (d) EMG sensor

Fig. 1. Sensors configuration [5].

Three lead ECG is recorded using four self-adhesive electrodes. Two electrodes are placed across the heart, below the collar-bones, a third one below the chest, and the grounding electrode in the middle chest (Fig. 1a).

Pulse is recorded thanks to a transmission Photoplethysmography sensor (PPG) from the right earlobe. Transmission PPG sensors detect light passed through the tissue and are therefore commonly used on peripheral sites such as fingers and earlobes. We chose the latter location since it is less sensitive to motion artefact and tissue alterations caused by both voluntary and involuntary movements as there is no muscle activity [5].

Electrodermal activity is recorded with sticker electrodes on the participant's non dominant hand. One electrode is placed on the palmar surface of the index medial phalange and the other on the palmar surface of the middle fingers' distal phalange.

For trapezius muscle activity, positive and negative electrodes are placed in parallel with the muscle fibres, near the centre of the right and left muscles, 2cm apart from each other. The reference electrode is placed at the elbow as an electrically neutral point of the body far from the muscle being measured [5].

3.2 Software and Stressors

For device and data management, we used SHIMMER'S software CONSENSYSPRO which is designed for adaptive human data collection and multi-sensor management. The software offers several functionalities such as sensors' configuration, data management and real-time streaming.

Besides, an application for the management of the experimental protocol has been developed to automatically store user related and behavioural data on a local SQL database. The application was developed on JavaFX.

First, it has a"Relaxation" window with an option to play a sound of our choice. A start and stop buttons are used to launch the relaxation session and store related timestamps in the SQL database for automatic signal segmentation.

The application has different serious games designed to induce stress during the experimental study. Four stress games have been selected based on literature and implemented in the application.

Stroop Color Word Test

A modified version of the SCWT is used in the application to induce stress. A screen with different cards in displayed. Each time, a specific card is framed in red and the subject has to select the first letter of the color in the framed card using the computer mouse. For an additional level of complexity, the letters in the color bar change color and position at a specific frequency.

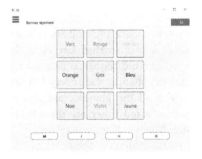

Mental Arithmetic

A series of arithmetic operation is displayed one after the other for the subject to perform using a keyboard. Each operation includes an addition, a subtraction, a multiplication as well as a division. We made sure all operations are of an attainable level of difficulty and the result is always an integer.

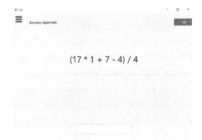

Table 1. Task duration for each stressor.

Age	Stressor	Duration	N° of questions
18–50 yo	SCWT	3 s	110
	Computer Work	15 s	21
	Mental Arithmetic	6 s	50
	Subtraction	5 s	60
50+ yo	SCWT	6 s	55
	Computer Work	20 s	16
	Mental Arithmetic	12 s	25
	Subtraction	10 s	30

Base Seven Subtractions

A second arithmetic task consisting of a series of subtractions of the number 7 from 1024.

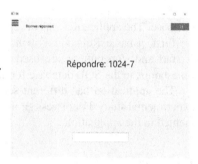

Speed and Concentration Game

A sequence of numbers is displayed on the screen above a virtual keyboard. Subject has to reproduce the sequence in a time period while numbers change place every few seconds.

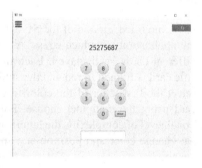

For all the games cited above, a score as well as a red timer are used to increase pressure. Moreover, the use of deceit helped induce a social-evaluative threat when failure or poor performance could be harmful to one's social esteem or social status [10]. Subjects were not aware that the objective is to induce stress. Instead, they were told an IQ score is computed based on their performance and this score is used to compare them to subjects of the same age.

Various tests were carried out to choose task's parameters including duration, update speed .... The goal was to reach a level of difficulty high enough to induce stress, but not too high so as not to cause a feeling of failure that would lead the subject to give up. Two options were selected depending on the age group of the subject as summarized in Table 1.

Using this design, we were able to provoke a stressful situation characterized by uncontrollability and social-evaluative threat [9, 10].

4   Eligibility Criteria and Participants

Subjects were selected in accordance with ethical criteria as well as the constraints related to the study itself. Volunteers were asked to fill a pre-selection questionnaire sent to them by email as part of selection process with four objectives [5] :

1. Exclude non eligible volunteers:
   Subjects were selected in order to have a statistically representative sample of the french population in terms of age and gender. Exclusion criteria included volunteers suffering from : cardiovascular diseases, chronic diseases (diabetes, hypertension and mental disorders (depression, dementia . . .) since these conditions may have an impact on the collected physiological data [5].
2. Build a subject profile:
   The pre-selection questionnaire was also used to collect general information about lifestyle elements that would potentially affect the stress response such as: the participant's level of physical activity, eating habits, sleeping habits, meditation, . . . These elements could be used in data interpretation [5].
3. Enunciate guidelines:
   Guidelines were given in the pre-selection questionnaire to check volunteer's acceptability to wear the biosensors and their willingness to respect some instructions. For example, selected subjects were asked to abstain from alcohol, caffeine/theine and tobacco, 12 h, 4 h and 2 h respectively before the experiment [5].
4. Measure Perceived Stress:
   The questionnaire also includes a PSS4 (Perceived Stress Scale) consisting of 4 questions. This scale assesses the state of perceived stress and measures the degree to which situations in one's life are appraised as stressful [5,37].

227 participants volunteered to take part of our study. 57 were rejected due to exclusion criteria and 74 healthy subjects were selected from the remaining volunteers. Our objective was to form a representative sample of the French population in terms of age and gender. Figure 2 summarizes the selection process.

5   Experimental Design

The goal of this experimental study is to elicit two affective states and identify characteristic patterns of mental stress in physiological signals. The study is performed under strict laboratory conditions in order to reduce the effect of environmental and behavioural noise to a minimum [5]. The experimental protocol is detailed below and depicted in Fig. 3 :

1. **Preparation:** Upon arrival at the study location and prior to the study, the participants read and signed a consent form. Then they were equipped with the sensors and a short sensor test was conducted. During this phase, questions were asked to verify compliance with the instructions including last caffeine, theanine, tobacco and alcohol consumption.

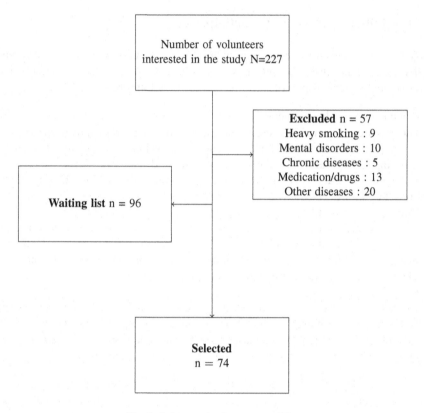

Fig. 2. Subject selection process [5].

2. **Relaxation/Meditation:** Subject is invited to relax during 15 min thanks guided meditation session instructed via an audio track. Subjects followed the instructions with closed eyes, while sitting in a comfortable position in a dark environment [5].
3. **Stress:** Subject performs various stressful tasks introduced above during 20 min.
4. **Recovery:** At the end of the protocol, data is recorded for an additional 10 min while subject is asked to stay seated with a calm music background.
   The purpose of this step is to evaluate how subjects recover from a stressful stimuli [5].

The study lasts for about 80 min including 40 min recording segmented as follows: 15 min relaxation, 20 min stress and 10 min recovery.

6   Protocol Validation and Labeling

Since the main purpose of this study is to use machine learning algorithms for stress recognition, we needed to validate our protocol beforehand in order to make sure subject's affective state matches the experimental protocol [5]. Two different measures are used as labels during to experiment :

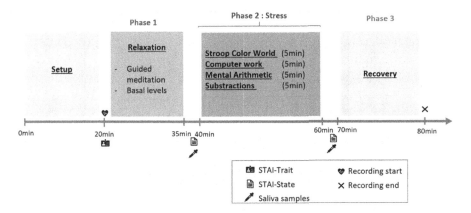

Fig. 3. Study experimental protocol [5].

– **Cortisol Samples:** Saliva samples are collected after the first and second phases (baseline and stress respectively). Since cortisol levels vary throughout the day with the highest peak reached few hours after waking up, all trials took place in the afternoon (after 2pm) to make sure the wake-up peak does not reverse the increase in cortisol levels from the first to the second sample [5,7,10].

– **STAI-S:** State-Trait Anxiety Inventory $(STAI)$ questionnaire comprises separate self-report scales for measuring two distinct anxiety concepts: trait anxiety $(STAI-T)$ and state anxiety $(STAI-S)$. Each scale is made up of 20 questions weighted from 0 to 4. Scores for both the S-Anxiety and the T-Anxiety scales can vary from a minimum of 20 to a maximum of 80. $(STAI-S)$ measures anxiety as an emotional state linked to a particular situation. It is used as a subjective label after each phase together with cortisol levels to validate our protocol [5].

Since cortisol is considered to be a stress hormone, we expect cortisol levels to be higher in the second sample taken after the stress phase with comparison to the first one. $STAI-S$ scores should also be higher if the subject was indeed stressed in the second phase. The combination of both physiological and subjective labels makes the validation process more reliable [5].

7 Collected Data

The 74 recruited healthy volunteers were 51% women and 49% men. The total 38 women were aged 19 to 63 years old with a mean age: 33 y.o $\pm$ 12.5 and the 36 men were aged 21 to 79 years old with a mean age : 35 y.o $\pm$ 13. Figure 4 shows age distribution for each gender.

Profile data was collected prior to the study through the pre-selection questionnaire such as subjects eating and sleeping habits.

Behavioural data related to the stress tasks as well as subject's self-evaluation scores were stored in the local SQL database linked to the application. Finally, physiological

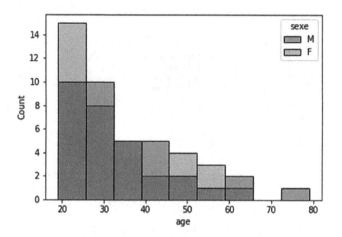

Fig. 4. Age & Gender distribution of the sample.

signals were recorded using Consensys Pro, Shimmer's platform, via Bluetooth and on the sensors SD card to avoid any undesired data losses.

Each signal was sampled at a rate appropriate for capturing the information contained in the signal. 512 Hz for ECG, PPG, EDA and 1000 Hz for EMG [5]. All the sensors are equipped with a three axis gyroscope for orientation and angular velocity.

Physiological signals cited above are recorded continuously for 40 min all along the study. Signal segmentation is achieved automatically using the timestamps from the SQL database. The first phase, *Relaxation phase*, is referred to as session 1, session 2 is the *Stress phase* and session 3 is the *Recovery*.

Each of the recorded parameters can be used either for data interpretation, classification or labeling depending on the end purpose. Some examples are presented but are not limited to Table 2 [5].

7.1 Signal Processing and Feature Extraction

As usual for biosignals, pre-pocessing steps have to be carried out prior to analysis and feature extraction. Pre-pocessing may include, down-sampling, filtering and artefacts removal. We used Python Toolboxes such as $Neurokit2$ [23], HRV: a Pythonic package for Heart Rate Variability Analysis [2] and $TSFEL$ [1] for the processing and feature extraction. Many tests have been carried out in order to choose the best parameters for each step.

Electrodemal Activity (EDA). EDA response consists of two characteristic components:

1. Tonic component: a slowly changing offset known as the skin conductance level (SCL).

Table 2. Types and potential use of collected data [5].

Type	Data	Use
Profile Data	Sex,age ... Eating and sleeping habits Exercising Meditation	Interpretation
Subjective/Psychological	PSS4 and STAI-T STAI-S	Interpretation Labeling
Behavioural	Responses Time Successes and failures in trials Task duration	Interpretation and/or segmentation
Physiological	Electrocardiogram (ECG) Photoplethysmogram (PPG) Electrodermal Activity (EDA) Electromyogram (EMG) Three axis gyroscope data **Salivary Cortisol Levels**	Data Analysis Classification Interpretation **Labeling**

2. Phasic component: a series of transient peaks known as skin conductance responses (SCRs) They usually occur in reaction to a stimuli but also spontaneously, in which case they are referred to as nonspecific (NS-SCR).

Since EDA's bandwidth is [0–3 Hz], the signal is down-sampled 32 Hz which is ten times the higher limit [6]. High frequency noise is removed thanks to a fourth order high-cut Butterworth filter. SCRs frequency in absence of any identifiable stimulus is 1 to 3 per minute (0.05 Hz). This is why we chose a cutoff frequency of 0.5 Hz for the Butterworth filter [8].

Extraction of phasic and tonic components of the EDA signal was achieved using the $nk.eda\_phasic$ [16] function from $Neurokit2$ Toolbox.

Heart Rate Variability (HRV). HRV is extracted from both PPG and ECG signals. ECG signals are filtered using a third-order bandpass Butterworth filter [5 Hz–150 Hz], a Discrete Wavelet Transform (DWT) Db4 with a *Hard tresholding* as well as a 50 Hz Notch filter to remove both high frequency noise and the power line. R peaks are extracted using an optimised Pan-Thompkins algorithm on Matlab [34].

PPG is filtered using a second-order Butterworth filter [0.5 Hz - 10 Hz] which removes both high frequency noises and the baseline drift [11]. Pulse detection was achieved using the Matlab function FIND PEAK.

Once HRV is extracted from ECG and PPG, it is preprocessed for ectopic beats RR <0.3 s and RR>1.3 s and missing data caused by transmission errors or false peaks detection [3]. Ectopic beats are deleted before using a Shape-preserving piece-wise cubic Hermit (Pchip) interpolation [4]. For the frequency domain analysis, HRV signal is resampled 8 Hz.

Finally, statistical, non linear, time and frequency domain features are computed from HRV and EDA signals on 5 min windows with 4 min overlap. Table 3 includes a non exhaustive list example of computed features in each domain. Exact formulas can be found at [1, 36].

Table 3. Examples of computed features from HRV and EDA.

Signal	Statistical	Time Domain	Frequency Domain	Non Linear
EDA	skewness, kurtosis, maximum, minimum, mean, standard deviation ...	slope, absolute energy, entropy, total energy ...	maximum frequency, spectral entropy, spectral variation, wavelet energy	
HRV	mean HR, minimum HR mean RR ...	RMSSD, SDNN, Pnn50, nn50, ...	LF power, HF power, LF/HF ...	SD1, SD2 ...

8   Statistical Analysis

For all the tests in this section, results are considered to be statistically significant at a critical threshold of 5% ($p\_value < 0.05$). First, an analysis of both subjective (STAI-S questionnaire) and physiological (cortisol) labels was carried out to validate the experimental protocol.

According to Table 4 and the box plots in Fig. 5, there seems to be a difference between the two conditions. Median values and scores variability are higher during the stress phase compared to relaxation. A two-tailed Wilcoxon Signed-Rank Test is used to check if the differences are significant. This non parametric test is designed to evaluate the difference between two conditions where the samples are correlated as is the case in this study. In particular, it is suitable for evaluating the data from a repeated-measures design in a situation where the prerequisites for a dependent samples t-test are not met.

1. The null hypothesis H0 asserts that Stai-State median scores before and after the stressors are identical.
2. The null hypothesis H0 asserts that cortisol median levels before and after the stressors are identical.

Table 4. Mean and Standard Deviation for STAI-S and cortisol levels during relaxation and stress phase.

Label	Condition			
	Stai-State (20–80)		Cortisol	
	μ	σ	μ	σ
Relaxation	28.74	7.58	5.51	4.26
Stress	39.97	11.27	6.51	4.39
p-value	< 0.00001		0.0004	

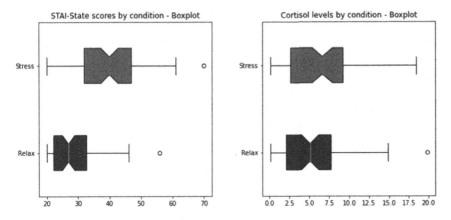

Fig. 5. Box plots comparing STAI-State and cortisol levels in stress and relaxation conditions.

Both p-values are under 0.05 which means median values for Stai-State and cortisol levels are significantly different before and after the stress phase. These results support the assumptions of the experimental design and prove the efficacy of the stressors.

Secondly, computed features from the recorded signals are analyzed and statistically compared. Kolmogorov-Smirnov test is used to study variable's distribution. For parametric variables, dependent t-test is used to compare the means through each phase. Features that do not meet validity conditions for parametric tests (distribution normality and equality of variances) are analyzed using non-parametric Wilcoxon Signed-Rank. We use $Scipy$ function $stats.wilcoxon$ on Python. Features are tested in paired classes, meaning Relaxation Vs Stress, Stress Vs Recovery and Relaxation Vs Recovery.

3. The null hypothesis H0 asserts that median EDA features before and after the stressors are identical across phases.
4. The null hypothesis H0 asserts that median HRV features before and after the stressors are identical across phases.

For most of the features, differences seem to be significant with a p-value under 0.05. Some examples are presented in Tables 5 and 6.

As can be seen from Tables 5 and 6, we would reject the null hypothesis at a confidence level of 5% for most of the features, concluding that there is significant differences between the phases. The non significant differences seem to be more frequent for Relaxation Vs Recovery comparison. In reality, these two phases can be similar for subjects who could not reach high relaxation. This may indeed explain the non significance for some features. Besides, these are preliminary results and further analysis using more advanced data analysis methods should be used for more founded results.

9   Case Study Strengths and Limitations

The strength of this study is that it explores new insights into continuous stress detection through various physiological signals. This paves the way for reliable stress

Table 5. P-values for examples of computed EDA features.

Feature	Relaxation VS Stress	Stress VS Recovery	Relaxation VS Recovery
Median Frequency	**0.006**	**0.013**	0.88
Absolute Energy	**<0.001**	**<0.001**	**<0.001**
Spectral Entropy	**<0.001**	**<0.001**	**<0.001**
Kurtosis	**<0.001**	**<0.001**	0.65
Median	**<0.001**	**<0.001**	**<0.001**
Minimum Tonic component	**<0.001**	**<0.001**	0.07
Mean Tonic component	**0.003**	0.056	0.149
Mean Phasic component	0.488	0.599	0.744

Table 6. P-values for examples of computed HRV features.

Feature	Relaxation VS Stress	Stress VS Recovery	Relaxation VS Recovery
Median Frequency	0.796	0.084	0.102
Kurtosis	**<0.001**	**<0.001**	0.872
Slope	**0.04**	**0.004**	0.272
LF/HF	**<0.001**	**0.017**	**<0.001**
Mean RR	**<0.001**	**<0.001**	**<0.001**
RMSSD	0.1	**<0.001**	**<0.001**
SDNN	0.491	**<0.001**	**<0.001**

monitoring systems for improved diagnosis and early treatment. Many physiological constrains and subject-specific variations were taken into consideration in the design of the study. Furthermore, the experimental protocol is validated with gold-standard stress measurements including both established psychological questionnaires and cortisol levels, which makes it reliable for analysis through AI algorithms.

It is worth mentioning that the evidence supporting this approach is, however, still experimental and further ambulatory data analysis needs to be carried out before it is possible to bring a product to market.

The relatively small (although one of the highest) sample size may limit the generalization of some results. Finally, a longitudinal study would be very interesting to explore stress patterns over time at an individual level, but time restrictions and subject's availability did not allow such experimental design.

Acknowledgements. Authors would like to thank Idex Sorbonne University for funding this experimental study as part of french state support for "Investissements d'Avenir program". Also thanks to all the subjects and to INSEAD lab for their expertise in participant recruitment and management which made the process extremely easier.

References

1. Barandas, M., et al.: TSFEL: time series feature extraction library. SoftwareX **11**, 100456 (2020)
2. Bartels, R., Peçanha, T.: HRV: a pythonic package for heart rate variability analysis. Github (2020). https://github.com/rhenanbartels/hrv/tree/0.2.8, https://doi.org/10.5281/zenodo.3960216. Accessed Oct 2021
3. Benchekroun, M., Chevallier, B., Istrate, D., Zalc, V., Lenne, D.: Preprocessing methods for ambulatory HRV analysis based on HRV distribution, variability and characteristics (DVC). Sensors **22**(5), 1984 (2022)
4. Benchekroun, M., Chevallier, B., Zalc, V., Istrate, D., Lenne, D., Vera, N.: Analysis of the impact of inter-beat-interval interpolation on real-time HRV feature estimation for e-health applications. In: JETSAN 2021-Colloque en Télésanté et dispositifs biomédicaux-8ème édition (2021)
5. Benchekroun, M., Istrate, D., Zalc, V., Lenne, D.: Mmsd: a multi-modal dataset for real-time, continuous stress detection from physiological signals. In: HEALTHINF, pp. 240–248 (2022)
6. Boucsein, W.: Principles of electrodermal phenomena. In: Electrodermal activity, pp. 121–122. Springer, Boston (2012). https://doi.org/10.1007/978-1-4614-1126-0_1
7. Colizzi, M., Costa, R., Todarello, O.: Transsexual patients' psychiatric comorbidity and positive effect of cross-sex hormonal treatment on mental health: results from a longitudinal study. Psychoneuroendocrinology **39**, 65–73 (2014)
8. Dawson, M.E., Schell, A.M., Filion, D.L.: The electrodermal system (2017)
9. Dickerson, S.S., Gruenewald, T.L., Kemeny, M.E.: Psychobiological responses to social self threat: functional or detrimental? Self identity **8**(2–3), 270–285 (2009)
10. Dickerson, S.S., Kemeny, M.E.: Acute stressors and cortisol responses: a theoretical integration and synthesis of laboratory research. Psychol. Bull. **130**(3), 355 (2004)
11. Elgendi, M., Jonkman, M., DeBoer, F.: Heart rate variability and the acceleration plethysmogram signals measured at rest. In: Fred, A., Filipe, J., Gamboa, H. (eds.) BIOSTEC 2010. CCIS, vol. 127, pp. 266–277. Springer, Heidelberg (2011). https://doi.org/10.1007/978-3-642-18472-7_21
12. Fink, G.: Chapter 1-stress, definitions, mechanisms, and effects outlined: lessons from anxiety. In: Fink, G. (ed.) Stress: Concepts, Cognition, Emotion, and Behavior, pp. 3–11 (2016)
13. Foley, P., Kirschbaum, C.: Human hypothalamus-pituitary-adrenal axis responses to acute psychosocial stress in laboratory settings. Neurosci. Biobehav. Rev. **35**(1), 91–96 (2010)
14. Giakoumis, D., et al.: Using activity-related behavioural features towards more effective automatic stress detection (2012)
15. Giannakakis, G., Grigoriadis, D., Giannakaki, K., Simantiraki, O., Roniotis, A., Tsiknakis, M.: Review on psychological stress detection using biosignals. IEEE Trans. Affect. Comput. **13**(1), 440–460 (2019)
16. Greco, A., Valenza, G., Lanata, A., Scilingo, E.P., Citi, L.: cvxEDA: a convex optimization approach to electrodermal activity processing. IEEE Trans. Biomed. Eng. **63**(4), 797–804 (2015)
17. Grossman, P.: Respiration, stress, and cardiovascular function. Psychophysiology **20**(3), 284–300 (1983)
18. Healey, J.A., Picard, R.W.: Detecting stress during real-world driving tasks using physiological sensors. IEEE Trans. Intell. Transp. Syst. **6**(2), 156–166 (2005)
19. Hoffmann, E.: Brain training against stress: theory, methods and results from an outcome study. Stress Rep. **4**(2), 1–24 (2005)

20. Karthikeyan, P., Murugappan, M., Yaacob, S.: Descriptive analysis of skin temperature variability of sympathetic nervous system activity in stress. J. Phys. Ther. Sci. **24**(12), 1341–1344 (2012)
21. Koelstra, S., et al.: DEAP: a database for emotion analysis; using physiological signals. IEEE Trans. Affect. Comput. **3**(1), 18–31 (2011)
22. Koldijk, S., Sappelli, M., Verberne, S., Neerincx, M.A., Kraaij, W.: The swell knowledge work dataset for stress and user modeling research. In: Proceedings of the 16th International Conference on Multimodal Interaction, pp. 291–298 (2014)
23. Makowski, D., et al.: NeuroKit2: a python toolbox for neurophysiological signal processing. Behav. Res. Methods **53**(4), 1689–1696 (2021)
24. Matousek, R.H., Dobkin, P.L., Pruessner, J.: Cortisol as a marker for improvement in mindfulness-based stress reduction. Complement. Ther. Clin. Pract. **16**(1), 13–19 (2010)
25. McDuff, D., Gontarek, S., Picard, R.: Remote measurement of cognitive stress via heart rate variability. In: 2014 36th Annual International Conference of the IEEE Engineering in Medicine and Biology Society, pp. 2957–2960. IEEE (2014)
26. Michels, N., et al.: Children's heart rate variability as stress indicator: association with reported stress and cortisol. Biol. Psychol. **94**(2), 433–440 (2013)
27. Nikula, R.: Psychological correlates of nonspecific skin conductance responses. Psychophysiology **28**(1), 86–90 (1991)
28. Onorati, F., Barbieri, R., Mauri, M., Russo, V., Mainardi, L.: Reconstruction and analysis of the pupil dilation signal: application to a psychophysiological affective protocol. In: 2013 35th Annual International Conference of the IEEE Engineering in Medicine and Biology Society (EMBC), pp. 5–8. IEEE (2013)
29. Pakarinen, T., Pietilä, J., Nieminen, H.: Prediction of self-perceived stress and arousal based on electrodermal activity. In: 2019 41st Annual International Conference of the IEEE Engineering in Medicine and Biology Society (EMBC), pp. 2191–2195. IEEE (2019)
30. Picard, R.W., Vyzas, E., Healey, J.: Toward machine emotional intelligence: analysis of affective physiological state. IEEE Trans. Pattern Anal. Mach. Intell. **23**(10), 1175–1191 (2001)
31. Qi, M., Gao, H., Guan, L., Liu, G., Yang, J.: Subjective stress, salivary cortisol, and electrophysiological responses to psychological stress. Front. Psychol. **7**, 229 (2016)
32. Scheirer, J., Fernandez, R., Klein, J., Picard, R.W.: Frustrating the user on purpose: a step toward building an affective computer. Interact. Comput. **14**(2), 93–118 (2002)
33. Schmidt, P., Reiss, A., Duerichen, R., Marberger, C., Van Laerhoven, K.: Introducing wesad, a multimodal dataset for wearable stress and affect detection. In: Proceedings of the 20th ACM International Conference on Multimodal Interaction, pp. 400–408 (2018)
34. Sedghamiz, H.: Complete Pan-Tompkins implementation ECG QRS detector. MATLAB Cent.: Commun. Profile 172 (2014). http://www.mathworks.com/matlabcentral/profile/authors/2510422-hooman-sedghamiz
35. Selye, H.: The evolution of the stress concept: the originator of the concept traces its development from the discovery in 1936 of the alarm reaction to modern therapeutic applications of syntoxic and catatoxic hormones. Am. Sci. **61**(6), 692–699 (1973)
36. Shaffer, F., Ginsberg, J.P.: An overview of heart rate variability metrics and norms. Front. Public Health **5**, 258 (2017)
37. Warttig, S.L., Forshaw, M.J., South, J., White, A.K.: New, normative, English-sample data for the short form perceived stress scale (PSS-4). J. Health Psychol. **18**(12), 1617–1628 (2013)
38. Yaribeygi, H., Panahi, Y., Sahraei, H., Johnston, T.P., Sahebkar, A.: The impact of stress on body function: a review. EXCLI J. **16**, 1057 (2017)

On the Use of WebAssembly for Rendering and Segmenting Medical Images

Sébastien Jodogne(✉)

Computer Science and Engineering Department (INGI), Institute of Information and Communication Technologies, Electronics and Applied Mathematics (ICTEAM), UCLouvain, 1348 Louvain-la-Neuve, Belgium
sebastien.jodogne@uclouvain.be
https://www.info.ucl.ac.be/~sjodogne/

Abstract. Rendering medical images is a critical step in a variety of medical applications, from diagnosis to therapy. There is a growing need for advanced viewers that can display the fusion of multiple layers, such as contours, annotations, doses, or segmentation masks, on the top of image slices extracted from volumes. Such viewers obviously necessitate complex software components. But desktop viewers are often developed using technologies that are different from those used for Web viewers, which results in a lack of code reuse and shared expertise between development teams. Furthermore, the rise of artificial intelligence in radiology calls for Web viewers that integrate deep learning models and that can be used outside of a clinical environment, for instance to evaluate algorithms or to train skilled workers. In this paper, we show how the emerging WebAssembly standard can be used to tackle these challenges by sharing the same code base between heavyweight viewers and zero-footprint viewers. Moreover, we introduce a fully functional Web viewer that is entirely developed using WebAssembly and that can be used in research projects or in teleradiology applications. Finally, we demonstrate that deep convolutional neural networks for image segmentation can be executed entirely inside a Web browser thanks to WebAssembly, without any dedicated computing infrastructure. The source code associated with this paper is released as free and open-source software.

Keywords: Medical Imaging · DICOM · Image segmentation · Web applications

1 Introduction

The volume of medical images that are generated worldwide is in constant growth. This can be explained by the fact that the treatment of an increasingly number of chronic diseases requires a longitudinal and multimodal exploitation of medical images. For a highly effective, personalized treatment, it is indeed often important to consider images that have been acquired throughout the entire life of the patient and to combine multiple cues produced by several types of imaging modalities. Artificial intelligence has enormous potential to assist radiologists in analyzing this growing body of imaging data [1].

© The Author(s), under exclusive license to Springer Nature Switzerland AG 2023
A. C. A. Roque et al. (Eds.): BIOSTEC 2022, CCIS 1814, pp. 393–414, 2023.
https://doi.org/10.1007/978-3-031-38854-5_20

The DICOM standard [21] specifies how medical images are encoded and exchanged. Fortunately, DICOM is nowadays adopted by any hospital dealing with digital medical images. Thanks to the fact that DICOM is an open standard, a large ecosystem of free and open-source software exists to handle medical images. For instance, when it comes to the need of storing, communicating and archiving DICOM images in full interoperability with the information systems of an hospital, free and open-source DICOM servers such as dcm4chee [30], Dicoogle [5] or Orthanc [10,11] can be used. Such free and open-source software can notably be used to deploy task-specific DICOM stores in the hospital that are dedicated to some medical specialisms or to some artificial intelligence application.

Obviously, once stored inside a DICOM server, the medical images must still be displayed. Various use cases exist for viewers of medical images: clinical review integrated within the electronic health records, specialized tools dedicated to one pathology or treatment, external access for the patient, quality control of modalities, second medical opinion, telemedicine, clinical trials... Moreover, the huge interest in artificial intelligence applied to medical imaging requires the development of advanced viewers that can be used to annotate or review regions of interest for the training of the algorithms, and to display the outputs of such algorithms (e.g. segmentation masks).

Depending on the clinical or pre-clinical scenario, one might either need a desktop software, a mobile application, or a Web platform to display the medical images. This led many community projects or commercial products to focus only on one of those three categories of platforms, or to have separate development teams working on distinct viewers for the several types of platforms. In the latter case, developing similar features in different languages depending on the target platform (JavaScript, C++, Java...) comes at a large cost because of non-shared source code. Furthermore, distinct code bases might suffer from different issues, or conversely might feature optimizations that are not available for the other platforms. Expertise is also less shared between development teams who are focused on different platforms and languages.

Two major open-source software libraries are currently used to render medical images. The first one is VTK [25], that is mature and mostly written in the C++ language. VTK is used by many heavyweight desktop viewers, including the 3D Slicer platform [15], the well-known OsiriX radiology application [24] and its fork Horos. Note that VTK is also often used for scientific visualization beyond medical imaging. The second library is Cornerstone3D [29], that is more recent and that is written in the JavaScript language to be used as a building block for higher-level Web applications. As it takes its roots in modern Web technologies, Cornerstone3D is at the core of many zero-footprint, lightweight Web viewers, notably OHIF [29], and is often encountered within cloud-based proprietary solutions.

The emerging WebAssembly standard (often abbreviated as "wasm") might be a game changer in this divided landscape between heavyweight and Web applications. WebAssembly is an open standard that defines a portable binary code (bytecode) for high-performance applications that can be run by Web browsers [8]. Its core specification was released as an official W3C recommendation in December 2019. WebAssembly is actively backed by the industry, and is now supported by the major Web browsers. Thanks to the Emscripten compiler, C++ source code can be transformed to WebAssembly bytecode, which can then be executed by Web browsers. This opens the path to the creation of C++ libraries that can be used both by native software (using a native compiler) and by Web platforms (using the Emscripten toolchain). Such C++ libraries could also be used by native mobile applications through Android NDK or an Objective-C wrapper for iOS. WebAssembly has thus an immense potential to improve code reuse in multi-platform developments, particularly in the field of medical imaging.

According to this discussion, the first main contribution of this paper is to propose a novel, free and open-source C++ library named "Stone of Orthanc," whose internal architecture was driven by the constraints of Web development while providing compatibility with the native compiler toolchains. The Stone of Orthanc library is designed to be as portable and versatile as possible, with a small footprint[1]. Historically, the Stone of Orthanc project started back in 2016 by leveraging the Google's PNaCl and Mozilla's asm.js technologies that are now superseded by WebAssembly. Additionally, this paper presents different applications for medical imaging that were built using the Stone of Orthanc library. In particular, the "Stone Web viewer" is introduced as a fully functional Web viewer for end users to review medical images.

A preliminary version of this paper appeared in the Proceedings of the 15th International Joint Conference on Biomedical Engineering Systems and Technologies (BIOSTEC 2022), which already introduced the Stone of Orthanc and the Stone Web viewer [14]. The present paper expands this preliminary work by exploring the topic of artificial intelligence algorithms applied to the automated segmentation of organs or biological structures in a Web environment.

Indeed, many clinical deployments of deep learning models require the medical images to be sent either to a dedicated on-premises server, or to a remote cloud infrastructure. The former on-premises paradigm requires a computation cluster to be deployed and maintained within the hospital, which is complex and costly for smaller facilities, whereas the latter cloud-based approach is often problematic with respect to the protection of clinical data, which requires careful legal agreements associated with an effective de-identification of the DICOM images. The complexity of this procedure also slows down the evaluation, and thus the adoption of artificial intelligence algorithms by hospitals. Furthermore, introducing skilled workers to artificial intelligence or making deep learning models available to researchers is difficult in practice, as such processes typically require the access to some professional clinical deployment of artificial intelligence.

In this paper, we introduce an extended version of the Stone Web viewer that can locally execute deep learning models directly inside Web browsers, without requiring any dedicated infrastructure or network communication. More precisely, this extended Web viewer was designed to apply U-Net architectures, that have proved to be remarkably successful on segmentation tasks for biomedical imaging [23]. This is made possible by implementing a platform-independent C++ code in the Stone of Orthanc library to apply CNN (Convolutional Neural Networks) models to 2D images. Thanks to the fact that the Stone of Orthanc library also offers primitives to render scenes composed of multiple layers, the Stone Web viewer can overlay the segmentation masks that are produced by the U-Net models, on the top of their input medical images. This novel

---

[1] This intimacy with the lightweight architecture of the Orthanc project for medical imaging [10, 11] explains the name of the Stone of Orthanc library, which is a tribute to the *palantír* that resides inside the tower of Orthanc in *The Lord of the Rings* by J. R. R. Tolkien.

contribution demonstrates that WebAssembly provides a new framework for rendering and segmenting medical images.

2   Stone of Orthanc

As explained in the Introduction, Stone of Orthanc is a C++ library to render medical images, with the goal of being compatible with WebAssembly. In the current section, we review how the high-level architecture of Stone of Orthanc has been engineered.

2.1   Motivations

The objective of creating a library that can be used by heavyweight software, by mobile applications as well as by Web platforms puts strong constraints on the architecture of the library. Most importantly, traditional native applications are multi-threaded and sequential, whereas Web applications are single-threaded and driven by asynchronous callbacks (closures). Stone of Orthanc was designed to accommodate with such extremely different platforms by adding different abstractions that will be explained in Sect. 2.2.

Besides this constrained computing architecture, the accurate rendering of medical images requires a careful mapping between pixel coordinates and 2D or 3D physical coordinates. The library must also be extensible to display the various kinds of overlays (such as segmentation masks or annotations) that might have been produced by artificial intelligence algorithms or manually added by physicians. Furthermore, medical specialties such as nuclear medicine, radiotherapy or protontherapy necessitate to display fusions of different layers (for instance, a dose over a CT-scan, or a contour over a PET signal). To fulfill such needs, the architecture of Stone of Orthanc integrates a portable 2D rendering engine for vectorized graphics with support of overlays that will be discussed in Sect. 2.3.

Figure 1 provides a summary of the software architecture of Stone of Orthanc. Because the goal of this paper is not to document the internal components of Stone of Orthanc, only the main concepts that drove the design of Stone of Orthanc are presented. The interested reader is kindly invited to dive into the source code of the project.

2.2   Loaders and Oracle

The Stone of Orthanc library provides developers with many primitives that are necessary to create medical imaging applications. In particular, the library offers facilities to download images from a DICOM server (notably using the DICOMweb standard, but a custom REST API can be used as well). In this way, Stone of Orthanc features C++ classes that contain 2D or 3D medical images, and that are filled by classes that are referred to as "Loaders." In the case of 3D dense volumes, the associated Loaders automatically sort the individual 2D slices of the volume with respect to their 3D location[2].

---

[2] The 3D location is determined by the "image position patient" (0x0020,0x0032) and "image orientation patient" (0x0020,0x0037) DICOM tags if available, or by the "instance number" (0x0020,0x0013) DICOM tag.

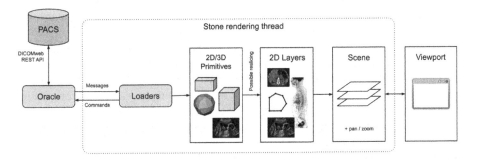

Fig. 1. High-level overview of the components of the Stone of Orthanc library [14]. The Oracle abstracts the runtime environment. The Loaders are responsible for loading the graphical primitives that have to be displayed. These graphical primitives are then converted into a set of 2D Layers (in particular, primitives corresponding to 3D volumes can be sliced along a cutting plane to extract a 2D Layer). The Layers are then superimposed to define a Scene that is finally composed onto the rendering surface of the Viewport. The user can interact with the Viewport to update the affine transform (pan/zoom) that is associated with the Scene.

However, as written above, the engines of JavaScript and WebAssembly are inherently single-threaded. Therefore, to be compatible with the Web runtimes, the core of the Stone of Orthanc library is not allowed to launch threads or to maintain a pool of threads for the Loaders to download the images, which contrasts with what would be done in a traditional C++ application. The solution adopted by Stone of Orthanc is to introduce a so-called "Oracle" singleton object that abstracts the way asynchronous operations such as downloads are processed on the target platform. The Oracle is the key component that enables the writing of source code that can be run indifferently by WebAssembly and by native applications.

The Stone of Orthanc library provides a different Oracle for the different target platforms. In the case of WebAssembly, the Oracle boils down to a wrapper that calls the primitives offered the Web browser itself using the Emscripten C headers. In the case of native applications, the Oracle abstracts the system SDK associated with the target platform: For instance, to handle downloads, the Oracle internally manages a set of worker threads connected to a shared queue of pending HTTP requests. Besides downloading DICOM instances, other examples of asynchronous operations implemented by the Oracles include reading files from the filesystem, or sleeping for a certain amount of time.

According to this discussion, the Oracle object receives a stream of "Command" objects that specify the asynchronous operations that must be carried on. Following the observer design pattern [7], each Command to be processed is associated with an "Observer" object that will receive a "Message" object that contains the result of the Command once it has been processed. For instance, in the case of the download of a DICOM instance from some REST API, the Command would contain the URL to download, the Observer would correspond to the Loader object that populates the target medical image, and the Message would contain the raw bytes of the DICOM instance. Sending a Command to the Oracle is a non-blocking operation, which reflects the asynchronous nature of the Oracle. The Observer is specified as a C++ "pointer to member function," with a slight use of C++ templates as syntactic sugar, and the Oracle invokes this member function upon completion of the Command.

The Oracle is part of the global context of the Stone of Orthanc library: Each class that executes asynchronous operations must keep a reference to the Oracle. In order to map the single-threaded aspect of WebAssembly into native environments supporting multi-threading, it is assumed that the global context is only accessed from one distinguished user thread that is responsible for the rendering. A mutex is included in the global context to prevent the Messages emitted by the Oracle from interfering with the rendering thread. Reference counting using shared pointers ensures that the Observer objects are not destructed before all the scheduled Commands they are receivers of have been processed[3].

It is worth noticing that the Oracle mechanism can be used as an accelerator for certain operations that can be time-intensive. For instance, Stone of Orthanc introduces a Command to download then parse DICOM instances as a single operation: In the case of a multi-threaded environment, this allows to offload the DICOM parsing to a thread without locking the mutex of Stone of Orthanc, which brings more concurrency in native environments[4]. This also allows to maintain a cache of parsed DICOM files.

2.3 Viewports and Layers

When it comes to the client-side rendering of medical images, the 2D operations of panning, zooming, and changing windowing must be as fast as possible. This calls for taking advantage of the 2D hardware acceleration that is provided by any GPU (graphics processing unit). To this end, both native applications and WebAssembly applications have access to the OpenGL API, the former through development libraries such as Qt or SDL, the latter through WebGL.

On the other hand, to reduce the network bandwidth in the presence of large images (typically 3D volumes), the developers of viewers might want to use streaming: In this scenario, a central server generates a stream of "screenshots" of a medical imaging scene, and those renderings are then sent to a thin client in charge of their actual display to the user. In the case of streaming, GPU is not necessarily available on the server, as multiple users might be connected to the same server. GPU might also be unavailable if printing an image, if generating a secondary capture image, or if the viewer runs on a low-power or embedded computer (such as the popular Raspberry Pi).

To accommodate with all such situations in a cross-platform and lightweight way, the architecture of Stone of Orthanc is designed to support both hardware acceleration (using straight OpenGL) and software rendering (using the widespread `cairo` drawing library). Furthermore, to maximize portability, the Stone of Orthanc library implements its own OpenGL shaders for the GPU-accelerated drawing of lines, texts, and bitmaps.

In Stone of Orthanc, each rendering surface (i.e. the application widget, the HTML5 canvas, or the memory buffer) is associated with a so-called "Viewport" abstract class

---

[3] The observer design pattern and reference counting are used elsewhere in Stone of Orthanc for sending messages from one object to another, and for broadcasting messages from one object to a set of Observers using a subscription mechanism.

[4] In the future, similar optimizations could be offered in the WebAssembly environment by leveraging Web workers.

that is responsible for the rendering of a 2D "Scene". A single application is allowed to manage multiple Viewports to show different Scenes.

The Scene is an object that encodes a superposition of "Layer" objects, each Layer being a 2D vectorized graphics with an alpha layer to allow for transparency. For instance, in a nuclear medicine application, a Scene would consist of three superimposed Layers, the foremost being the contours (a set of 2D polygons stored in a DICOM RT-STRUCT instance), the second being the texture associated with the PET-scan signal (with a heat colormap providing an alpha value for transparency), and the background being the CT-scan slice (a texture containing floating-point values expressed in Hounsfield units). Besides its constituting Layers, the Scene also contains a 2D-to-2D affine transform that maps the coordinates of Layers to the Viewport coordinates. Altering this transform is used to pan and zoom the Scene onto the Viewport.

Each Scene and Layer is agnostic of the actual rendering surface: It is up to the Viewport to compose the Scene as a bitmap, before putting it onto the rendering surface. Depending on the type of their associated rendering surface, Viewport objects will use a different algorithm to render a Scene, following the strategy design pattern [7]. This separation of concerns between Viewports and Scenes, is like the one between the Oracle and Commands. If a Layer containing a bitmap must be rendered, the Viewport is also responsible for the proper conversion of the pixel values (that typically correspond to floating-point numbers or 16 bit integers) to a bitmap that is suitable for the rendering surface (in general, red/green/blue/alpha values in 8 bits per pixel). This conversion must take into account the windowing parameters of the Layers, if any.

Summarizing, the rendering engine of Stone of Orthanc is inherently oriented toward 2D vectorized graphics. This choice is similar to that of the original Cornerstone.js library, but contrasts with the VTK library, that is more 3D-oriented. The advantage of focusing on 2D rendering is to make the rendering of multi-layer scenes more natural to the developers than if 3D must also be considered. Importantly, just like the Oracle/Commands/Observers architecture, this Viewport/Scene/Layers architecture is compatible with both native applications and WebAssembly applications. It is also worth noticing that Stone of Orthanc could be used as a rendering engine for vectorized graphics in native, mobile or Web applications out of the field of medical imaging.

Viewers for medical imaging need to display 3D volumes, not just 2D images. Section 2.2 explained how Loaders are used to download 3D images and store them into RAM. To render 3D volumes, Stone of Orthanc introduces the concept of "VolumeReslicer" that is an abstract class taking as its inputs one 3D image and one cutting 3D plane, and producing a 2D slice as its output. This 2D slice can then be injected as a Layer into the Scene to be rendered. Volume reslicers are currently implemented for MPR (Multiplanar Reconstruction, cf. Sect. 5.1) and for reslicing along an arbitrary cutting plane (cf. Sect. 5.2). To maximize the portability of Stone of Orthanc, the reslicing of volumes is done entirely using the CPU. Additional reslicers will be implemented in the future for MIP (Maximum Intensity Projection) rendering, possibly using the Oracle as an accelerator for the computations.

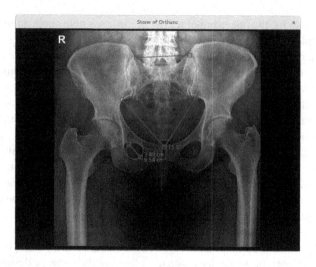

Fig. 2. Simple 2D viewer displaying a radiography image [14]. In this case, the Viewport is a SDL window, with one background Layer containing a 16bpp bitmap. The windowing can be changed using the mouse. The viewer can be used to take measures of lines, circles and angles in physical coordinates. These measures are geometric primitives stored in the foreground Layers of the Scene.

2.4   Sample Desktop Viewer

The distribution of the Stone of Orthanc library comes with the source code of a sample, basic viewer that provides an example about how Stone of Orthanc can be used to display one 2D slice of a DICOM instance downloaded from an Orthanc server. This viewer is a standalone desktop application that is started from the command line by providing the URL of the Orthanc REST API, together with the identifier of the DICOM instance to be displayed. This example uses SDL to manage its window, making it eminently cross-platform.

A screenshot of this application can be found in Fig. 2. Zooming, panning, and windowing are supported, as well as taking measures. The mouse interactions are handled by a dedicated abstract class called "ViewportInteractor" that is responsible for tracking mouse events, and that is part of the Stone of Orthanc library. Interestingly, because the DICOM image is downloaded from the Orthanc server, it is decoded server-side, which frees the viewer from handling the various transfer syntaxes of the DICOM standard, hereby simplifying the source code. The full application only consists of 700 lines of code.

3   Stone Web Viewer

The so-called "Stone Web viewer" is currently the main application that leverages the Stone of Orthanc library. The Stone Web viewer is a fully functional teleradiology solution, as depicted in Fig. 3. It can simultaneously display multiple DICOM series, and it implements some advanced features such as measurements, synchronized

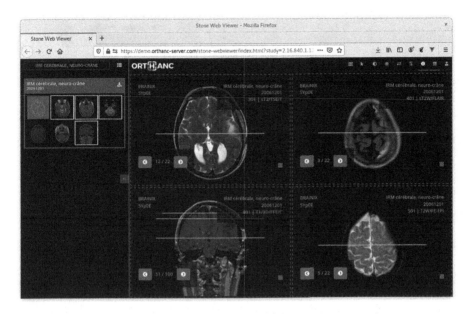

Fig. 3. Screenshot of the Stone Web viewer [14].

browsing, 3D cross-hair, and 3D reference lines. The Stone Web viewer communicates with a DICOM server using the DICOMweb protocol, making it theoretically compatible with any PACS (Picture Archiving and Communication System) environment supporting DICOMweb.

To the best of our knowledge, the Stone Web viewer is the first viewer of medical images that entirely relies on WebAssembly. Most of its source code is written in C++ and compiled using the Emscripten toolchain. The buttons and the HTML5 canvas are managed by a small Vue.js application that calls the WebAssembly bytecode using an automatically generated JavaScript wrapper. Contrarily to the sample desktop viewer described in Sect. 2.4, the Stone Web viewer does not rely on the remote server to decode the DICOM files: It embeds the DCMTK library in the WebAssembly bytecode to this end.

The Stone Web viewer is a client-side application that is entirely run by the Web browser. Because its binary assets consist of a mere set of static resources (HTML files, JavaScript sources and WebAssembly bytecode), the Stone Web viewer can be served by any HTTP server (such as nginx, Apache or Microsoft IIS). To fulfill the same-origin security policy, the HTTP server must be configured as a reverse proxy to map the REST API of the DICOMweb server next to the assets of the Stone Web viewer. The configuration file of the Stone Web viewer has an option to provide the root of the DICOMweb API to this end.

However, this manual configuration of a HTTP server might sound complex to users without a background in network administration. To ease the deployments, a plugin for Orthanc has been developed to directly serve the assets of the Stone Web viewer using the embedded HTTP server of Orthanc. Thanks to this Stone Web viewer plugin and thanks to the DICOMweb plugin for Orthanc, it is extremely easy to start the Stone Web

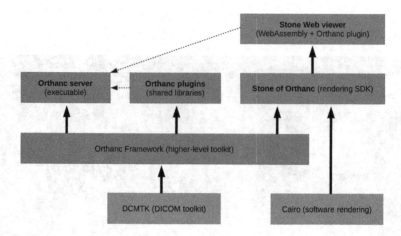

Fig. 4. Overview of the high-level architecture of the Stone Web viewer [14]. The green boxes indicate the major third-party libraries, the blue boxes represent components provided by the Orthanc project [10], and the red boxes correspond to the Stone of Orthanc project. (Color figure online)

viewer. Furthermore, this plugin is readily available in the Docker images, the Microsoft Windows installers and the macOS packages provided by the Orthanc project[5].

Figure 4 provides the big picture of the different components that are involved in the Stone Web viewer. The Stone Web viewer is a high-level application that is built on the top of the Stone of Orthanc library. As can be seen, the Stone of Orthanc library reuses some classes from the Orthanc project that are referred to as the "Orthanc Framework." The Stone Web viewer can either be served from a HTTP server or be run as a plugin to the main Orthanc server.

4   Client-Side Segmentation Using Deep Learning

Thanks to the flexibility of the Stone of Orthanc library, the Stone Web viewer can be extended in many ways. As explained in Sect. 2.3, Stone of Orthanc can notably render stacks of superimposed Layers. It is thus possible to overlay a segmentation mask on the top of a medical image. In this section, this capability will be used to apply a deep learning model for lung segmentation to the slice that is currently displayed by the Stone Web viewer, then to display the output of this segmentation. The segmentation mask will be computed locally, entirely inside the Web browser, thanks to WebAssembly.

4.1   U-Net Architecture

U-Net is a remarkably successful deep learning architecture for bioimaging segmentation [23]. Contrarily to the sliding-window approach, in which all the possible patches of a fixed size in an image are scanned by a CNN producing one binary output for each

---

[5] An online demo of the Stone Web viewer plugin is also available at: https://demo.orthanc-server.com/.

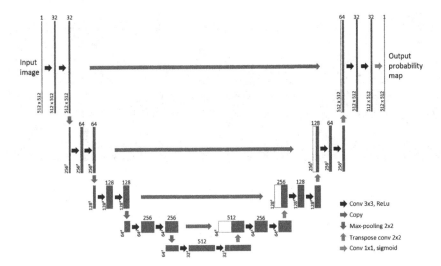

Fig. 5. The U-Net architecture that is used in this paper. The main differences with respect to the original U-Net architecture [23] are the size of the input and output images (both 512×512 pixels), the number of filters used for the convolutions (it ranges from 32 to 512 filters), and the zero-padding that is used in convolutions (which preserves the image sizes throughout the network). The same architecture was used in our recent work related to federated learning for the segmentation of the heart [20]. The resulting U-Net models contain exactly 7,759,521 floating-point parameters.

patch [3], the U-Net architecture considers the input image as a whole. U-Net models first apply a contraction path to generate high-level features, then apply an expansion path to output the segmentation mask, resulting in the typical "U" shape that is depicted in Fig. 5. This architecture allows for the global spatial structure of the medical images to be considered. Generating a segmentation mask given an input image is also much faster than using the sliding-window approach.

In this work, the U-Net models were trained on the individual 2D axial slices of segmented CT-scan images to minimize a smoothed version of the Dice loss function [28], that is defined as:

$$\mathcal{L}(\hat{Y}, Y) = -\frac{2\left(\sum_{(x,y)} \hat{Y}(x,y)Y(x,y)\right) + \epsilon}{\left(\sum_{(x,y)} \hat{Y}(x,y)\right) + \left(\sum_{(x,y)} Y(x,y)\right) + \epsilon},$$

where $Y(x,y) \in \{0,1\}$ (resp. $\hat{Y}(x,y)$) denotes the expected binary value in the segmentation mask (resp. the actual prediction of the U-Net) of the pixel at coordinates (x,y), and where ϵ is a coefficient that prevents divisions by zeros as well as vanishing gradients induced by the slices that do not contain any pixel belonging to the segmentation mask.

4.2 Dataset for Lung Segmentation and Data Augmentation

A U-Net model for the segmentation of the lungs was trained on the *Lung CT Segmentation Challenge 2017* (LCTSC) dataset [31,32] provided by *The Cancer*

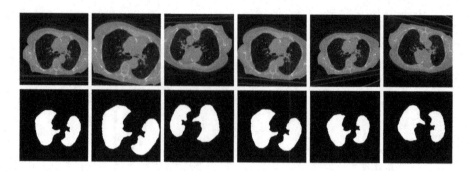

Fig. 6. A illustrative set of training slices (top) together with their segmentation mask of the lungs (bottom), as obtained through data augmentation. The first column shows the original slices from the LCTSC dataset, and the other columns some of their augmented versions. Those images were all generated by REST API calls to the rendering plugin.

Imaging Archive project [4]. This dataset contains DICOM CT-scan images together with the delineation of both lungs encoded as DICOM RT-STRUCT instances. The latter DICOM RT-STRUCT format is routinely used by radiotherapy and nuclear medicine departments to encode the contours of organs and tumors. The LCTSC dataset contains 60 DICOM studies, each study corresponding to one 3D CT-scan, and is divided in 36 studies for the train set and 24 studies for the test set. This defines 3393 training 2D slices and 2063 testing 2D slices. A validation set containing 20% of the train set was retained. This validation set was used for the early stopping of the training to avoid overfitting.

Importantly, data augmentation was used to improve the performance of the model while reducing overfitting [26]: This well-known technique consists in artificially increasing the size of a dataset using random label-preserving transformations, such as rotations, offsets, flips or zooms. An illustration of data augmentation applied to the LCTSC dataset is shown in Fig. 6. Most research works dealing with CNN include a preprocessing pipeline that consists in converting the source DICOM images to a set of files in dedicated folders that can easily be opened as NumPy arrays, possibly including data augmentation, before carrying on the actual training of the models in Python.

In this paper, we preferred to use the Orthanc PACS server as the sole source for the training data. The DICOM instances of the LCTSC dataset were rapidly stored and indexed in Orthanc using the folder indexer plugin [13]. Secondly, we developed a so-called "rendering plugin" for the Orthanc server that generates NumPy arrays on-the-fly through REST API requests. The latter requests specify the DICOM identifier of their CT-scan slice or their RT-STRUCT instance of interest, as well as the parameters for possible data augmentation. This plugin was developed on the top of the primitives offered by the Stone of Orthanc library. Thanks to this plugin, the training process can be entirely isolated from the rendering of the augmented training images. This approach facilitates the data management by providing a robust training environment, and it avoids the duplication of the training data on the filesystem. The resulting training pipeline does not contain any preprocessing step.

4.3   Training

The U-Net model for lung segmentation was trained in Python using Keras with the TensorFlow back-end [2]. The Adam optimizer was used, with random initial weights, a learning rate of $2 \cdot 10^{-5}$ and a batch size of 1. Note that this batch size of 1 corresponds to the value that was used in the original U-Net paper [23]. Four dropout layers [27] were introduced at the four max-pooling layers (cf. Figure 5) to prevent overfitting. The smoothing parameter ϵ of the Dice loss function $\mathcal{L}(\hat{Y}, Y)$ was set to 10.

Online data augmentation was applied through Keras data generators calling the REST API of the rendering plugin, which means that the augmented images were different at each epoch. The following transformations for data augmentation were experimentally found to provide good results: rotations between $-10°$ and $10°$, zoom-in and zoom-out up to 5%, displacements up to 5 pixels in both axes, flips along both axes, and slight modifications of the Hounsfield values of the CT-scan up to 1%.

The training took 7 h on a standard desktop computer (Intel Core i7-9700 CPU equipped with a NVIDIA GeForce GTX 1650 GPU). The resulting Dice score was 95%, which indicates average performance. Note that the objective of this paper was not to train the best-performing U-Net model. Instead, our goal was to train a sensible U-Net model on an average computer, to release open-source code for other people to independently reproduce this result, then to release the U-Net model in open-access to demonstrate its use in the context of WebAssembly. Further development could release better U-Net models in open-access, for instance by taking advantage of recent meta-optimization techniques such as nnU-Net [9].

4.4   U-Net Models in the Stone Web Viewer

Once the U-Net model for lung segmentation is available, it still must be applied to some slice displayed in the Stone Web viewer. This implies that the model generated by Keras must somehow be executed by WebAssembly, without any access to Python.

To this end, we implemented inside the Stone of Orthanc library, a highly portable sub-library written in plain C++ to apply CNN models. Our CNN toolkit is focused on 2D images, not on generic tensors, which implies that both its footprint and its complexity are small. This library provides a reference implementation for all the distinct types of layers that are encountered in the U-Net architecture (cf. Fig. 5). The library is currently single-threaded to match the constraints of WebAssembly, and it only uses the CPU for maximum portability. Future work will improve its performance by leveraging multi-threading and GPU. It is nonetheless worth noticing that convolution layers are already implemented as matrix products, which is a well-known technique to improve the locality of the data, hereby greatly speeding up the convolutions.

Another difficulty lies in the complex file format that is used by Keras to save the parameters of the CNN models. To alleviate this problem, we decided to convert the models to a simpler binary format using Google's Protocol Buffers (Protobuf) library. A conversion script written in Python uses the Keras API to explore the parameters of the various layers in the trained model, then to save them using the Protobuf format. Protobuf being a highly portable library, it can be cross-compiled to WebAssembly. Altogether, this provides a pipeline to load Keras models into the Stone Web viewer.

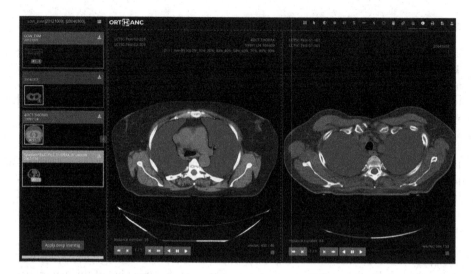

Fig. 7. Segmentation using U-Net models in the Stone Web viewer, applied to two test slices of the LCTSC dataset. The user launches the segmentation by clicking on the "*Apply deep learning*" button at the bottom left of the Web interface. Then, a green progress bar below the button provides feedback about the computation by the Web worker. The segmentation mask is finally rendered as a red, semi-transparent overlay on the top the slice of the CT-scan.

Combining these different elements, Fig. 7 shows an extended version of the Stone Web viewer that supports deep learning for lung segmentation. The CNN toolkit applies the U-Net model in a dedicated Web worker, which amounts to running the segmentation in a separate thread, as Web workers are the official HTML way of executing tasks in the background of a Web application. This use of a Web worker avoids to freeze the user interface while applying the U-Net model. The full deep learning pipeline can be found in Fig. 8. On a standard laptop computer equipped with an Intel i7-1165G7 CPU, applying the U-Net model of Fig. 5 necessitates 18 s, which is only twice longer than the same code executed as a native executable. As indicated above, future work will try and reduce this execution time. The key point here is that U-Net models can be applied through WebAssembly directly in a teleradiology application, without resorting to any dedicated computing cluster or to any cloud infrastructure. The diffusion in open-access of U-Net models usable directly in a free and open-source Web viewer may have an impact on the teaching and research related to artificial intelligence in medical imaging.

5   Other Applications

The core features of the Stone of Orthanc library were explained in Sect. 2. Section 3 introduced the Stone Web viewer as a full teleradiology solution that was extended with deep learning in Sect. 4. In this section, several other higher-level applications that were built using the Stone of Orthanc library are reviewed.

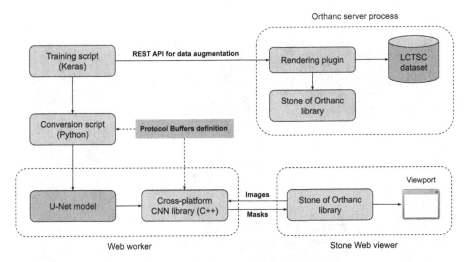

Fig. 8. The full deep learning pipeline for U-Net models. Data files are highlighted in green, whereas the blue boxes indicate the software components. Google's Protocol Buffers are used as an intermediate binary file format between Keras and the Stone Web viewer. The U-Net model is applied in a dedicated Web worker, asynchronously of the Stone Web viewer, because this is a time-consuming operation that would freeze the user interface. Evidently, the training and conversion scripts are executed offline, prior to the use of the U-Net model in the Stone Web viewer. (Color figure online)

5.1 Rendering Oncology Images

In the context of nuclear medicine, radiotherapy and protontherapy, patients rarely have the opportunity to view the images of their own treatment plan from home. This is because the Web portals used in hospitals are mostly focused on the radiology work-flow, and thus are typically unable to display advanced information such as contours or dose delivery. Yet, viewing one's own treatment plan might have positive impact on the empowerment of the patient and on the reduction of stress during the treatment.

In collaboration with the radiotherapy department of the University Hospital of Liège, we have developed a simple radiotherapy viewer as a cross-platform desktop application built using the Qt toolkit and the Stone of Orthanc library. This viewer was used in a controlled randomized clinical trial to evaluate the feasibility of using a viewer of radiotherapy plans in the context of patient education [16]. In this clinical trial, the patients received a USB key containing their own images and the viewer application, after a personal meeting with their oncologist and with a nurse who explained how to use the viewer.

The user interface of the viewer is depicted in Fig. 9. It is designed to be as simple as possible. It displays the fusion of the simulation CT-scan, the planned dose (DICOM RT-DOSE), and the different contours (DICOM RT-STRUCT) following a MPR layout. The user can select which contours are displayed.

Following the terminology of Sect. 2.3, the user interface of this application is made of three different Scene objects: one for the axial projection, one for the sagittal

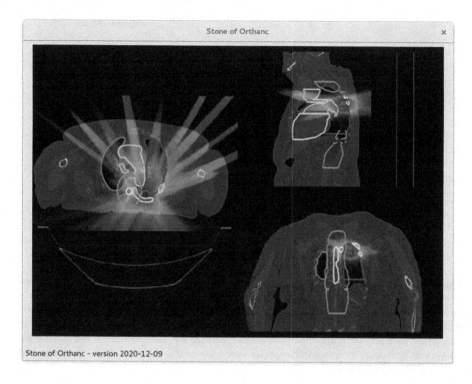

Fig. 9. Desktop application for patient education in the context of external radiotherapy [14,16].

projection, and one for the coronal projection. In turn, each of these three Scene objects contains three Layer objects: The foremost Layer contains the polygons that correspond to the contours of the delineated structures, the central Layer displays a colorized version of the slice of the dose (with an alpha channel for transparency), and the backward Layer shows the CT-scan slice. The multimodal fusion is then obtained by blitting the three 2D Layer objects of each Scene onto the corresponding drawing surface.

From an algorithmic point of view, the surface rendering of the 3D contours is done by reading the content of one DICOM RT-STRUCT instance. In such an instance, the contours of each structure are specified as a list of polygons on the individual axial slices. Consequently, the rendering of one specific slice in the axial projection simply consists in drawing the polygons that are contained in this slice of interest. The sagittal and coronal projections are more complex to deal with. We first select the polygons that intersect the given sagittal or coronal slice. Each of those intersections define a 2D box in the plane of interest. The final rendering is done by drawing a set of polygons that corresponds to the union of all those 2D boxes. Well-known, efficient computational geometry algorithms based on the sweep line paradigm are available to compute such unions of rectangles [19,22].

On the other hand, the extraction of an axial, sagittal or coronal slice out of the CT-scan volume stored in RAM whose voxels are indexed by (i, j, k) integers is straightforward: It consists in setting i, j or k to the value of interest, then implementing two

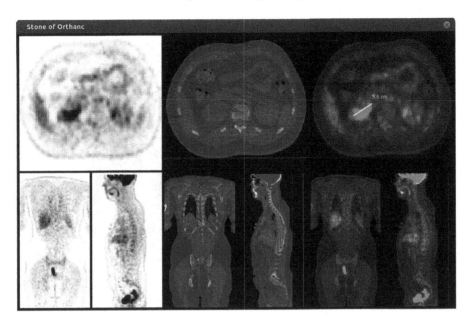

Fig. 10. Desktop application for the rendering of PET-CT-scans according to a clinical-like layout [14].

nested loops over the two other dimensions. The same algorithm can be applied to the PET-scan volume, if its axes are aligned with those of the CT-scan volume. If the two volumes are not aligned, the PET-scan volume can be resliced, a process that will be described in Sect. 5.2.

Note that besides radiotherapy, the Stone of Orthanc library can be used to render similar oncology images in the field of nuclear medicine. For instance, Fig. 10 illustrates another desktop application that provides an advanced rendering of a PET-CT-scan using a layout that is commonly encountered in professional applications. Those two applications could be ported to Web environments thanks to WebAssembly.

5.2   Real-Time Volume Reslicing

As indicated at the end of Sect. 2.3, Stone of Orthanc does not use the GPU if extracting one slice out of a 3D volume along an arbitrary cutting plane: Volume reslicing is done entirely in RAM by the CPU. This technical choice was motivated by simplicity and portability, but it raises concerns related to performance. To evaluate the performance, a simple WebAssembly application was developed that is depicted in Fig. 11. The mouse was used to change the orientation of the cutting plane.

From an algorithmic point of view, the cutting plane is specified by one 3D point indicating the origin of the plane, and by two orthonormal 3D vectors indicating the directions of the X and Y axes in the plane. The intersection of the source volumetric image (which is a rectangular cuboid) with the cutting plane is first computed. If non-empty, this intersection defines a polygon containing between 3 and 6 vertices in

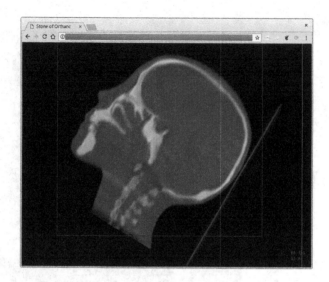

Fig. 11. Real-time reslicing of a 3D volume by a Web browser [14].

the cutting plane [6, Figure 39-6]. Secondly, the bounding box of this polygon in the reference system of the cutting plane defines the physical extent of the 2D image to be generated. The width and height of the extracted bitmap is derived from the desired pixel spacing. Finally, the extracted bitmap is filled by looping over its pixels, looking for the value of the voxel in the source volume that is the closest to the coordinates of each 2D pixel on the 3D cutting plane. Bilinear or trilinear interpolation can also be applied to improve the visual quality of the reslicing.

On a standard computer (Intel Core i7-3770 at 3.4 GHz), the rendering of one slice of size $512 \times 512 \times 502$ voxels in 16bpp takes about 25 ms (40 frames per second), which is fully compatible with real-time requirements. On an old, entry-level smartphone (Samsung Galaxy A3 2017) running the Mozilla Firefox browser, the same rendering takes about 100 milliseconds (10 frames per second), which is still usable in practice.

5.3 Digitally Reconstructed Radiographs

The Stone of Orthanc library also features some computational geometry primitives to deal with volume rendering. It notably contains C++ classes to generate a digitally reconstructed radiograph (DRR) from a CT volume, which is frequently used in the context of radiotherapy or protontherapy to position the patient in the treatment machine. The DRR is the 2D radiograph that would be imaged using a virtual X-ray camera centered at a given 3D point with a given focal length.

DRR can be computed by raytracing each voxel of the CT volume according to the perspective transform, which is a costly computation because it involves divisions. Stone of Orthanc optimizes this computation by using the so-called "shear-warp transform" [17, 18]. The intuitive idea behind shear-warp is to postpone as much as possible

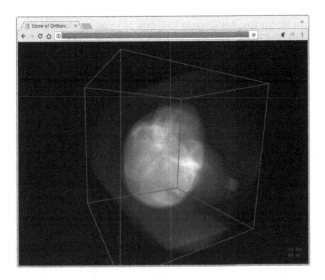

Fig. 12. Web rendering of a digitally reconstructed radiograph (DRR) from a CT-scan [14]. The projection is computed client-side by the Web browser in near-real-time (a few frames per second).

the application of the perspective transformation, and to apply it only once to a single *"intermediate image"* (this is the "warp" step). This intermediate image is created from the summation of the individual slices of the volume after the application of an affine transform in which the X and Y axes are left uncoupled, which enables a fast computation (this is the "shear" step that is separately applied to each slice). The shear-warp transform provides an efficient algorithm for CPU-based volume rendering.

Figure 12 shows a WebAssembly application that computes a DRR in near-real-time. On a standard computer, the full rendering of a $512 \times 512 \times 502$ volume in 16bpp takes about 1 s. While moving the virtual camera, the number of slices used for the rendering can be reduced to improve speed, thus enhancing the user experience. The GPU could be used to speed up this computation by implementing an appropriate Oracle command. Besides DRR, the shear-warp algorithm could also be applied to compute MIP rendering by putting the virtual camera at infinity, and by replacing the summation with a "max" operation in the intermediate image.

6 Conclusions

This paper introduces Stone of Orthanc as a library to render medical images, in a way that is compatible with desktop, mobile and Web applications. Stone of Orthanc is fully written in C++, and leverages the emerging WebAssembly standard if targeting Web applications. Sample applications of Stone of Orthanc are described as well. In particular, the Stone Web viewer is introduced as the first free and open-source teleradiology solution entirely developed using WebAssembly. As shown in this paper, WebAssembly can be used to maximize code reuse in medical imaging, which should also be true in many other scientific fields that involve numerical computations.

This paper also demonstrates how U-Net models can be executed client-side by Web browsers to segment images in a teleradiology solution, without running the computation on a dedicated server, and without having to transfer the medical images to a remote cloud infrastructure. This contribution could notably help the teaching of artificial intelligence for medical imaging by sharing technical knowledge about deep learning to a much larger audience, as it avoids the need to resort to proprietary solutions that are not available outside of large-scale clinical environments.

The source code of the Stone of Orthanc library is publicly released under the LGPL license, and the Stone Web viewer is licensed under the AGPL. The whole Stone of Orthanc project currently contains more than 70,000 lines of code[6].

Future work will pursue the exploitation of Stone of Orthanc for artificial intelligence applications in medical imaging. We notably plan to design applications supporting the "AI Results (AIR)" IHE profile that is designed to standardize how the inputs and outputs of artificial intelligence algorithms are exchanged. The integration of MPR layout, MIP rendering and whole-slide imaging [12] directly within the Stone Web viewer will also be investigated. Finally, as far as client-side deep learning is concerned, we plan to improve the performance of our deep learning toolkit, to establish an open-access library of traceable U-Net models, and to extend the Stone Web viewer to other types of deep learning networks beyond image segmentation (such as image classification and object detection).

Acknowledgments. The author wants to thank Benjamin Golinvaux, Alain Mazy and Osimis for their contributions to the development of the Stone of Orthanc project.

References

1. Cheng, P.M., et al.: Deep learning: an update for radiologists. Radiographics **41**(5), 1427–1445 (2021). https://doi.org/10.1148/rg.2021200210
2. Chollet, F., et al.: Keras (2015). https://github.com/fchollet/keras
3. Ciresan, D., Giusti, A., Gambardella, L., Schmidhuber, J.: Deep neural networks segment neuronal membranes in electron microscopy images. In: Pereira, F., Burges, C.J.C., Bottou, L., Weinberger, K.Q. (eds.) Advances in Neural Information Processing Systems, vol. 25. Curran Associates, Inc. (2012). http://papers.nips.cc/paper/by-source-2012-1292
4. Clark, K., et al.: The cancer imaging archive (TCIA): maintaining and operating a public information repository. J. Digit. Imaging **26**(6), 1045–1057 (2013). https://doi.org/10.1007/s10278-013-9622-7
5. Costa, C., Ferreira, C., Bastião, L., Ribeiro, L., Silva, A., Oliveira, J.L.: Dicoogle - an open source peer-to-peer PACS. J. Digit. Imaging **24**(5), 848–856 (2011). https://doi.org/10.1007/s10278-010-9347-9
6. Fernando, R.: GPU Gems: Programming Techniques, Tips and Tricks for Real-Time Graphics. Pearson Higher Education (2004)
7. Gamma, E., Helm, R., Johnson, R., Vlissides, J.M.: Design Patterns: Elements of Reusable Object-Oriented Software, 1st edn. Addison-Wesley Professional (1994)

---

[6] The source code is located at: https://hg.orthanc-server.com/orthanc-stone/.

8. Haas, A., et al.: Bringing the Web up to speed with WebAssembly. In: Cohen, A., Vechev, M.T. (eds.) Proceedings of the 38th ACM SIGPLAN Conference on Programming Language Design and Implementation, PLDI 2017, Barcelona, Spain, 18–23 June 2017, pp. 185–200. ACM (2017). https://doi.org/10.1145/3062341.3062363

9. Isensee, F., Jaeger, P.F., Kohl, S.A.A., Petersen, J., Maier-Hein, K.H.: nnU-net: a self-configuring method for deep learning-based biomedical image segmentation. Nat. Methods **18**(2), 203–211 (2021). https://doi.org/10.1038/s41592-020-01008-z

10. Jodogne, S.: The orthanc ecosystem for medical imaging. J. Digit. Imaging **31**(3), 341–352 (2018). https://doi.org/10.1007/s10278-018-0082-y

11. Jodogne, S., Bernard, C., Devillers, M., Lenaerts, E., Coucke, P.: Orthanc - a lightweight, RESTful DICOM server for healthcare and medical research. In: Proceedings of the IEEE International Symposium on Biomedical Imaging: from Nano to Macro, pp. 190–193 (2013). https://doi.org/10.1109/ISBI.2013.6556444

12. Jodogne, S., et al.: Open implementation of DICOM for whole-slide microscopic imaging. In: VISIGRAPP (6: VISAPP), pp. 81–87 (2017). https://doi.org/10.5220/0006155100810087

13. Jodogne, S.: Importing and serving open-data medical images to support artificial intelligence research. In: EuSoMII Annual Meeting, vol. 13(S1). SpringerOpen (2021). https://doi.org/10.1186/s13244-022-01168-w

14. Jodogne, S.: Rendering medical images using WebAssembly. In: Proceedings of the 15th International Joint Conference on Biomedical Engineering Systems and Technologies, vol. 2, pp. 43–51 (2022). https://doi.org/10.5220/0000156300003123

15. Kikinis, R., Pieper, S.D., Vosburgh, K.G.: 3D slicer: a platform for subject-specific image analysis, visualization, and clinical support. In: Jolesz, F.A. (ed.) Intraoperative Imaging and Image-Guided Therapy, pp. 277–289. Springer, New York (2014). https://doi.org/10.1007/978-1-4614-7657-3_19

16. Kirkove, D., et al.: Étude de faisabilité: utilisation de l'imagerie médicale en éducation thérapeutique en radiothérapie. Cancer/Radiothérapie (2022). https://doi.org/10.1016/j.canrad.2022.04.004

17. Lacroute, P.: Fast volume rendering using a shear-warp factorization of the viewing transformation. Ph.D. thesis, Stanford University (1995). Technical report CSL-TR-95-678

18. Lacroute, P., Levoy, M.: Fast volume rendering using a shear-warp factorization of the viewing transformation. In: Proceedings of the 21st Annual Conference on Computer Graphics and Interactive Techniques, pp. 451–458. SIGGRAPH 1994. ACM, New York (1994). https://doi.org/10.1145/192161.192283

19. Lipski, W., Preparata, F.P.: Finding the contour of a union of ISO-oriented rectangles. J. Algorithms **1**(3), 235–246 (1980). https://doi.org/10.1016/0196-6774(80)90011-5

20. Misonne, T., Jodogne, S.: Federated learning for heart segmentation. In: 2022 IEEE 14th Image, Video, and Multidimensional Signal Processing Workshop (IVMSP), pp. 1–5 (2022). https://doi.org/10.1109/IVMSP54334.2022.9816345

21. National Electrical Manufacturers Association: ISO 12052/NEMA PS3, Digital Imaging and Communications in Medicine (DICOM) standard (2021). http://www.dicomstandard.org

22. Preparata, F.P., Shamos, M.I.: Computational Geometry: An Introduction. Texts and Monographs in Computer Science. Springer, Heidelberg (1985). https://doi.org/10.1007/978-1-4612-1098-6

23. Ronneberger, O., Fischer, P., Brox, T.: U-net: convolutional networks for biomedical image segmentation. In: Navab, N., Hornegger, J., Wells, W.M., Frangi, A.F. (eds.) MICCAI 2015, Part III. LNCS, vol. 9351, pp. 234–241. Springer, Cham (2015). https://doi.org/10.1007/978-3-319-24574-4_28

24. Rosset, A., Spadola, L., Ratib, O.: OsiriX: an open-source software for navigating in multidimensional DICOM images. J. Digit. Imaging 17(3), 205–216 (2004). https://doi.org/10.1007/s10278-004-1014-6

25. Schroeder, W., Martin, K., Lorensen, B.: The Visualization Toolkit: An Object-oriented Approach to 3D Graphics, 4th edn. Kitware Inc. (2006)

26. Shorten, C., Khoshgoftaar, T.M.: A survey on image data augmentation for deep learning. J. Big Data 6(1), 1–48 (2019). https://doi.org/10.1186/s40537-019-0197-0

27. Srivastava, N., Hinton, G., Krizhevsky, A., Sutskever, I., Salakhutdinov, R.: Dropout: a simple way to prevent neural networks from overfitting. J. Mach. Learn. Res. 15(56), 1929–1958 (2014)

28. Sudre, C.H., Li, W., Vercauteren, T., Ourselin, S., Jorge Cardoso, M.: Generalised dice overlap as a deep learning loss function for highly unbalanced segmentations. In: Cardoso, M.J., et al. (eds.) DLMIA/ML-CDS -2017. LNCS, vol. 10553, pp. 240–248. Springer, Cham (2017). https://doi.org/10.1007/978-3-319-67558-9_28

29. Urban, T., et al.: LesionTracker: extensible open-source zero-footprint web viewer for cancer imaging research and clinical trials. Can. Res. 77(21), e119–e122 (2017). https://doi.org/10.1158/0008-5472.CAN-17-0334

30. Warnock, M.J., Toland, C., Evans, D., Wallace, B., Nagy, P.: Benefits of using the DCM4CHE DICOM archive. J. Digit. Imaging 20(Supp. 1), 125–129 (2007). https://doi.org/10.1007/s10278-007-9064-1

31. Yang, J., et al.: Data from lung CT segmentation challenge (2017). https://doi.org/10.7937/K9/TCIA.2017.3R3FVZ08

32. Yang, J., et al.: Autosegmentation for thoracic radiation treatment planning: a grand challenge at AAPM 2017. Med. Phys. 45(10), 4568–4581 (2018). https://doi.org/10.1002/mp.13141

Referable Diabetic Retinopathy Detection Using Deep Feature Extraction and Random Forest

Chaymaa Lahmar[1] and Ali Idri[1,2(✉)]

[1] Software Project Management Research Team, ENSIAS, Mohammed V University in Rabat, Rabat, Morocco
ali.idri@um5.ac.ma, ali.idri@um6p.ma
[2] Modeling, Simulation and Data Analysis, Mohammed VI Polytechnic University Benguerir, Ben Guerir, Morocco

Abstract. Diabetic retinopathy (DR) is the most common eyes complication of diabetes worldwide; it can cause vision loss and blindness. The early diagnosis can significantly help in assuring an effective treatment. The computer vision techniques are playing an important role in improving the diagnosis results. This paper proposes a hybrid architecture that combines: four of the most recent deep learning techniques for feature extraction (DenseNet_201, MobileNet_V2, VGG16 and VGG19) with a random forest classifier for referable diabetic retinopathy detection over the APTOS, Kaggle DR and Messidor-2 datasets. The study evaluated and compared: (1) the random forest models with their base learners, (2) the designed random forest models with the same feature extractor over different number of trees, (3) the decision tree classifiers with the best random forest models and (4) the best random forest models of the four feature extractors to each other. The empirical evaluations used: four classification performance criteria (accuracy, sensitivity, precision and F1-score), 5-fold cross-validation, Scott Knott statistical test, and Borda Count voting method. The best model was constructed using a random forest classifier of 9 trees with MobileNet_V2 for feature extraction, it was trained over the APTOS dataset, and it achieved an accuracy value of 82.12%. The experimental results demonstrated that combining random forest with deep learning models is effective for referable diabetic retinopathy detection using fundus images.

Keywords: Diabetic retinopathy · Random forest · Transfer learning · Classification

1 Introduction

Diabetic retinopathy (DR) is the most severe ocular complication of diabetes; it is caused by high blood sugar levels damaging the retina [1]. DR remains the leading cause of visual impairment and blindness among working-age adults in the world. Globally, the prevalence of diabetic retinopathy in individuals with diabetes is expected to be 35%, corresponding to nearly 100 million people worldwide [2]. The early detection of DR can help in assuring successful diagnosis and effective treatment [3].

Medical image analysis using computer vision techniques is an active area of research. Recently, more attention is paid to imaging modalities using Machine Learning (ML) and Deep Learning (DL) in cardiology, breast cancer and diabetic retinopathy [4–11]. Multiple systems have been developed to automatically detect DR, knowing that ophthalmologists usually focus on the presence of some typical lesions associated with DR such as hard exudates, micro-aneurysms, red lesions, and abnormal blood vessels from fundus images [12]. The end-to-end DL techniques showed good performance in DR detection by extracting the most important features from the images, and provided high accurate results [13, 14].On the other hand, classical ML techniques gave accurate results for DR classification, and they are less time consuming and require fewer parameter tuning compared to DL ones. Many researchers designed hybrid architectures where they combined the strengths of deep learning techniques for feature extraction and classical machine learning for classification [15–17]. For instance, in our previous work [18], we developed and evaluated twenty-eight hybrid architectures combining seven of the most popular DL techniques for feature extraction (DenseNet201, Inception_V3, InceptionResNet_V2, MobileNet_V2, ResNet50, VGG16, and VGG19), and four classifiers (MLP, SVM, DT, and KNN) for a binary classification of referable diabetic retinopathy, and we compared them to seven end-to-end DL architectures over the APTOS dataset. The hybrid architecture designed using the SVM classifier and MobileNet_V2 for feature extraction was the top performing with an accuracy equal to 88.80%. However, two limitations have been identified in [18]: (1) only one dataset was used to evaluate the deep hybrid architectures, and (2) lack of use of ensemble methods. A common way to improve the performances of the hybrid architectures is to use ensemble-based methods [19]. Ensemble learning methods were originally developed to improve the prediction power and stability of the classification model by combining several learners [20]. In fact, theoretical and empirical studies have demonstrated that an ensemble of classifiers is typically more accurate than a single classifier [21]. The widely-used ensemble classification methods include bagging, boosting and stacking [22].

This paper proposes a hybrid architecture that combines pre-trained DL techniques for feature extraction and ensemble learning through bagging using random forest (RF) for referable diabetic retinopathy classification over the APTOS, Kaggle DR and Messidor-2 datasets. The main objective is to develop, evaluate and compare the hybrid RF models that are designed using four of the most recent DL techniques for feature extraction: DenseNet201, MobileNet_V2, VGG16, and VGG19 over different number of trees (3, 5, 7 and 9). Breiman [23] developed the concept of bagging in 1994 to improve classification by combining predictions of randomly generated training sets, the results proved that most of the improvement is obtained with unstable base models using only 10 bootstrap replicates, for that reason, the present study varies the number of trees between 3 and 9. The ML classifier that is frequently used to construct homogeneous ensembles is decision tree (DT), thus RF was used for classification [24]. The four DL techniques (DenseNet_201, MobileNet_V2, VGG16 and VGG19) were selected based on their performances as feature extractors for diabetic retinopathy detection over the APTOS, Kaggle DR and Messidor-2 datasets [18, 25, 26]. All the empirical evaluations used: four classification performance criteria (accuracy, sensitivity, precision and

F1-score), 5-fold cross-validation, Scott Knott (SK) statistical test to select the best cluster of the outperforming models[27], and Borda Count voting system to rank the best performing ones[28]. The present study discusses four research questions (RQs):

- (RQ1): Do hybrid RF models perform better than their trees?
- (RQ2): What is the best number of trees for each hybrid RF model over each feature extractor?
- (RQ3): Do hybrid RF models perform better than the DT classifiers?
- (RQ4): What is the best hybrid RF model for each dataset and over the three datasets?

The main contributions of this paper are the following:

1. Designing four DT models using different DL techniques as feature extractors: DenseNet201, VGG16, VGG19 and MobileNet_V2.
2. Designing sixteen hybrid RF models (4 models with a different number of trees for each DL architecture).
3. Evaluating the sixteen hybrid RF models over the APTOS, Kaggle DR and Messior-2 datasets.
4. Comparing the performances of the sixteen hybrid RF models using SK clustering test and Borda Count voting method.
5. Comparing the performances of the sixteen hybrid RF models with their base learners (trees) using SK clustering test and Borda Count voting method.
6. Comparing the performances of the best hybrid RF model for each feature extractor with the DT classifier and to each other using SK clustering test and Borda Count voting method.

The remaining sections of this paper are provided as follows. Section 2 presents an overview of the techniques used for feature extraction and classification. Section 3 describes the related work. Section 4 presents the data preparation. Section 5 describes the methodology followed throughout this paper. Section 6 discusses the empirical results. Section 7 presents the threats of validity of the study. Section 8 outlines conclusions and future works.

2 Background

In the present study, we used four pre-trained DL techniques: VGG16, VGG19, DenseNet_201 and MobileNet_V2 as feature extractors with a random forest classifier to design the hybrid architectures. We used transfer learning for feature extraction and homogeneous ensemble learning through bagging for classification. This subsection gives a summary of the different methods and techniques used in this work.

2.1 Deep Learning Techniques for Feature Extraction

Transfer learning is a ML technique that transfers the knowledge of a model from a related source task to a second related task. Transfer learning only works in DL if the model features learned from the first task are general [29]. This method optimizes its modeling by allowing rapid progress and improved performance. Compared with training from scratch, using a pre-trained CNN model on a target dataset can significantly improve the performance, while compensating for the lack of sufficient training data in the target task [30]. Transfer learning is widely used in computer vision, the models for image classification that result from a transfer learning approach based on pre-trained CNNs are usually composed of two parts: The convolutional base, which performs feature extraction, and the classifier, which classifies the input image based on the features extracted by the convolutional base. In this work, we used four pre-trained models as feature extractors. We used the convolutional base of the pre-trained model in its original form and then we used its outputs to feed the classifier. The four pre-trained models used for feature extraction are:

- **VGG16 and VGG19:** VGG16 is a convolution neural network (CNN) architecture which was used to win ILSVR (ImageNet) competition in 2014 [31]. It is composed of convolution layers blocks of 3x3 filters with a stride 1 and always used the same padding and maxpooling layer of 2x2 filters of stride 2. It has 3 fully connected layers (FC) and a softmax for the output. All hidden layers are equipped with the rectified linear unit (ReLU) non-linearity. The 16 in VGG16 refers to 16 layers of the model and the 19 in the VGG19 refers to 19 layers.

- **DenseNet201:** is a CNN architecture that is 201 layers deep. It is composed of dense blocks that are densely connected together: Each layer receives in input all previous layers output feature maps [32]. A Dense block is composed of a Batch Normalization, ReLU activation, 3x3 convolutions and zero padding. And a transition layer is composed of Batch Normalization, 1x1 convolution and average pooling. Traditional CNNs with L layers have L connections when DenseNets have $L(L + 1)/2$ direct connections. DenseNets have several compelling advantages: they alleviate the vanishing-gradient problem, encourage feature reuse, strengthen feature propagation and substantially reduce the number of parameters.

- **MobileNet_V2:** is a CNN based on an inverted residual structure where the residual connections are between the bottleneck layers. It contains 53 layers and it is a lightweight architecture that performs a single convolution on each color channel rather than combining all three and flattening it [33].

2.2 Classification Techniques

Bagging or "Bootstrap aggregating" is a homogenous ensemble method that improves the accuracy by decreasing the variance and reducing the overfitting [34]. This method generates sample subsets (bootstrap) by randomly sampling from the training dataset with or without replacement, in the first case many of the original examples of the training dataset may be repeated while others may be left out. The base learners are then trained on the generated subsets (bags) and their predictions are combined to get an aggregated prediction. The aggregation averages over the results of the base learners when predicting a numerical outcome and does a majority vote when predicting a class. The training is performed in a parallel manner and the accuracy increases if perturbing the learning set causes major changes in the predictor built [23, 35]. The ML classifier that is frequently used to construct homogeneous ensembles is decision tree [24], thus we used random forest for the classification:

- **Decision Tree (DT):** is the most frequently used supervised machine learning model. It is used for both classification and regression problems. In the tree structures, each node represents a feature from the data pattern, each branch represents a decision rule, and each leaf node represents an output depending on the problem [36].
- **Random Forest (RF):** is a bagging ensemble that uses multiple DTs that will be used to obtain a better prediction performance through majority vote [37]. Each DT node uses a subset of attributes randomly selected from the whole original set of attributes, and each tree uses a different bootstrap sample data. RF classifier has been attracting increasing attention due to its excellent classification accuracy and high efficiency; It is a computationally efficient technique that can operate quickly over large datasets [38].

3   Related Works

Motivated by the success of DL in computer vision, various studies used deep learning based hybrid architectures for diabetic retinopathy detection [14, 18, 26]. For instance, the study [39] proposes a deep learning-based architecture, for the classification and grading of diabetic retinopathy images. The authors used the CNN pre-trained model ResNet50 for feature extraction and Random Forest for classification. The proposed architecture achieved an accuracy of 96% and 75.09% over the Messidor-2 and EyePACS datasets, respectively. In [40], the authors presented a novel CNN model for features extraction from retinal fundus images, the output features are used as input for different machine learning classifiers (SVM, Naive Bayes, J48, AdaBoost and Random Forest). The evaluations were over three datasets IDRiD, MESSIDOR, and KAGGLE and the classifiers were compared in terms of specificity, precision, recall, False Positive Rate (FPR), Kappa-score, and accuracy. The results showed that the CNN feature extractor with the J48 classifier outperformed all the other classifiers over MESSIDOR, IDRiD, and KAGGLE datasets. In the study [41], the authors created a fully automated algorithm for DR detection in fundus photographs. All information learned in the model was visualized readily through an automatically generated abnormality heatmap. For the features extraction the authors used a customized CNN, for the classification they used the Decision Tree algorithm and for the visualization of the learning procedure of the network, they implanted a convolutional visualization layer at the end of the network, encapsulating all previous information into a large layer at the end of the network. Finally, for the evaluation of the performance of the model they used the ROC curve, sensitivity and specificity. The results showed the importance of combining the DT classifier with the CNN feature extractor for diabetic retinopathy detection. The study [42] aims to develop a new approach for DR classification using multiple CNNs for feature extraction and random forest for classification over the Messidor-2 dataset. The authors evaluated their proposed method in terms of specificity, sensitivity, negative predictive value, area under the curve (AUC), and their confidence intervals (CIs). The results showed the importance of using the hybrid architectures for diabetic retinopathy detection since the sensitivity of the model achieved 96.8% when the specificity was 87%.

4 Data Preparation

This section presents the data preparation process we followed for the three datasets, which consists of data acquisition, data pre-processing and augmentation.

4.1 Data Acquisition

In this subsection, we present the three publicly available datasets used in all the empirical evaluations carried out in this study: APTOS, Kaggle DR and Messidor-2. Note that DR is usually classified into five stages: no DR, mild, moderate, severe non proliferative diabetic retinopathy, and proliferative diabetic retinopathy.

APTOS (Asia Pacific Tele Ophthalmology Society) dataset: it was collected by Aravind Eye Hospital in India, it contains 3662 images with the grades of DR on a scale of 0 to 4; the images were gathered from multiple clinics using a variety of cameras[43].

Kaggle DR Dataset: a public dataset of retinal images provided by EYEPACS platform for the Diabetic Retinopathy Detection competition which was sponsored by the California Healthcare Foundation. It is the largest public dataset for DR classification. It contains a total of 35,126 fundus images. It contains the grades of DR on a scale of 0 to 4. The images were taken using a variety of digital cameras [44]. Note that for the Kaggle DR Dataset we have used more than 5000 images for the training and evaluation of our models.

Messidor-2 Dataset: is an extension of the Messidor dataset. It contains 1058 of the images of the original Messidor dataset which were collected by 3 ophthalmology departments, in France, between 2005 and 2006, as well as 690 additional images that were collected between 2009 and 2010 in the Ophthalmology department of Brest University Hospital, France. The images were taken with approximately 44% of pupil dilation. It contains the grades of DR on a scale of 0 to 4, and the stages of maculopathy or DME on a scale from 0 to 1 [45, 46, 47, 48].

4.2 Data Preprocessing and Augmentation

In order to improve the quality of the images, several pre-processing methods were applied since the images of low quality can produce inaccurate results [49]. The target variable of our study is the referable DR; therefore, we started by relabeling the three datasets from a scale of 0 to 4, to a scale of 0 to 1 where 0 stands for no referable DR and 1 stands for referable DR. Note that referable DR was defined as a diabetic retinopathy severity level of moderate non proliferative diabetic retinopathy or worse and/or diabetic macular edema. Then, we cropped the largest square image inscribed in the retina in order to remove the black space areas in the fundus images. After that, all the images were resized to 224 × 224 in accordance with the input requirement of the four DL techniques used as Feature extractors. And, we applied the algorithm of Graham to make the blood vessels as well as the lesion areas in the images more explicit [50]. Then, in order to remove the noise from the images, we normalized the data by converting the pixel values of images from [0, 255] to [0, 1]. Finally, we applied data augmentation techniques in the three datasets, since the number of images in each category (rDR and No rDR) is imbalanced, more than half of images in the three datasets were labeled with

No rDR class. We resampled the images of the datasets by generating three or four new images from each single input image with different augmentation techniques such as shifting, flipping, and rotating. Therefore, the total number of samples was increased by 2.

5 Experimental Process

Figure 1 shows the methodology we followed to carry out the empirical evaluations of this experiment. It consists of eight steps and is similar to methodologies used in [25, 51–59]. The evaluation process involves:

1) For each dataset and feature extractor, assess the performance of the DT classifier in terms of accuracy, sensitivity, precision and F1-score.
2) For each dataset and each feature extractor construct 9 bags, and for each bag assess the performance of the DT classifier in terms of accuracy, precision, sensitivity and F1-score, those models are called base learners.
3) For each dataset and feature extractor construct 4 hybrid RF models depending on four numbers of trees (3, 5, 7 and 9) using the bags constructed before.
4) For each dataset and feature extractor compare the hybrid RF models, constructed in the previous step, with their base learners, constructed in the step 2, using the SK test based on accuracy and Borda count to rank the models of the best SK cluster based on accuracy, precision, sensitivity and F1-score.
5) For each dataset and each feature extractor, compare the 4 hybrid RF models with different number of trees to each other using the SK test and the Borda count voting method.
6) For each dataset and each feature extractor, compare the best hybrid RF models with the DT classifier, constructed in the step 1, using the SK test and the Borda count voting method.
7) For each dataset compare the best hybrid RF models of each feature extractor to each other using the SK test and the Borda count voting method.
8) Compare the best hybrid RF models of each dataset to each other using the SK test and the Borda count voting method.

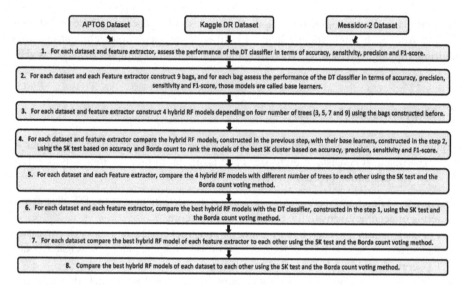

Fig. 1. Experimental design.

6   Results and Discussion

This section presents and discusses the results of the empirical evaluations over the three datasets: APTOS, Kaggle DR and Messidor-2. Python 3 was used with the two DL frameworks Keras and TensorFlow as DL backend and OpenCV for image pre-processing.

6.1   (RQ1): Do Hybrid RF Models Perform Better than Their Trees?

This subsection evaluates and compares the hybrid RF models with their base learners (trees). For each feature extractor over the three datasets, the hybrid RF models were first compared in terms of accuracy with the single trees used to construct them. Thereafter, the SK statistical test was used to determine the best cluster, and finally the Borda Count was used to rank the models belonging to the best SK cluster. Figure 2 shows the difference in % between the accuracy values of the hybrid RF models and the mean accuracy value of their trees over the three datasets. The number 3, 5, 7 or 9 refers to the number of trees that construct each RF model. We observe that:

- For the three datasets, the accuracy of the hybrid RF models is always better than the mean accuracy of their trees. And the difference of accuracies increases with the number of trees that construct them.
- For the APTOS dataset, the highest difference value was equal to9.2% with a RF of 9 trees using DenseNet201 for feature extraction while the lowest one was equal to 1.96% with a RF of 3 trees, usingMobileNet_V2 for feature extraction.
- For the Kaggle DR dataset, the highest difference value was equal to 10.24% with a RF of 9 trees using DenseNet201 for feature extraction while the lowest one was equal to5% with a RF of 3 trees usingVGG19 for feature extraction.

- For the Messidor -2 dataset, the highest difference value was equal to 7.16% with a RF of 9 trees using MobileNet_V2 for feature extraction while the lowest one was equal to 2.27% with a RF of 3 trees usingVGG16for feature extraction.

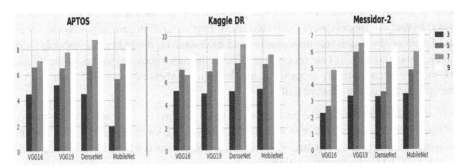

Fig. 2. The difference between the accuracy of the hybrid RF models and their trees over the three datasets.

Thereafter, the SK statistical test was used to determine the best cluster and to compare the performances of the hybrid RF models with their base learners (trees) in terms of accuracy. We observe that:

- For the APTOS dataset, we obtained more than one cluster for each feature extractor where the best cluster contains only the hybrid RF model except when using the MobileNet_V2 with the RF of 3 trees and the VGG16 with the RF of 5, 7 and 9 trees, the best cluster contains the hybrid RF model and at least one of its trees.
- For the Kaggle DR dataset, we obtained one cluster except when using the DenseNet201, MobileNet_V2 with 5, 7 and 9 trees and the VGG19 with 7 and 9 trees, we obtained more than one cluster where the best cluster contains only the hybrid RF model.
- For the Messidor-2 dataset, we obtained more than one cluster for each feature extrac- tor where the best cluster contains only the hybrid RF model except when using the DenseNet201 and MobileNet_V2with the RF of 3 and 5 trees and the VGG19 with the RF of 3 trees, the best cluster contains the hybrid RF model and at least one of its trees.

In order to identify the best model for the cases where the SK test identified in the best clusters the hybrid RF model with at least one its trees, the models of each dataset and feature extractor were ranked by using the Borda Count voting system based on accuracy, sensitivity, F1-score and precision. The results of the Borda Count voting method show that the hybrid RF models are always ranked first. To conclude, the hybrid RF models outperformed their trees and the difference of accuracies between them and their trees is relatively important. Note that the reason why the RF hybrid models outperformed their trees is that that the trees of each RF classifier protect each other from their individual errors. While some trees may be wrong, many others will be right, so as a group the trees are able to make the right predictions [60].

6.2 (RQ2): What Is the Best Number of Trees for Each Hybrid RF Model over Each Feature Extractor?

This subsection evaluates and compares the hybrid RF models implemented with the same feature extractor over different number of trees (3, 5, 7 or 9) for each dataset, in order to identify the number of trees that gives the best performance. The performances of the hybrid RF models were evaluated using four criteria: accuracy, precision, recall and F1-score. For each feature extractor and each dataset, the hybrid RF models were first compared in terms of accuracy. Fig. 3 shows the mean accuracy values of the hybrid RF models of each feature extractor using the four numbers of trees (3, 5, 7 or 9) over the three datasets. We observe that:

- For the APTOS dataset, the best accuracy value reached 82.12% and it was obtained using a RF classifier of 9 trees with the MobileNet_V2 for feature extraction, and the worst accuracy value reached 77.04% and it was obtained with a RF of 3trees using the VGG19 for feature extraction.
- For the Kaggle DR dataset, the best accuracy value reached 81.36% and it was obtained using a RF classifier of 9trees with the MobileNet_V2 for feature extraction, and the worst accuracy value reached 74.89% and it was obtained using a RF of 3 trees with the VGG19 for feature extraction.
- For the Messidor-2 dataset, the best accuracy value reached 78.68% and it was obtained using a RF classifier of 9 trees with the MobileNet_V2 for feature extraction, and the worst accuracy value reached 70.39% and it was obtained using a RF of 3 trees with the VGG19 for feature extraction.

Thereafter, the SK statistical test was used to determine the best cluster, and finally Borda Count was used to rank the hybrid RF models belonging to the best SK cluster. We found that the ranks are ascending: the hybrid RF models constructed using 9 trees are the best performing followed by the models constructed using 7, 5 and 3 trees respectively.

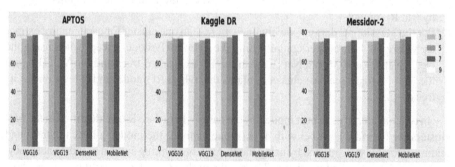

Fig. 3. Mean accuracy values of the hybrid RF models using different number of trees over the three datasets.

6.3 (RQ3): Do Hybrid RF Models Perform Better than the DT Classifiers?

This subsection evaluates and compares the first ranked hybrid RF model found in RQ2 with the DT classifier over each dataset and feature extractor. Figure 4 shows the comparison of the mean accuracy values of the best hybrid RF models of each feature extractor and the DT classifier designed using the same feature extractor while Table 1 summarizes the accuracy values of the best hybrid RF models and the DT classifier using each feature extractor over the three datasets. We observe that:

- For the APTOS dataset, the best accuracy value was obtained using the hybrid RF model of 9 trees with the MobileNet_V2 and it achieved 82.12% while the worst accuracy value was obtained using the DT classifier with the VGG19 and it achieved 69.99%.
- For the Kaggle DR dataset, the best accuracy value was obtained using the hybrid RF model of 9 trees with the MobileNet_V2 and it achieved 81.36% while the worst accuracy value was obtained using the DT classifier with the VGG19 and it achieved 69.61%.
- For the Messidor-2 dataset, the best accuracy value was obtained using the hybrid RF model of 9 trees with the MobileNet_V2 and it achieved 78.68% while the worst accuracy value was obtained using the DT classifier with the VGG19 and it achieved 64.61%.

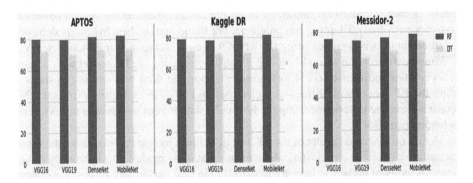

Fig. 4. Mean accuracy values of the best hybrid RF models of each feature extractor and the DT classifier designed using the same feature extractor over the three datasets.

Thereafter, we used the SK test to compare the hybrid RF models and the DT classifier trained over each feature extractor and dataset. We obtained two clusters where the first cluster was always represented by the hybrid RF model and the second one with the DT classifier.

To sum up, the hybrid RF model outperformed the DT classifier over the three datasets since the RF classifier integrates multiple decision trees into a forest through the idea of ensemble learning to get a more accurate prediction value [61]. The RF algorithm has an excellent ability to process large data with accuracy [62]. Different from decision trees, RF generates decision trees randomly and avoids overfitting by using random subsets of features to create smaller trees [62, 63].

Table 1. Mean accuracy values of the best hybrid RF model and the DT classifier over the three datasets.

Classifier	Dataset	FE			
		VGG16	VGG19	DensNet201	MobileNet_V2
RF	APTOS	80.12	79.75	81.51	82.12
	Kaggle DR	78.99	78.11	80.98	81.36
	Messidor-2	75.87	74.73	76.56	78.68
DT	APTOS	72.21	69.99	72.87	73.16
	Kaggle DR	71.40	69.61	70.32	72.22
	Messidor-2	70.04	64.61	68.76	74.33

6.4 (RQ4): What Is the Best Hybrid RF Model for Each Dataset and over the Three Datasets?

This subsection evaluates and compares the best hybrid RF models of the four feature extractors for each dataset and over the three datasets. Figure 5 shows the results of the SK test of the best hybrid RF models for each feature over each dataset. We observe that one cluster was obtained over the three datasets. The hybrid RF models of the best SK cluster of each dataset were ranked by using the Borda Count voting system based on accuracy, sensitivity, F1-score and precision. We found that the best hybrid model over the three datasets is designed using the RF of 9 trees as a classifier and MobileNet_V2 as feature extractor, the second-best one is constructed using the RF model with 9 trees as a classifier and DenseNet201 as feature extractor, the third best one is constructed using the RF model with 9 trees as a classifier and VGG16 as feature extractor. The fourth ranked one is designed using the RF model with 9 trees as classifier and VGG19 as feature extractor.

Figure 6 shows the results of the SK test of the best hybrid RF models of the three datasets. We obtained one cluster, which means that these models are statistically indifferent in terms of accuracy. In order to identify the best performing model, we ranked the models using the Borda Count voting system based on accuracy, sensitivity, F1-score and precision. Table 2 presents the ranking results of the three models. We found that the best hybrid RF model was trained over the APTOS dataset, followed by the models trained over the Kaggle DR and Messidor-2 datasets.

To sum up, the best hybrid model over the three datasets is designed using the RF of 9 trees as a classifier and MobileNet_V2 as feature extractor. In general, the MobileNet_V2 model is widely used for diabetic retinopathy detection [14, 18, 25, 26], and it has many advantages over the other deep models because it is based on an inverted residual structure where the residual connections are between the bottleneck layers. The intermediate expansion layer uses lightweight depth-wise convolutions to filter features as a source of non-linearity which provides robust feature extraction with a reduced number of parameters [33]. As for the classification task, the RF model is also widely used in diabetic retinopathy classification using fundus images [14] and it has been

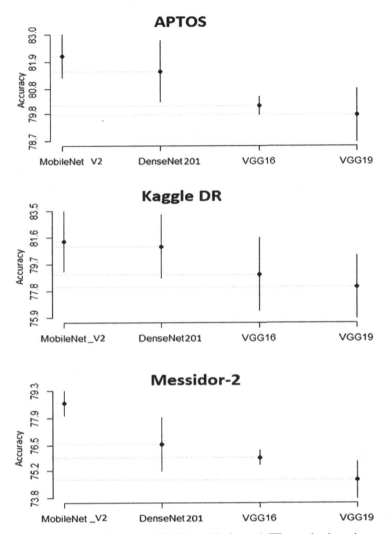

Fig. 5. SK Results of the best hybrid RF models for each FE over the three datasets.

demonstrated to be a robust predictor for both small sample sizes and high dimensional data [62].

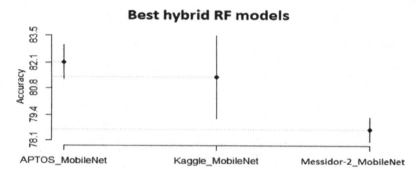

Fig. 6. SK Results of the best hybrid RF models of the three datasets

Table 2. Borda Count ranking of the best hybrid RF models over the three datasets.

Dataset	Feature extractor	Accuracy (%)	Sensitivity (%)	Precision (%)	F1-score (%)	Rank
APTOS	MbileNet_V2	82.12	75.98	86.95	81.78	1
Kaggle DR	MbileNet_V2	81.36	62.73	94.11	74.93	2
Messidor-2	MbileNet_V2	78.68	83.22	76.45	79.65	2

7 Threats of Validity

This section presents the threats to this paper's validity with respect to external and internal validity.

Internal Validity: This paper used the 5-fold cross validation method for evaluation. The main reason to use the 5-fold cross validation is that cross validation gives more stable estimations [64]. Another internal threat for this experiment is the use of transfer learning to extract the features of the fundus images over the APTOS, Kaggle DR and Messidor-2 datasets, using the most powerful DL techniques for DR detection.

External Validity: This study used three public datasets of fundus images which was helpful to compare the performance of the different models and feature extractors over each dataset. However, it would be interesting to study if the robustness of the models holds with different datasets with the same type of images. It will this study be a good benefit to redo this study using other DL techniques, or different type of CNN models such us auto encoders with other publicly or private datasets in order to confirm or refute the findings of this study.

Construct Validity: For the reliability of the classifier performances obtained, this paper focused on four classification metrics (accuracy, recall, precision and F1-Score). The main reasons behind the choice of these performance criteria are: (1) most of the studies used them to measure the classification performance [14], and (2) the type of the data is balanced. Moreover, the conclusion was drawn by using the SK test and Borda count voting system with equal weights using these four performance criteria.

8 Conclusion and Future Work

This paper presented and discussed the results of an empirical comparative study of forty-eight hybrid RF models constructed using the random forest classifier with four different number of trees (3, 5, 7 or 9) and four DL techniques for feature extraction (VGG16, VGG19, DenseNet201 and MobileNet_V2) for referable DR classification over three datasets. All the empirical evaluations used four performance criteria (accuracy, precision, sensitivity and F1-score), SK statistical test, and Borda Count to assess and rank these models over the APTOS, Kaggle DR and Messidor-2 datasets. The results showed that the hybrid RF models with the highest number of trees are the best performing over the three datasets in terms of accuracy, precision, sensitivity and F1-score, and they also outperformed the base learners (tress) that construct them as well as the DT classifiers. Therefore, we recommend the use of the random forest classifier with the MobileNet_V2feature extractor for referable diabetic retinopathy classification, since it gave good results over the three datasets and it outperformed its DT classifier and the base learners used to construct it over the three datasets.

Ongoing works focuses on implementing hybrid bagging ensembles using other classifiers as base learners to possibly improve the accuracy and comparing them with the hybrid RF models.

References

1. Diabetic retinopathy - NHS. https://www.nhs.uk/conditions/diabetic-retinopathy/. Accessed 20 Nov 2021
2. Zheng, Y., He, M., Congdon, N.: The worldwide epidemic of diabetic retinopathy. Indian J. Ophthalmol. **60**(5), 428–431 (2012). https://doi.org/10.4103/0301-4738.100542
3. Vashist, P., Singh, S., Gupta, N., Saxena, R.: Role of early screening for diabetic retinopathy in patients with diabetes mellitus: an overview. Indian J. Community Med. **36**(4), 247–252 (2011). https://doi.org/10.4103/0970-0218.91324
4. Raju, M., Pagidimarri, V., Barreto, R., Kadam, A., Kasivajjala, V., Aswath, A.: Development of a deep learning algorithm for automatic diagnosis of diabetic retinopathy. Stud. Health Technol. Inform. **245**, 559–563 (2017). https://doi.org/10.3233/978-1-61499-830-3-559
5. Zeng, X., Chen, H., Luo, Y., Ye, W.: Automated diabetic retinopathy detection based on binocular siamese-like convolutional neural network. IEEE Access **7**, 30744–30753 (2019). https://doi.org/10.1109/ACCESS.2019.2903171
6. García, G., Gallardo, J., Mauricio, A., López, J., Del Carpio, C.: Detection of diabetic retinopathy based on a convolutional neural network using retinal fundus Images. In: Lintas, A., Rovetta, S., Verschure, P.F.M.J., Villa, A.E.P. (eds.) ICANN 2017. LNCS, vol. 10614, pp. 635–642. Springer, Cham (2017). https://doi.org/10.1007/978-3-319-68612-7_72
7. Zerouaoui, H., Idri, A.: Reviewing machine learning and image processing based decision-making systems for breast cancer imaging. J. Med. Syst. **45**(1), 1–20 (2021). https://doi.org/10.1007/s10916-020-01689-1

8. Gupta, P., Garg, S.: Breast cancer prediction using varying parameters of machine learning models. Procedia Comput. Sci. **171**, 593–601 (2020). https://doi.org/10.1016/j.procs.2020.04.064

9. Kourou, K., Exarchos, T.P., Exarchos, K.P., Karamouzis, M.V., Fotiadis, D.I.: Machine learning applications in cancer prognosis and prediction. Comput. Struct. Biotechnol. J. **13**, 8–17 (2015). https://doi.org/10.1016/j.csbj.2014.11.005

10. Wong, K.K., Fortino, G., Abbott, D.: Deep learning-based cardiovascular image diagnosis: a promising challenge. Future Gener. Comput. Syst. **110**, 802–811 (2020). https://doi.org/10.1016/j.future.2019.09.047

11. Litjens, G., et al.: State-of-the-art deep learning in cardiovascular image analysis. JACC Cardiovasc. Imaging **12**(8P1), 1549–1565 (2019). https://doi.org/10.1016/j.jcmg.2019.06.009

12. Ahmad, A., Mansoor, A.B., Mumtaz, R., Khan, M., Mirza, S.H.: Image processing and classification in diabetic retinopathy : a review. In 2014 5th European Workshop on Visual Information Processing (EUVIP), pp. 1–6 (2014)

13. Asiri, N., Hussain, M., Al Adel, F., Alzaidi, N: Deep learning based computer-aided diagnosis systems for diabetic retinopathy: a survey. arXiv, no. Dl (2018)

14. Islam, M.M., Yang, H.C., Poly, T.N., Jian, W.S., Li, Y.C.J.: Deep learning algorithms for detection of diabetic retinopathy in retinal fundus photographs: A systematic review and meta-analysis. Comput. Methods Programs Biomed. **191**, 105320 (2020). https://doi.org/10.1016/j.cmpb.2020.105320

15. Zhang, W., et al.: Automated identification and grading system of diabetic retinopathy using deep neural networks. Knowl.-Based Syst. **175**, 12–25 (2019). https://doi.org/10.1016/j.knosys.2019.03.016

16. Mookiah, M.R.K., Acharya, U.R., Chua, C.K., Lim, C.M., Ng, E.Y.K., Laude, A.: Computer-aided diagnosis of diabetic retinopathy: a review. Comput. Biol. Med. **43**(12), 2136–2155 (2013). https://doi.org/10.1016/j.compbiomed.2013.10.007

17. Tsiknakis, N., et al.: Deep learning for diabetic retinopathy detection and classification based on fundus images: a review. Comput. Biol. Med. **135**, 104599 (2021). https://doi.org/10.1016/j.compbiomed.2021.104599

18. Lahmar, C., Idri, A.: Classifying diabetic retinopathy using CNN and machine learning. In: Proceedings of the 15th International Joint Conference on Biomedical Engineering Systems and Technologies - BIOIMAGING, pp. 52–62 (2022). https://doi.org/10.5220/0010851500003123

19. Bagui, S.C.: Combining Pattern Classifiers: Methods and Algorithms, vol. 47, no. 4 (2005)

20. Sagi, O., Rokach, L.: Ensemble learning: a survey, Wiley Interdiscip. Rev. Data Min. Knowl. Discov. **8**(4), e1249 (2018). https://doi.org/10.1002/WIDM.1249

21. Maclin, R., Opitz, D.: Popular ensemble methods: an empirical study. J. Artif. Intell. Res. **11**, 169–198 (2011). https://doi.org/10.1613/jair.614

22. Wang, G., Hao, J., Ma, J., Jiang, H.: A comparative assessment of ensemble learning for credit scoring. Expert Syst. Appl. **38**(1), 223–230 (2011). https://doi.org/10.1016/j.eswa.2010.06.048

23. Breiman, L.: Bagging predictors. Mach. Learn. **24**, 123–140 (1996)

24. Hosni, M., Abnane, I., Idri, A., de Gea, J.M.C., Alemán, J.L.F.: Reviewing ensemble classification methods in breast cancer. Comput. Methods Programs Biomed. **177**, 89–112 (2019). https://doi.org/10.1016/j.cmpb.2019.05.019

25. Lahmar, C., Idri, A.: On the value of deep learning for diagnosing diabetic retinopathy. Health Technol. (Berl) **12**(1), 89–105 (2022). https://doi.org/10.1007/S12553-021-00606-X/FIGURES/11

26. Lahmar, C., Idri, A.: Deep hybrid architectures for diabetic retinopathy classification. Comput. Methods Biomech. Biomed. Eng.: Imaging Vis. **11**(2), 166–184 (2023). https://doi.org/10.1080/21681163.2022.2060864

27. Jelihovschi, E.G., Faria, J.C.: ScottKnott : a package for performing the scott-knott clustering algorithm in R, pp. 1–6 (2000)
28. García-Lapresta, J.L., Martínez-Panero, M.: Borda count versus approval voting: a fuzzy approach. Public Choice **112**(1), 167–184 (2002). https://doi.org/10.1023/A:1015609200117
29. Guo, Y., Shi, H., Kumar, A., Grauman, K., Rosing, T., Feris, R.: Spottune: transfer learning through adaptive fine-tuning. In: Proceedings of the IEEE Computer Vision Pattern Recognition, pp. 4800–4809 (2019). https://doi.org/10.1109/CVPR.2019.00494
30. Pan, S.J., Yang, Q.: A survey on transfer learning. IEEE Trans. Knowl. Data Eng. **22**(10), 1345–1359 (2010). https://doi.org/10.1109/TKDE.2009.191
31. Simonyan, K., Zisserman, A.: Very deep convolutional networks for large-scale image recognition. In: 3rd International Conference Learning Representation ICLR 2015 - Conference Track Proceedings, pp. 1–14 (2015)
32. Huang, G., Liu, Z., Van Der Maaten, L., Weinberger, K.Q.: Densely connected convolutional networks. In: Proceedings - 30th IEEE Conference on Computer Vision and Pattern Recognition, CVPR 2017, pp. 2261–2269 (2017). https://doi.org/10.1109/CVPR.2017.243
33. Sandler, M., Howard, A., Zhu, M., Zhmoginov, A., Chen, L.C.: MobileNetV2: inverted residuals and linear bottlenecks. In: Proceedings of the IEEE Conference on Computer Vision and Pattern Recognition, pp. 4510–4520 (2018). https://doi.org/10.1109/CVPR.2018.00474
34. Liang, G., Zhu, X., Zhang, C.: An empirical study of bagging predictors for different learning algorithms. In: Proceedings of the National Conference on Artificial Intelligence, vol. 2, pp. 1802–1803 (2011)
35. Bühlmann, P., Yu, B.: Analyzing bagging. Ann. Stat. **30**(4), 927–961 (2002). https://doi.org/10.1214/aos/1031689014
36. Poolsawad, N., Kambhampati, C., Cleland, J.G.F.: Balancing class for performance of classification with a clinical dataset. Lect. Notes Eng. Comput. Sci. **1**(November), 237–242 (2014)
37. Cutler, A., Cutler, D.R., Stevens, J.R.: Random forests. Ensemble Mach. Learn., 157–175 (2012). https://doi.org/10.1007/978-1-4419-9326-7_5
38. Oshiro, T.M., Perez, P.S., Baranauskas, J.A.: How many trees in a random forest? In: Perner, P. (ed.) MLDM 2012. LNCS (LNAI), vol. 7376, pp. 154–168. Springer, Heidelberg (2012). https://doi.org/10.1007/978-3-642-31537-4_13
39. Yaqoob, M.K., Ali, S.F., Bilal, M., Hanif, M.S., Al-Saggaf, U.M.: ResNet based deep features and random forest classifier for diabetic retinopathy detection. Sensors **21**(11), 3883 (2021). https://doi.org/10.3390/S21113883
40. Gayathri, S., Gopi, V.P., Palanisamy, P.: A lightweight CNN for diabetic retinopathy classification from fundus images. Biomed. Signal Process. Control **62**, 102115 (2020). https://doi.org/10.1016/J.BSPC.2020.102115
41. Gargeya, R., Leng, T.: Automated identification of diabetic retinopathy using deep learning. Ophthalmology **124**(7), 962–969 (2017). https://doi.org/10.1016/j.ophtha.2017.02.008
42. Abràmoff, M.D., et al.: Improved automated detection of diabetic retinopathy on a publicly available dataset through integration of deep learning. Invest. Ophthalmol. Vis. Sci. **57**(13), 5200–5206 (2016). https://doi.org/10.1167/iovs.16-19964
43. APTOS 2019 Blindness Detection I Kaggle (2019). https://www.kaggle.com/c/aptos2019-blindness-detection. Accessed 24 June 2021
44. Diabetic Retinopathy Detection I Kaggle. https://www.kaggle.com/c/diabetic-retinopathy-detection/data. Accessed 24 June 2021
45. Messidor - ADCIS. https://www.adcis.net/fr/logiciels-tiers/messidor-fr/. Accessed 24 June 2021
46. Messidor-2 - ADCIS. https://www.adcis.net/fr/logiciels-tiers/messidor2-fr/. Accessed 24 June 2021

47. Decencière, E., et al.: Feedback on a publicly distributed image database: the Messidor database. Image Anal. Stereol. **33**(3), 231–234 (2014). https://doi.org/10.5566/ias.1155

48. MESSIDOR-2 DR Grades | Kaggle. https://www.kaggle.com/google-brain/messidor2-dr-grades. Accessed 24 June 2021

49. Razzak, M.I., Naz, S., Zaib, A.: Deep learning for medical image processing: overview, challenges and the future. In: Dey, N., Ashour, A.S., Borra, S. (eds.) Classification in BioApps. LNCVB, vol. 26, pp. 323–350. Springer, Cham (2018). https://doi.org/10.1007/978-3-319-65981-7_12

50. Diabetic Retinopathy Detection | Kaggle. https://www.kaggle.com/c/diabetic-retinopathy-detection/discussion/15801. Accessed 24 June 2021

51. Idri, A., Hosni, M., Abran, A.: Improved estimation of software development effort using classical and fuzzy analogy ensembles. Appl. Soft Comput. J. **49**, 990–1019 (2016). https://doi.org/10.1016/j.asoc.2016.08.012

52. Mittas, N., Angelis, L.: Ranking and clustering software cost estimation models through a multiple comparisons algorithm. IEEE Trans. Softw. Eng. **39**(4), 537–551 (2013). https://doi.org/10.1109/TSE.2012.45

53. Bony, S., Pichon, N., Ravel, C., Durix, A., Balfourier, F., Guillaumin, J.J.: The relationship between mycotoxin synthesis and isolate morphology in fungal endophytes of Lolium perenne. New Phytol. **152**(1), 125–137 (2001). https://doi.org/10.1046/j.0028-646X.2001.00231.x

54. Sharma, J., Zettler, L.W., Van Sambeek, J.W., Ellersieck, M.R., Starbuck, C.J.: Symbiotic seed germination and mycorrhizae of federally threatened Platanthera praeclara (Orchidaceae). Am. Midl. Nat. **149**(1), 104–120 (2003). https://doi.org/10.1674/0003-0031(2003)1490104:SSGAMO.2.0.CO;2

55. Azzeh, M., Nassif, A.B., Minku, L.L.: An empirical evaluation of ensemble adjustment methods for analogy-based effort estimation. J. Syst. Softw. **103**, 36–52 (2015). https://doi.org/10.1016/j.jss.2015.01.028

56. Idri, A., Abnane, I., Abran, A.: Missing data techniques in analogy-based software development effort estimation. J. Syst. Softw. **117**, 595–611 (2016). https://doi.org/10.1016/j.jss.2016.04.058

57. Idri, A., Abnane, I., Abran, A.: Evaluating Pred(p) and standardized accuracy criteria in software development effort estimation. J. Softw. Evol. Process **30**(4), 1–15 (2018). https://doi.org/10.1002/smr.1925

58. Idri, A., Abnane, I.: Fuzzy analogy based effort estimation: an empirical comparative study. In: IEEE CIT 2017 - 17th IEEE International Conference on Computer and Information Technology, pp. 114–121 (2017). https://doi.org/10.1109/CIT.2017.29

59. Zerouaoui, H., Idri, A.: Deep hybrid architectures for binary classification of medical breast cancer images. Biomed. Signal Process. Control **71**, 103226 (2022). https://doi.org/10.1016/J.BSPC.2021.103226

60. Random Forest® — A Powerful Ensemble Learning Algorithm - KDnuggets. https://www.kdnuggets.com/2020/01/random-forest-powerful-ensemble-learning-algorithm.html. Accessed 26 June 2022

61. Carvalho, T.P., Soares, F.A., Vita, R., Francisco, R.D.P., Basto, J.P., Alcalá, S.G.: A systematic literature review of machine learning methods applied to predictive maintenance. Comput. Ind. Eng. **137**, 106024 (2019). https://doi.org/10.1016/j.cie.2019.106024

62. Biau, G., Scornet, E.: A random forest guided tour. TEST **25**(2), 197–227 (2016). https://doi. org/10.1007/s11749-016-0481-7

63. Breiman, L.: Random forests. Mach. Learn. **45**, 5–32 (2001)

64. Xu, Y., Goodacre, R.: On splitting training and validation set: a comparative study of cross-validation, bootstrap and systematic sampling for estimating the generalization performance of supervised learning. J. Anal. Test. **2**(3), 249–262 (2018). https://doi.org/10.1007/s41664-018-0068-2

Author Index

A. C. A. Roque et al. (Eds.): BIOSTEC 2022, CCIS 1814, pp. 435–436, 2023.
https://doi.org/10.1007/978-3-031-38854-5

Printed in the United States
by Baker & Taylor Publisher Services